The White Book of Neurologic Examination

A Beginner's Essential

The White Book
of Neurologic
Examination
A Beginner's Essential

You-Jiang Tan

National Neuroscience Institute, Singapore

World Scientific

NEW JERSEY · LONDON · SINGAPORE · BEIJING · SHANGHAI · HONG KONG · TAIPEI · CHENNAI · TOKYO

Published by

World Scientific Publishing Co. Pte. Ltd.

5 Toh Tuck Link, Singapore 596224

USA office: 27 Warren Street, Suite 401-402, Hackensack, NJ 07601

UK office: 57 Shelton Street, Covent Garden, London WC2H 9HE

British Library Cataloguing-in-Publication Data
A catalogue record for this book is available from the British Library.

THE WHITE BOOK OF NEUROLOGIC EXAMINATION
A Beginner's Essential

ISBN 978-981-123-923-6 (hardcover)
ISBN 978-981-123-983-0 (paperback)
ISBN 978-981-123-924-3 (ebook for institutions)
ISBN 978-981-123-925-0 (ebook for individuals)

For any available supplementary material, please visit
https://www.worldscientific.com/worldscibooks/10.1142/12342#t=suppl

Contents

Introduction

Neurology can appear daunting to the uninitiated. With a deeper appreciation of neurology, however, it is often realized that this fear is unfounded. Through the elegant demonstrations of physical signs and the incisive gathering of clinical history, doctors can find joy in the mental gymnastics that go into the evaluation of patients with symptoms that are often hopelessly non-specific.

You become more than a doctor as you don the hat of a seasoned detective, dissecting through seemingly unimpressive clues with cursory help from imaging studies and mechanical adjuncts to arrive at that fabled eureka moment.

Alas, after spending years in medical school performing well-oiled examination routines without knowing the underlying rationale and often ending up more confused than enlightened, a junior doctor like yourself may find it hard to shake off your neurophobia.

With well-packaged and easy-to-understand information, it is hoped that this book — while far from being the panacea to that fear — may equip junior doctors with simple tools to approach common neurological conditions, make sense of the seemingly bland signs and symptoms, and appreciate neurology as a whole with all its romantic beauty and seductive charm.

To help our long-suffering peers build strong foundations and prepare for their professional exams, the coming chapters will include tips and pointers that are appropriate for MBBS/MD and MRCP PACES which can help improve examination finesse and bring clarity to the neuro-localisation processes. I have picked these up over the years whilst tutoring students, and being tutored by various esteemed seniors and peers of mine, many whom I cannot possibly thank enough, and I cannot wait to share them with you."

I hope you will find joy using this book!

1

Getting Started

A. Getting Started — Preparatory Work

A meaningful neurologic examination requires the examiner to adopt the psyche of a crime scene investigator. You are no longer a doctor but a detective, searching for and piecing together clues that can help you find the culprit. Because the eyes see only what the mind is prepared to comprehend, examining a patient without knowing what to look for will likely be a waste of precious time.

Before you examine a patient, pay attention to the patient's symptoms. Very often, the localisation process begins here. You should, as best as you can, answer the following **5 questions** which can be easily remembered with the mnemonic "**SPOOF**".

- **S**ymptoms
- **P**attern of involvement
- **O**ther important symptoms
- **O**nset and duration
- **F**unctional status (premorbidly and presently)

	Questions	Examples
1.	**What are the symptoms?**	Domains involved: • Cranial nerves • Motor or sensory or sensorimotor • Autonomic • Cerebellar This will help you plan your physical examination, focusing on the symptomatic regions first.
2.	**What is the pattern of involvement?**	Pattern of symptomatic involvement: • Appendicular vs. axial • Proximal vs. distal • Monolimbic vs. tetra- vs. hemi- vs. paraparesis • Facial, bulbar

(*Continued*)

(Continued)

	Questions	Examples
3.	Are there other important symptoms?	Systemic diseases may hide behind seemingly benign neurologic complaints. Look out for symptoms that may suggest an underlying systemic disease, e.g.: • Unintentional weight loss • Loss of appetite • Gastrointestinal symptoms • Rheumatologic symptoms (i.e., joints, skin, nails and eyes, etc.)
4.	Onset, progression, and duration of symptoms	**Tempo** of onset and duration: • Acute vs. insidious • Recent onset vs. chronic process **Progression**: • Static • Progressive • Relapsing, remitting For example: "Mr. X was previously independent in his daily activities, but for the past two weeks, he has been confined to a chair and requires assistance with his daily needs."
5.	Functional status • Baseline • Present	Do ask the patient if he/she requires assistive devices for mobility, feeding, and toileting, e.g.: • Walking sticks, walking frames, or wheelchairs • Nasogastric tube or PEG tubes • Diapers or urinary catheters

After answering the "SPOOF" questions, you will have a better idea of what to look out for in your patient. You are now ready to begin examining your patient.

Tips for Examination Candidates

It is impossible to make learned localisation attempts without prior information on the presenting symptoms. In the artificial setting of professional examinations, take some time to read the question stems or case vignettes provided and attempt to answer the "SPOOF" questions before examining the patient.

I once observed a candidate who examined a "wheelchair-bound patient with frequent falls". Upon detecting mild weakness in his legs (MRC grade 4+), he confidently attributed the patient's woes solely to his motor deficits ignoring the fact that the mild weakness did not explain why the patient had significant impairment in mobility.

There was a mismatch between his clinical impression and the patient's functional status.

The patient turned out to have spinocerebellar ataxia, and his impaired mobility was the result of cerebellar dysfunction rather than the weakness alone. This case highlights the importance of paying due attention to the presenting symptoms so as to get a better sense of your examination findings.

2

Basics of the Neurological Examination

A. Preparatory Work — Pay Attention to the Symptoms

The neurologic assessment of a patient is a lengthy process. Every shred of detail may provide vital clues. Paying attention to the patient's **symptoms** (see **Chapter 1**) is the quintessential first step of the neurolocalisation process.

- What neurologic deficits are you likely to encounter in your patient? Do they correlate with the predominant symptoms?
- How chronic are the patient's complaints? Do you expect to find features of chronicity on the patient?
- How functionally impaired is the patient? Are the patient's clinical deficits severe enough to explain the degree of impairment?

B. The Setting

The environmental setting and patient's position should be optimised to facilitate the clinical examination:

- The room should be adequately bright.
- Ensure that you have the necessary clinical equipment.
- The patient should be positioned appropriately for the examination of interest.

Clinical Examination	Patient's Position
Cranial nerves	• Seated upright in a chair
Upper limbs	• Seated in a chair • Lying at a 45° incline
Lower limbs	• Lying supine

C. Exposing the Patient

Proper exposure is necessary when inspecting for scars, deformities and muscle atrophy. In the artificial setting of a professional examination, it is wise to expose other pertinent areas beyond the regions of interest. When examining the upper limbs, for example, concurrently exposing the lower limbs will provide you with additional clues pertaining to the extent of the deficits. The presence of co-existing abnormalities over the lower limbs may refine your list of diagnoses towards a generalised rather than a focal disease process. Exposure should be as adequate as necessary for a thorough examination whilst preserving the patient's modesty.

Examination	Areas to Expose	Comments

Examination of cranial nerves	Neck, shoulders and upper limbs	When examining the cranial nerves, expose the following areas:
		• **Neck and shoulders:**
		  ○ The **sternocleidomastoid** and **trapezius** muscles are innervated by the accessory nerve (CN XI).
		  ○ The neck and shoulder muscles are often affected in muscular dystrophies.
		• **Upper limbs**
		  ○ **Horner's syndrome:** co-existing wasted hands may localise the lesion along the sympathetic pathway's second-order neuron.
		  ○ **Cranial nerve deficits:** the presence of unilateral sensorimotor or cerebellar deficits over the upper limbs suggests the presence of "long-tract signs", localising the lesion within the brainstem (Chapter 6). Examples include Weber's syndrome and Millard-Gublers syndrome.

Examination of the upper limbs	Expose the arms from the shoulders to the fingers. Additionally, expose the lower limbs as best as the scenario allows.	Exposing the lower limbs may provide important clues which when present may suggest a more extensive involvement of the underlying disorder.

(Continued)

Examination	Areas to Expose	Comments
Examination of the lower limbs	The legs should ideally be exposed from the inguinal regions to the toes. However, exposure from the proximal thighs downward is an accepted compromise. The upper limbs should also be exposed as best as the scenario allows.	Using the example of an upper limb examination, squaring of shoulders with concomitant atrophy of both thighs may hint at a generalised disease process affecting the proximal musculature (e.g., proximal myopathy), a conclusion that is difficult to draw without the additional findings over the upper limbs.

The ideal extent of exposure may not be appropriate for some patients (e.g., having a lady remove her shirt to expose her shoulders). Always explain to the patient what you intend to do and seek his/her permission before proceeding.

D. Inspection

We should spend at least **10 seconds** inspecting the patient **from the foot of the bed**. The findings from the inspective process alone can provide vital clues regarding the nature of the underlying neurologic disorder, its pattern of involvement, and its chronicity. Additionally, pay attention to the patient's surroundings, where the presence of mobility aids may hint at the patient's existing functional impairments. A good inspection helps guarantee a good finish. These steps will launch you in the right direction in your neurolocalisation process.

Phases	Comments

Inspecting from the foot of the bed or couch	**Observe the patient** for:
	• Features of chronic lower motor neuron (LMN) disease:
	  o Atrophy
	  o Deformities such as claw toes, hammer toes
	  o Neuropathic skin changes
	• Features of chronic upper motor neuron (UMN) disease:
	  o Contractures
	• Functional aids:
	  o Nasogastric tube
	  o Percutaneous Endoscopic Gastrostomy (PEG) tube
	  o Diapers
	  o In-dwelling catheters
	  o Suprapubic catheters
	  o Calf compressive devices

(Continued)

(Continued)

Phases	Comments

	• Other adjuncts:
	   ○ Arm slings
	   ○ Ankle-foot orthoses
	
	Observe the surroundings for the following:
	• Non-invasive ventilators
	• Dietary thickeners
	• Mobility aids

Inspecting up-close	**Observe the patient for:**
	1. Fasciculations
	2. Scars
	3. Additional abnormalities suggestive of other systemic diseases, e.g.:
	   • Heliotrope rash of dermatomyositis
	   • Neurofibroma
	   • Diabetic dermopathy
	   • Xanthelasma

E. Screening Tests

Having a set of screening tests at the start of a neurologic examination can help guide the neurologic examination thereafter. The table below is a summary of better-described tests which you may find useful in your practice.

Examination of the Upper Limbs		
Description of the Test	**Clinical Findings**	**Comments**
Have the patient stretch out his/her arms with the palms facing skywards. The fingers should be **straightened** and **adducted,** and the forearms should be well-**supinated**. Have the patient close his/her eyes.	• Pronator drift • Abnormal upward or lateral movements • Abduction of the little finger (Wartenberg's sign, finger escape sign, and digiti quinti sign*)	A pronator drift hints at an UMN disease process. Abnormal sway of the limb hints at underlying ataxia.

*Wartenberg sign:[2] The Wartenberg sign describes the involuntary abduction of the little finger in ulnar neuropathy due to the unopposed action of the extensor digiti minimi (innervated by the radial nerve). **Digiti quinti sign:**[3] Best examined with the palms facing downwards, the abduction of the little finger suggests an underlying UMN pathology.

(Continued)

(Continued)

Examination of the Upper Limbs		
Description of the Test	**Clinical Findings**	**Comments**
With his/her eyes opened, instruct the patient to pronate his/her outstretched arms and extend both wrists and fingers.	• Weakness of the wrist and/or finger extensors	This quickly screens for "wrist-drop" and "finger-drop", which in the right setting may respectively indicate a proximal or distal radial neuropathy respectively.
(Optional) Have the patient flex his/her elbow to 90° and resist you while you exert a strong pulling force at his/her wrist. Release your grip suddenly and observe.[1]	• Holme's rebound test** (not the same as the Holme's rebound phenomenon)	In cerebellar disorders, the patient is unable to control the unexpected flexor contraction upon the release of your grip, resulting in the exaggerated flexion of the elbow.[1]
Have the patient clench both fists strongly for 5 seconds, then have him/her unclench them quickly.	• Grip myotonia	This is a useful screening test for grip myotonia in professional examinations due to the likelihood of encountering patients with myotonic dystrophy, but less so in routine clinical practice unless a myotonic disorder is suspected.
Examination of the Lower Limbs		
Description of the Test	**Clinical Findings**	**Comments**
Instruct the patient to extend both ankles.	• Unilateral or bilateral foot-drop	A unilateral foot-drop in the right clinical context may lateralise the disease process to that side.

**Holme's rebound test and Holme's rebound phenomenon: These two distinct entities have been erroneously regarded by many as the same. Holme's rebound test is described above. Holme's rebound phenomenon, however, is demonstrated on the patient's outstretched arms through the application and sudden release of a downward force at the patient's wrists.[1] A normal limb rebounds slightly in the opposite direction. This response is exaggerated by spasticity, and is absent in cerebellar diseases.[1]

F. Tone Assessment

Tone assessment involves the qualitative evaluation of the degree of muscle tension or resistance to an externally applied movement. The **fully relaxed** limb is **passively moved** through its **full range of motion** about a joint. The following three "rules" are helpful when assessing the tone:

Rules	Comments
1. Assess across one joint at a time	Isolating the joints allows you to accurately assess the tone across that particular joint. If tone is assessed across two or more joints (e.g. the wrist and the elbow concurrently), the tone across one joint may confound the assessment of the other.
2. Vary the speed of movement	Because **spasticity is velocity-dependent** while rigidity is not, varying the speed of passive movement allows further characterisation of the tone.
3. Move the limb through its full range of motion	Mild spasticity is best appreciated at the end range of motion (modified Ashworth scale).[4] Failure to do so may mask subtle spasticity.

A patient's tone may be categorised into one of these **three groups**:

Tone	Comments		
Normotonia	Normal muscle tone.		
Hypotonia	Decreased tone, suggestive of a LMN pathology.		
Hypertonia	A state of increased tone, it can be further classified into three groups:		
	Hypertonia	**Description**	
	Rigidity	<ul><li>Rigidity is **independent of the velocity** of the externally applied movement, and also displays the same degree of resistance throughout.</li><li>There are two clinical subtypes:<ul><li>○ **Cogwheel rigidity:** there is intermittent increase in tone during movement due to concomitant hypertonia and tremors.</li><li>○ **Lead-pipe rigidity:** sustained resistance to passive movement, without the intermittent fluctuations seen in cogwheel rigidity.</li></ul></li></ul>	

(Continued)

Tone		Comments

	Spasticity	Spasticity is **dependent on the velocity** of the externally applied movement, and is best detected when moving the limb about its joint at greater speeds. It affects the upper and lower limbs in distinct patterns, due to build-up of excitation bias towards the antigravity muscles. As such, spasticity is best detected in the following muscle groups:
		• Upper limbs
		  ○ Elbow flexors
		  ○ Wrist flexors
		  ○ Forearm pronators
		• Lower limbs
		  ○ Hip adductors
		  ○ Knee extensors
		  ○ Ankle plantarflexors
		
		The spastic "catch" is assessed by moving the limb passively through its **full range of motion**, as the "catch" is often best appreciated at the motion's end range. The "catch" is the physical manifestation of a **hyperexcitable stretch reflex** seen in UMN disorders.
		
		Clasp-knife rigidity is a common finding in a spastic limb, and is distinct from the spastic "catch" phenomenon described above. It is the physical manifestation of a **hyperexcitable Golgi tendon reflex**, also seen in UMN pathologies. A protective feedback mechanism, it monitors the tension at the tendons, kicking in before excessive mechanical stress can result in damage and causing the muscle to abruptly relax. It is exaggerated by UMN disorders. To demonstrate clasp-knife rigidity:
		• Passively flex the patient's elbow.
		• As elbow flexion continues, the triceps brachii muscle is increasingly stretched.
		• At a certain point of tension, the hyperexcitable Golgi tendon reflex kicks in.
		• The resistance to elbow flexion abruptly ceases, manifesting as a "sudden give".

	Paratonia	Paratonia describes a pseudo-voluntary aberration of tone in response to passive movement of the limbs, and is associated with psychiatric and cognitive disorders: • **Oppositional (gegenhalten) paratonia** — pseudo-voluntary resistance against passive movements of the limb, with any attempt met with an equally strong opposing force.

(Continued)

(Continued)

Tone		Comments
		• **Facilitatory (mitgehen) paratonia** — pseudo-voluntary assistance facilitating the movements administered on the limb.

G. Deep Tendon Reflexes

The deep tendon reflex (DTR) is an involuntary muscle contraction in response to a stretching force applied on a tendon, usually by the tendon hammer. The vivacity of the DTR depends on the tendon's length and tension. It is important to note that the Babinski reflex is not a deep tendon reflex.

DTRs are clinically and qualitatively graded as **hyporeflexic, normoreflexic**, or **hyperreflexic**. Hyporeflexic DTRs suggest an underlying LMN lesion, while brisk or hyperreflexic DTRs suggest an UMN disorder.

Reflexes	Grading	Character
Absent	0	Hyporeflexic
Trace, present only with reinforcement	1	
Normal	2	Normoreflexic
Hyperactive or brisk	3	Hyperreflexic
Clonus	4	
Sustained clonus	5	

The following tips may be helpful when assessing the DTRs:

Tips	Comments
Avoid striking the tendon through clothing	Striking through clothing may dampen the force applied on the tendon, adversely affecting the grade of reflex response.
Strike with a consistent force	The grade of reflex response depends on the striking force. A consistent force should thus be applied so that the elicited reflexes may be accurately interpreted.
The limbs should be similarly positioned	The grade of reflex response depends on the initial stretch and tension of the tendon, i.e., striking the biceps brachii tendon of a fully extended elbow will falsely attenuate the reflex. As such, positioning the limbs similarly will allow you to compare the reflexes between them.
Reinforcement manoeuvres	When reflexes are difficult to elicit, reinforcement manoeuvres allow for better characterisation of the reflex. Commonly used manoeuvres include having the patient clench his/her teeth, and the Jendrassik manoeuvre (Figure 2.1).

(Continued)

Movement	Main Muscles	Nerve	Myotome[5,6]
Abduction of fingers	Dorsal interossei Abductor digiti minimi	Ulnar nerve	T1
Hip flexion	Iliopsoas Quadriceps (contributory)	L1–L3 root (iliopsoas)	L1, L2 and L3
Hip extension	Gluteus maximus	Inferior gluteal nerve	L5, S1
Hip abduction	Gluteus medius, gluteus minimus and tensor fasciae latae	Superior gluteal nerve	L5
Hip internal rotation	Gluteus medius, gluteus minimus and tensor fasciae latae	Superior gluteal nerve	L5
Knee extension	Quadriceps femoris muscles[+]	Femoral nerve	L3, L4
Knee flexion	Hamstring muscles[++]	Sciatic nerve	S1
Ankle dorsiflexion	Tibialis anterior	Deep peroneal nerve	L4, L5
Hallux extension	Extensor hallucis longus	Deep peroneal nerve	L5
Ankle eversion	Peroneus longus and brevis	Superficial peroneal nerve	L5, S1
Ankle plantar flexion	Gastrocnemius Soleus	Tibial nerve	S1
Ankle inversion	Tibialis posterior, and tibialis anterior	Tibial and deep peroneal nerves	L4

[+]The quadriceps (four-headed) femoris group of muscles consist of four separate muscles: vastus medialis, vastus intermedius, vastus lateralis and rectus femoris.

[++]Hamstring muscles consist of two pairs of muscles: the long and short heads of the biceps femoris on the lateral aspect of the thigh, and the semitendinosus and semimembranosus medially.

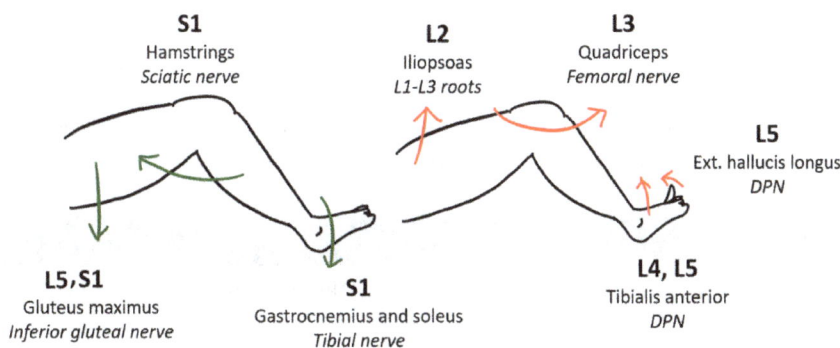

Figure 2.2. Movements of the lower limbs, with their corresponding myotomes, muscles and nerves. DPN: deep peroneal nerve.

I. Assessment of the Sensory Systems

Assessment of the sensory systems involves evaluating the **spinothalamic** and **dorsal column-medial lemniscus (DCML) modalities**, providing further neurolocalisation clues. Although both tracts convey sensory information to the sensory cortices, they have very different neuroanatomy. The character and pattern of sensory deficits can help to answer the following questions:

Questions	Comments
What sensory modalities are affected?	Due to their neuroanatomical differences (Figures 2.3 and 2.4), the involvement of these tracts can help characterise the underlying disorder. Using tabes dorsalis as an example, its predilection for the posterior columns through which the DCML tracts run results in significant impairment of proprioception and fine touch, whilst sparing the spinothalamic modalities (pain and temperature).

What is the extent of sensory deficits?	The pattern of sensory deficits has neurolocalisation implications, such as:
	• **Focal, single limb:**
	  ○ Single or multiple dermatomes: suggests a radiculopathic process.
	  ○ Sensory territory of a single nerve: e.g., median, ulnar, or radial neuropathies.
	  ○ Sensory territories of multiple nerves: suggestive of a plexopathy, or concurrent neuropathies of multiple nerves.
	• **Sensory level:** suggestive of disorders within the spinal cord, conus medullaris, or the cauda equina.
	• **Distal, length-dependent pattern ("gloves and stockings"):** peripheral neuropathy.
	• **Dissociated sensory loss (see below):** incomplete spinal cord syndromes (e.g., Brown-Sequard syndrome, Tabes Dorsalis, etc.) and brainstem syndromes (e.g., lateral medullary syndrome).
	
	Dissociated sensory loss describes the selective loss of either spinothalamic or DCML modalities, whilst sparing the other. This is only possible due to the neuroanatomical differences of the tracts (Figures 2.3 and 2.4).

To better assess the sensory tracts, a degree of familiarity is important. Here, we will describe the pertinent sensory tracts and the examination techniques involved.

Sensory Tracts	Description
Spinothalamic tract	The spinothalamic tract is responsible for the following sensory modalities: 1. Pain 2. Temperature 3. Crude (non-discriminative) touch and pressure

(Continued)

Sensory Tracts	Description
	The spinothalamic tract consists of **lateral** and **anterior** (or ventral) pathways. The lateral spinothalamic tract conveys temperature and pain sensation, while the anterior spinothalamic tract carries information on non-discriminative touch. The tract is arranged in a somatotopic fashion, with the cervical, thoracic, lumbar, and sacral segments organised from the medial-most to the lateral-most positions, respectively. The **first-order neurons** join the spinal cord via the Lissauer's tract, where they ascend one or two nerve segments and synapse with the **second-order neurons**. The **second-order neurons** decussate within the spinal cord via the anterior commissure before ascending within the spinothalamic tract located at the anterior and lateral aspects of the cord. The **second-order neurons** enter the brainstem ventromedially at the medulla, progressing upwards to reach the **ventral posterior lateral nucleus of the thalamus** where they synapse with the **third-order neurons**. These neurons will then depart for the somatosensory cortices (see Figure 2.3). 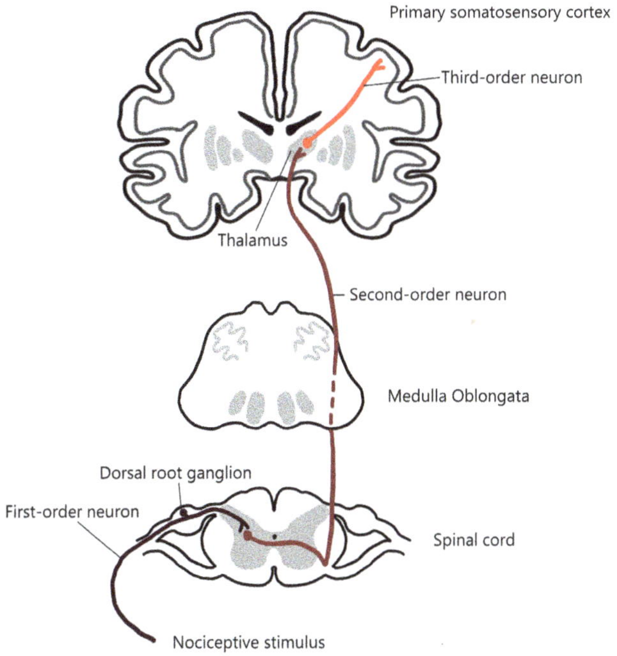

Figure 2.3.   Schematic drawing of the spinothalamic tract.

(Continued)

(Continued)

Sensory Tracts	Description

Spinothalamic tract	**Domain assessed:** Perception of pain.
	
	Equipment: Sharp end of a pin, toothpick, or equivalent device.
	
	Reference point: The forehead.
	It is not recommended to use the sternal angle as the reference point when examining the upper and/or lower limbs, as it prematurely assumes that the cervical cord and roots are normal. In patients with cervical pathologies, the sensation over the sternal angle may be abnormal, rendering it an inadequate reference point.
	
	Technique:
	There are different methods to examine the limbs:
	• By dermatomal distribution vs. by nerve distributions.
	• From distal to proximal vs. from proximal to distal.
	The choice of approach should be guided by the clinical suspicion at that point of time. For example, if the working diagnosis is peripheral neuropathy, it will be more meaningful to begin sensory assessment distally and proceed proximally.
	
	You should:
	• Begin by telling the patient what you are about to do.
	• Gently touch the reference point (the forehead) with the device and ask if the patient can feel the stimulus and appreciate its "pointedness".
	• Instruct the patient to close his or her eyes.
	• **Lightly touch** the area of interest with a device and ask the patient if he or she could:
	  ○ Feel the prick.
	  ○ Appreciate the "pointedness" when compared to the reference point.
	• Compare the sensation between the assessed limbs and against the reference point.
	
	During the assessment:
	• Do not scratch or stroke the patient's skin with the device.
	• Do not apply injurious force on the patient with the device.
	• Do not reuse disposable equipment (e.g., toothpick, broken wooden spatula).

DCML	The DCML tracts are responsible for the following sensory modalities: 1. Fine/discriminative touch 2. Vibration sense 3. Proprioception: position sense and kinaesthesia (sense of motion)

(Continued)

Sensory Tracts	Description
	First-order neurons enter the spinal cord and ascend in the ipsilateral dorsal column. The neurons from the lower half of the body join the dorsal column medially, ascending within the fasciculus gracilis, while those from the upper half of the body (inclusive of the upper limbs) join the column laterally, ascending within the fasciculus cuneatus. These **first-order neurons** from the fasciculus gracilis and fasciculus cuneatus synapse at the ipsilateral **nucleus gracilis** and **nucleus cuneatus** respectively at the **caudal medulla**.

Second-order neurons then decussate as the internal arcuate fibres and ascend within the **medial lemniscus** before synapsing at the contralateral **ventral posterior lateral nucleus** of the thalamus.

Third-order neurons leave the thalamus to ascend to the primary somatosensory cortices (see Figure 2.4). In actuality, the DCML pathways are complex, with different pathways serving proprioception, fine touch, and sense of vibration to varying degrees.

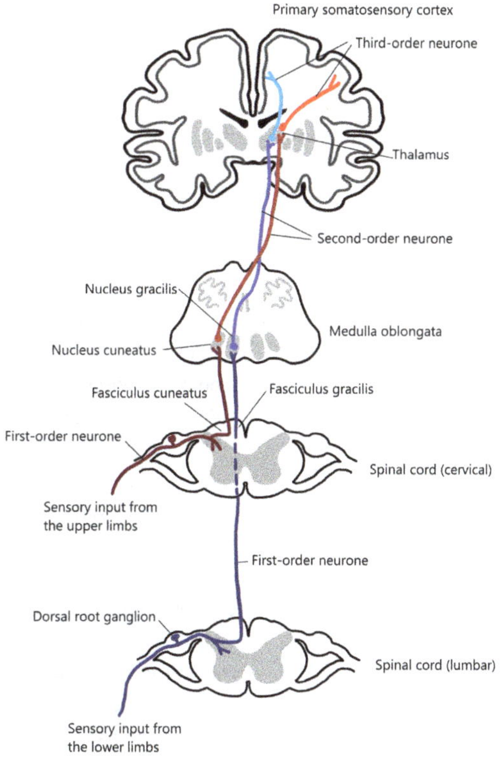

Figure 2.4.   Schematic drawing of the DCML tract.

(Continued)

Sensory Tracts	Description
	Assessing the DCML Tract

Proprioception, fine touch, and vibration sense are commonly assessed DCML domains. Vibration sense is lost early in diabetic peripheral neuropathy, and its assessment is imperative if diabetic neuropathy is suspected.

Domain	Vibration Sense	Position Sense	Fine Touch
Equipment	128 Hz tuning fork	None	Cotton ball 10g monofilament

Vibration	Vibration is a sensitive modality as it accurately and quickly senses, transmits, and processes rapidly changing stimuli. In the initial stages of disease, the ability to follow a train of stimuli is often impaired, resulting in a diminishing or loss of vibration sense and reflecting the ill-health of the peripheral nervous system or the posterior columns.	
	Equipment: 128 Hz tuning fork	
	Reference Point: The forehead	

	Technique
	• Tap the tuning fork gently against a firm surface (e.g., heel of your palm or a tendon hammer) and apply the base of the fork onto a bony surface **after the ringing is no longer audible**.
	• Begin at the reference point:
	  ○ Inform the patient that he or she will experience a buzzing sensation.
	  ○ Be specific and precise. Avoid ambiguous questions like "can you feel this?" The patient may misinterpret that the desired sensation is that of the base of the tuning fork touching his skin.
	• Repeat the above step, but with a non-vibrating tuning fork. This allows the patient to appreciate the difference between a vibrating and a non-vibrating tuning fork.
	• Instruct the patient to close his or her eyes before proceeding to assess the limb of interest:
	  ○ Strike the tuning fork against a hard surface.
	  ○ Apply the base of the tuning fork onto a bony surface **after** the ringing noise is no longer audible and ask if the patient is able to appreciate the vibration.	

(Continued)

Sensory Tracts	Description
	○ Instruct the patient to immediately indicate to you when the vibration has stopped. Begin distally, noting the patient's perception of the vibration, and progress proximally if the responses are diminished or absent. Compare between the left- and right-sided limbs. The common sites to place the tuning fork are as follows:

Upper Limbs	• Distal and proximal interphalangeal joints • Metacarpophalangeal joints • Radial and ulnar styloids • Olecranon process • Clavicles
Lower Limbs	• Interphalangeal joint of the big toe • Medial or lateral malleoli of the ankle • Anterior superior iliac spine

Sensory Tracts		Description
		Another method of assessing vibration sense involves shifting a still-vibrating tuning fork to a contralateral, homologous bony prominence as soon as the patient ceases to detect the vibration at the initial site. If the patient is able to sense vibration at the second site, the patient is deemed to have asymmetrical loss of vibration sense. However, this method is vulnerable to errors, as vibration may be briefly sensed when the tuning fork is moved from one side to another due to normal sensory adaptive mechanisms. I do not recommend this method.
	Position sense (proprio-ception)	**Equipment:** none **Technique:** • Begin by telling the patient what you are about to do. • Have the patient look at the appendage of interest (e.g., the big toe or thumb) while you gently and slowly move the appendage about their joints in small and slow deflections. • Instruct the patient to verbalise the new position of the appendage as he or she felt it to be. • Allow the patient some time to understand the instructions and seek clarification if needed.

(Continued)

(Continued)

Sensory Tracts	Description	
	• Instruct the patient to close his or her eyes and repeat the above steps.	
	Upper Limbs	• Begin at the distal phalanx of the thumb. • Stabilise the interphalangeal joint by holding it gently between two fingers. • Move the distal phalanx about the interphalangeal with your fingers holding the phalanx at the sides. • Avoid applying pressure over the thumb's pulp and nail.
	Lower Limbs	• Begin at the distal phalanx of the big toe. • Stabilise the interphalangeal joint by holding it gently between two fingers. • Move the distal phalanx about the interphalangeal joint using two fingers, holding the phalanx at the sides rather than applying pressure over the big toe's pulp and nail.
	Our proprioceptors are highly sensitive to changes in position and can detect displacements as small as 1–2 degrees. To improve the reliability of this test, ensure that the **deflections are small and slow**. Small movements will allow you to detect mild proprioceptive loss, while slow movements avoid confounding the assessment with kinesthesia. Additionally, a patient with profound proprioceptive loss can statistically guess the correct response 50% of the time if he or she is allowed only "up" or "down" responses, limiting the sensitivity of the assessment. This may be avoided with the following steps: • Allow the patient three possible responses: "up", "down", or "I don't know, please repeat again". • The patient should be instructed against guessing his or her responses. • If the patient hesitates, it is safe to assume that he or she was guessing the answers. This should prompt you to repeat the test.	

(*Continued*)

Sensory Tracts	Description	
	Fine touch	**Equipment:** 10g monofilament (gold standard) or a cotton bud/ball (alternative). **Reference Point:** The forehead. It is not recommended to use the sternal angle as the reference point when examining the upper and/or lower limbs, as this prematurely assumes that the cervical cord and roots are normal. In patients with cervical pathologies, sensation over the sternal angle may be affected, rendering it an inadequate reference point. **Technique:** There are many different methods to examine the limbs: • By dermatomal distribution vs. by nerve distributions. • From distal to proximal vs. from proximal to distal. The choice of approach should be guided by the clinical suspicion at that point of time. For example, if the working diagnosis is peripheral neuropathy, it will be more meaningful to begin sensory assessment distally and proceed proximally. If a monofilament is used: • Begin by telling the patient what you are about to do. • Lightly touch or dab the reference point with the monofilament and ask if he or she can feel the stimulus. • **Do note stroke** the skin with the monofilament. • The patient should then be instructed to close his or her eyes. • Lightly touch the area of interest with the device and ask the patient if he or she could feel the stimulus. • Compare side-to-side, distal-to-proximal, and against the reference point. If a cotton bud is used, you may twirl the edge into a wisp of cotton and dab the skin to test the patient's sensation of light touch.

(*Continued*)

(*Continued*)

Sensory Tracts	Description
	During the assessment, you should ensure the following: • Do not scratch or stroke the patient with the device. • Do not apply injurious force. • Do not reuse disposable equipment (i.e., the cotton buds). • Clean the monofilament with an alcohol swab so that it may be reused later on another patient.

As each patch of skin is served by specific nerves and dermatomes, the pattern of sensory deficits yields significant neurolocalisation clues. The dermatomes of the upper and lower limbs are discussed separately in **Chapters 3 and 4.**

J. Assessment of the Cerebellar System

Cerebellar examination usually follows sensory testing. The complete assessment of the cerebellar system requires you to examine the patient's eyes, speech, trunk, upper limbs and lower limbs. The features of cerebellar dysfunction are summarised below:

Anatomical Regions	Findings Suggestive of Cerebellar Dysfunction
Eyes	• Multi-directional nystagmus • Dysmetric saccades • Jerky pursuit

Speech	• Ataxic dysarthria
	    ○ Scanning speech
	    ○ Staccato speech

Upper limbs	• Holme's rebound test: demonstration of impaired check response • Dysmetria • Dysdiadochokinesia
Trunk	• Truncal ataxia
Lower limbs	• Heel-shin dysmetria • "Pendular" knee jerk (the leg continues to swing more than 4 times after the initial knee jerk) due to hypotonia
Gait[6,7]	• Unsteady, broad-based gait • Irregularity of steps • Reduced cadence • Lateral veering

A detailed description of a cerebellar examination is described further in **Chapters 3 and 4.**

K. Conclusion

In summary, the examination of a patient's limbs involves the following components:

- Setting
- Positioning the patient
- Exposure
- Inspection
- Tone
- Deep tendon reflexes
- Motor assessment
- Sensory assessment
- Cerebellar assessment
- Assessment of gait and function

It is only after these have all been confidently assessed that you can make learned and appropriate use of the localisation principles discussed later in this book.

Tips for Examination Candidates

Exposure and inspection of the patient will yield many important clues on the nature and character of the culprit pathology. A learned candidate can generate a reasonable list of differential diagnoses from the initial steps alone. As such, committing time and attention to these clues will set the stage towards success in your neurolocalisation adventure!

References

1. Campbell W, Barohn R. (2020) *DeJong's The Neurologic Examination*, 8th ed. Lippincott Williams & Wilkins, Philadelphia.
2. Wilkinson I, Lennox G. (2005) *Essential Neurology*, 4th ed. Wiley-Blackwell, Chicester.
3. Digiti Quinti: Alter M. (1973) The digiti quinti sign of mild hemiparesis. *Neurology* **23**(5): 503–505.
4. Pandyan AD, Johnson GR, Price CI, Curless RH, Barnes MP, Rodgers H. (1999) A review of the properties and limitations of the Ashworth and modified Ashworth Scales as measures of spasticity. *Clin Rehabil* **13**(5): 373–383.
5. Polkey CE. (1977) Book reviews. *Br Med Bull* **33**(2): 182.
6. Lim E, Tey HL. (2009) *The Black Book of Clinical Examination*, 1st ed. McGraw-Hill, Singapore.
7. Stolze H, Klebe S, Petersen G, Raethjen J, Wenzelburger R, Witt K, Deuschl G. (2002) Typical features of cerebellar ataxic gait. *J Neurol Neurosurg Psychiatry* **73**(3): 310–312.

3

Neurological Examination of the Upper Limbs

A. Introduction

The neurological assessment of the upper limbs requires the same basic steps of most neurologic examinations, from inspecting the patient, to assessing for functional impairment. Generally, the flow of the examination follows the sequence below:

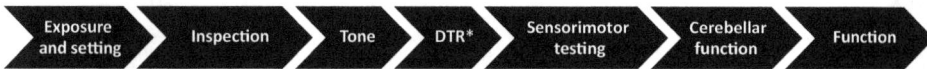

Exposure and setting → Inspection → Tone → DTR* → Sensorimotor testing → Cerebellar function → Function

*DTR: deep tendon reflex

This chapter aims to provide a step-by-step approach to the neurological examination of the upper limbs, aided by pictorial representations of a model (a kind volunteer and good colleague of mine). With the model's modesty and comfort in mind, he was kept attired in most of the pictures. In actual examinations and in clinical practice, however, the patient should be adequately exposed throughout. The deep tendon reflexes and their root levels, and the limb movements with their corresponding nerves and myotomes, are detailed in separate tables in **Chapter 2**.

Examination Steps

| Exposure, setting, and inspection | 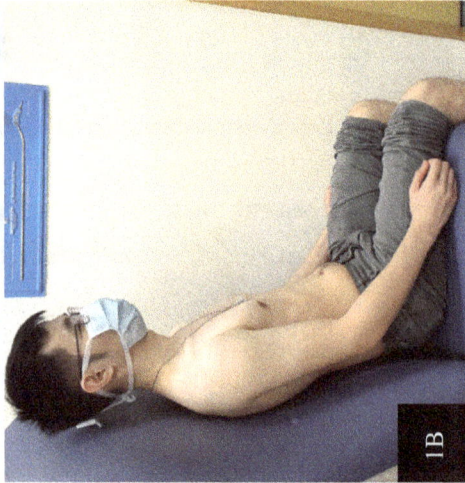 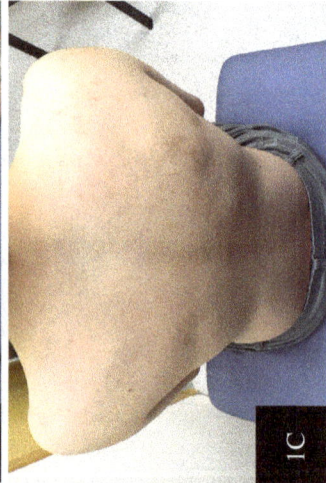 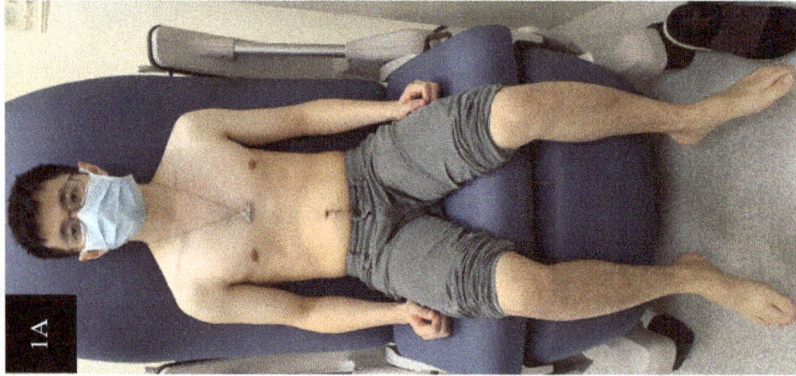 | When examining the upper limbs, the patient should be seated upright or at a 45° incline (**1A**). The following areas should be exposed:

• Upper limbs
• Neck and shoulders
• Chest and back

Additionally, exposing the lower limbs allows you to look for concomitant abnormalities of the legs, which when present may hint at a more diffuse disease process.

Begin inspecting the patient from his front, then proceed to his sides and back (**1A–C**). Observing for:

• Muscle wasting of the:
  ○ Neck and shoulders
  ○ Arms, forearms and the hands
• Scars and deformities, especially over the back and the upper limbs.

Abnormal posture, e.g., kyphoscoliosis, camptocormia, torticollis, etc. |

| Screening tests | 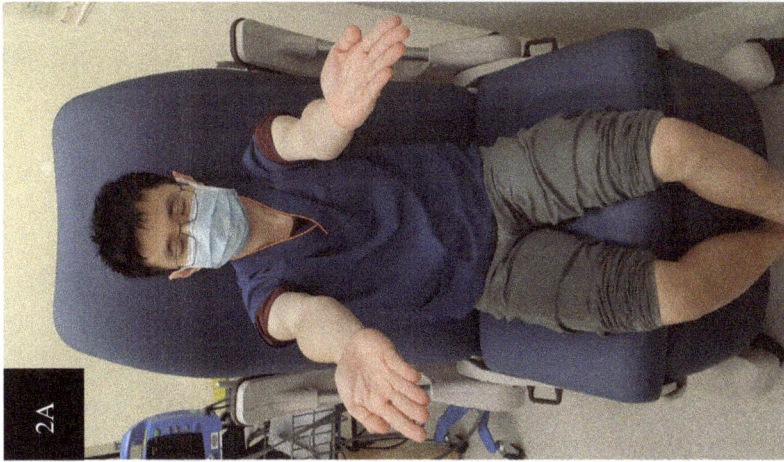 2A   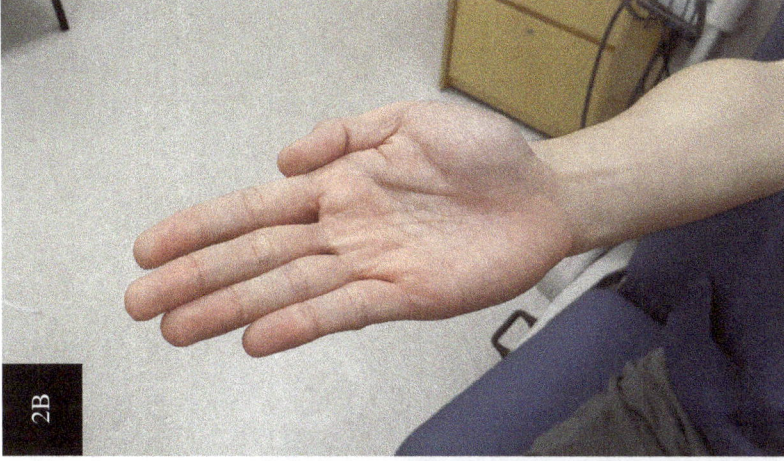 2B | Begin by testing for **pronator drift** (2A). Instruct the patient to close his/her eyes with outstretched arms. Ensure that the forearms are well-supinated, with fingers kept adducted and straightened **(2B)**. |

(Continued)

(Continued)

Examination Steps

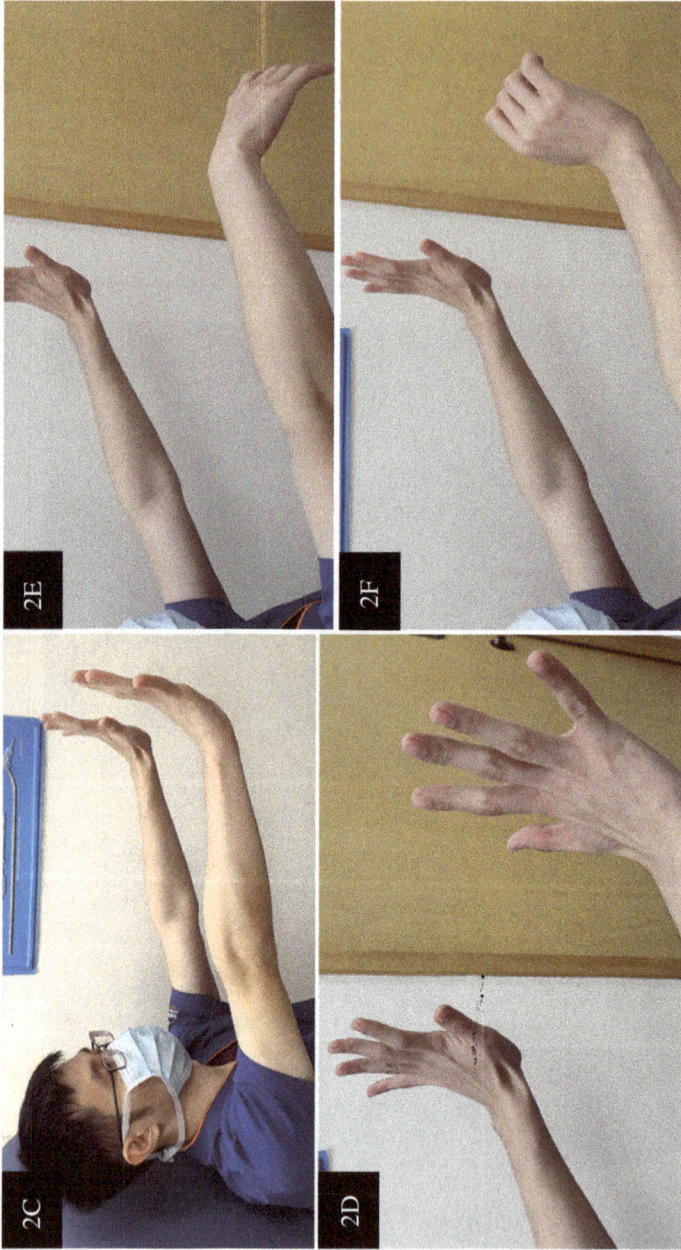

Next, have the patient **extend the wrists and fingers (2C, 2D)**. This allows to rapidly screen for weakened wrist extensors (wrist drop sign, **2E**) and finger extensors (finger drop sign, **2F**).

Screen for **grip myotonia** by asking the patient to clench his/her fists tightly for 3–5 seconds, then unclenching them as fast as possible (**2G, 2H**).

The inclusion of this test is important in both undergraduate and postgraduate examinations, during which patients with myotonic dystrophy are not infrequently encountered. The early suspicion of myotonic dystrophy will allow you to plan your examination, so that some time may be set aside to demonstrate the non-neurologic features of myotonic dystrophy.

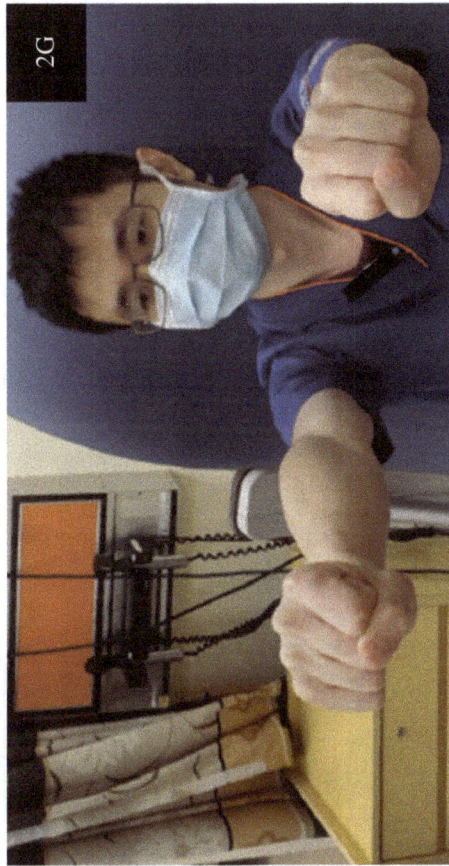

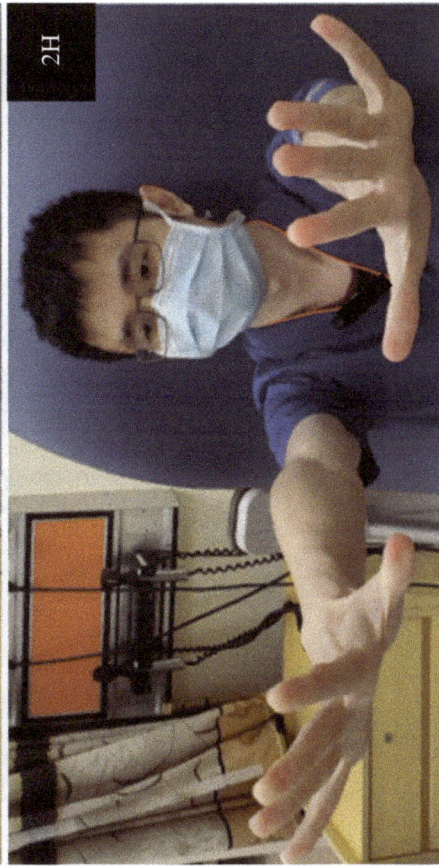

2G

2H

(Continued)

(Continued)

Examination Steps	

Tone

The tone of the upper limb is assessed over the elbow and wrists. A good assessment requires the following:

- Assess one joint at a time
- Move the joint through its full range of motion
- Vary your speed, so as to distinguish rigidity from spasticity

Passively flex and extend the elbows first (**3A, 3B**), then the wrists (**3C, 3D**). Rigidity at the wrist, when with superimposed wrist tremors, can be described as "**cogwheeling**". Spasticity at the wrist is demonstrated by administering quick flick of the wrist (**3D**), during which a sudden increase in tone is experienced.

When testing for "**pronator catch**", ensure that the elbow is flexed at 90° to relax the pronator teres. Fully pronate the forearm (**3E**), and then, in quick motion, supinate the forearm (**3F**) to quickly and fully stretch the pronator teres.

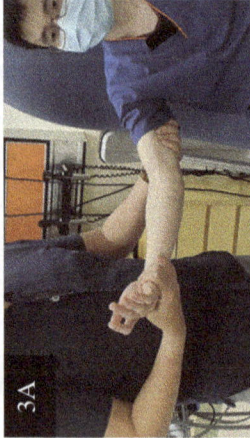

3A

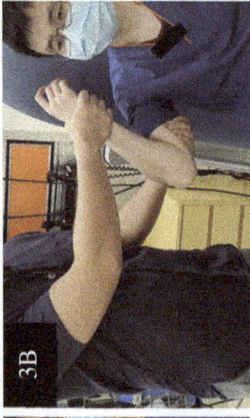

3B

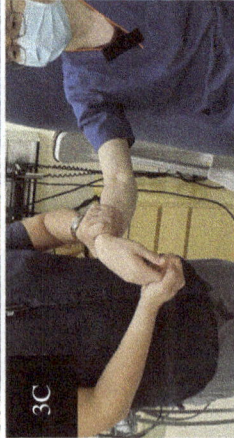

3C

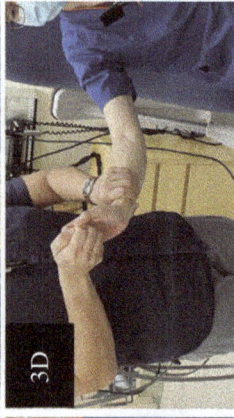

3D

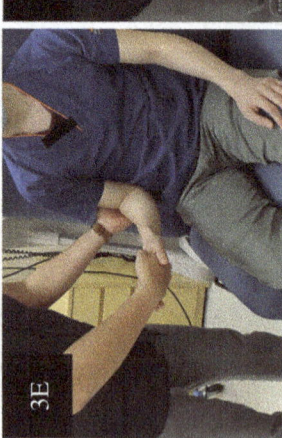

3E

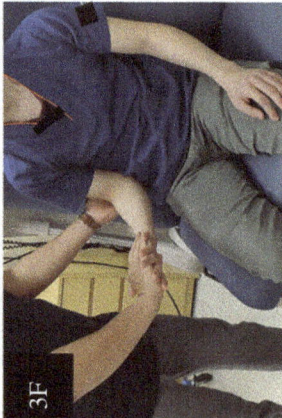

3F

DTR		
4A	4B 4C	Position the patient's arms as illustrated (**4A**), and ensure that the patient is fully relaxed. The corresponding cervical spinal roots of the DTRs are described in **Chapter 2**. Begin by striking the patient's biceps brachii tendons as shown (**4B**, **4C**).

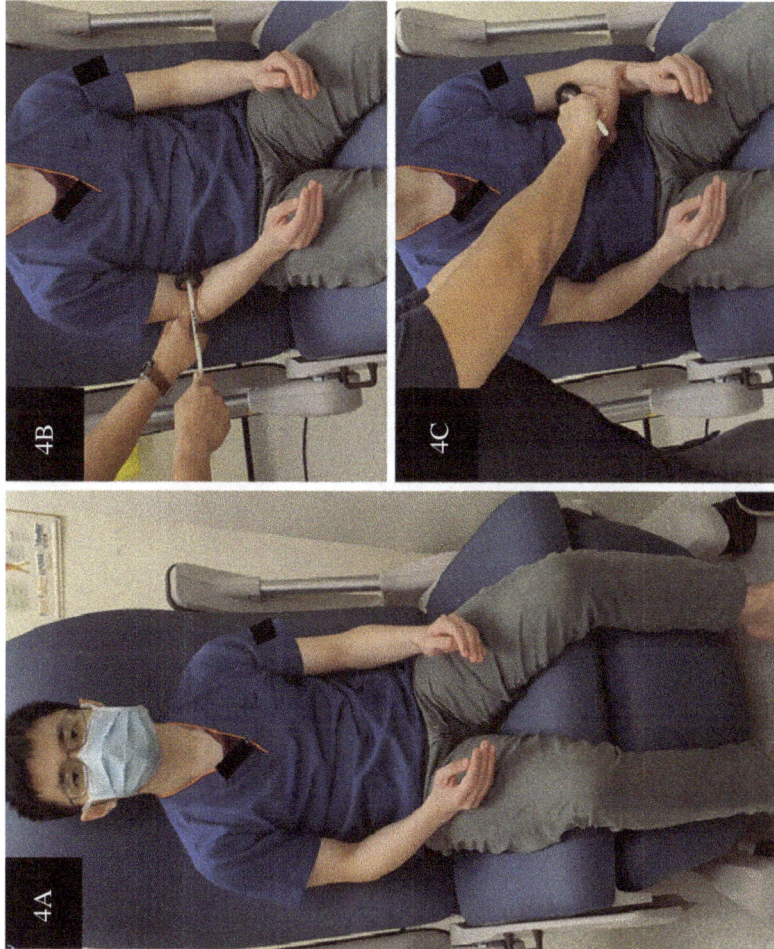

(Continued)

(Continued)

Examination Steps

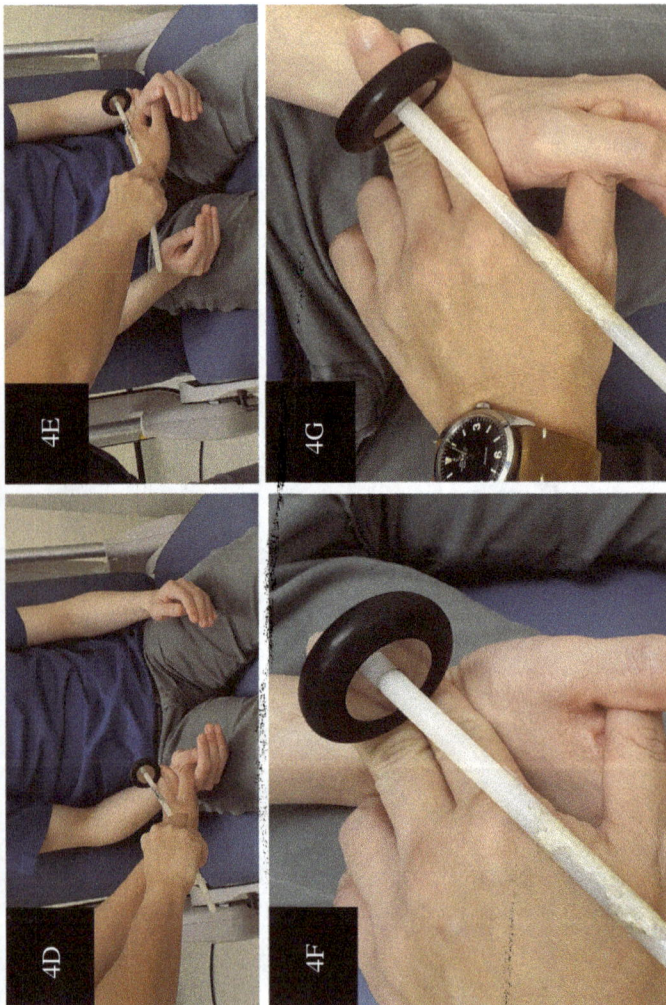

Next, proceed to the brachioradialis tendon at the **radial styloid process (4D, 4E)**. Keeping the wrists in their neutral positions with the thumb mildly adducted out of the way of the fingers, you can better demonstrate the flexion of fingers (**4F, 4G**). An **"inverted supinator reflex"** (not shown) describes the diminished contraction of the elbow flexors, and a hyperactive flexion response of the fingers. Its presence localizes the lesion at C5/6 level of the spinal root and cord (i.e., C5/6 myeloradiculopathy).

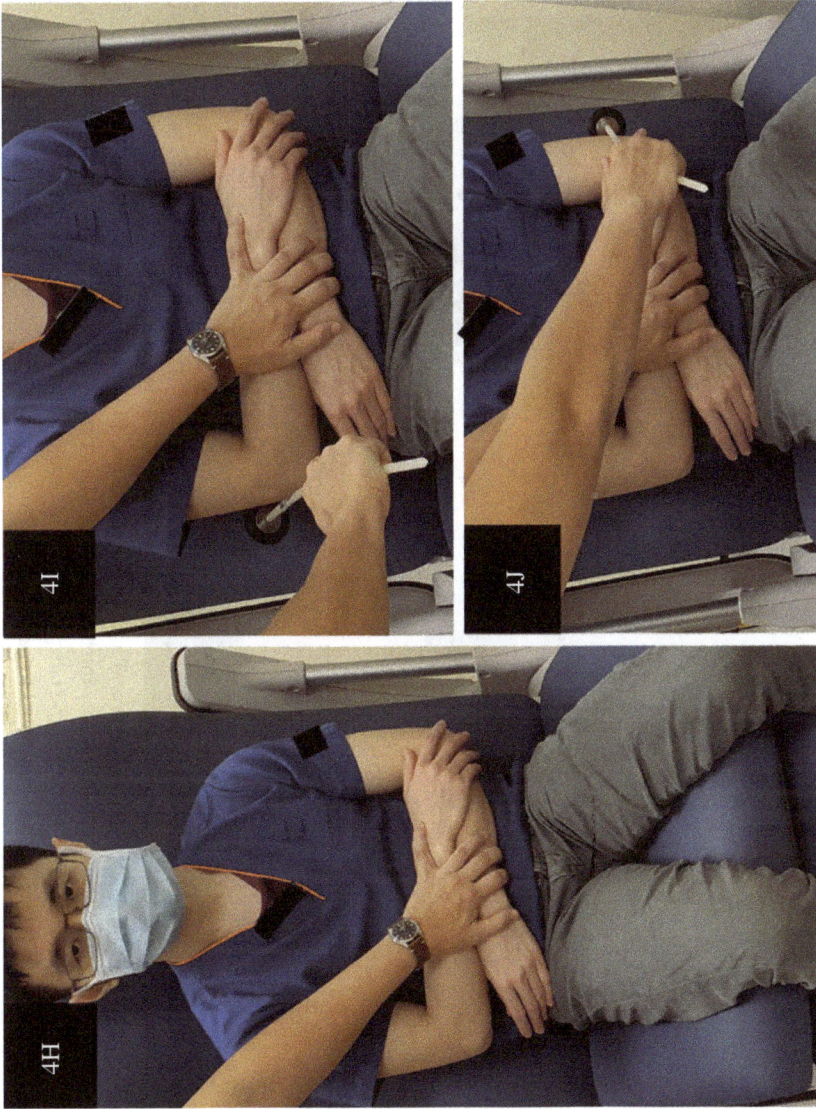

Finally, position the patient's arms as shown (**4H**), ensuring that the patient is fully relaxed. Proceed to strike the triceps brachii at its tendon (**4I**, **4J**).

(*Continued*)

(Continued)

Motor strength	Examination Steps
	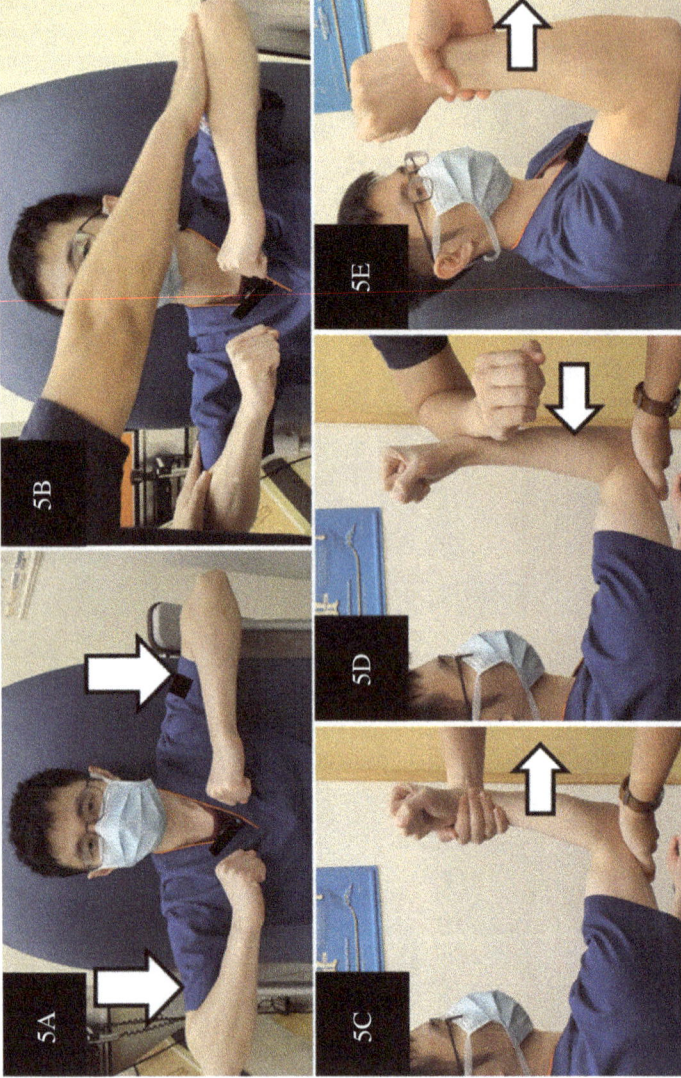 **5A and 5B** show the testing of shoulder abductors. When testing the **elbow flexors and extensors**, position the shoulders as shown in **5C–E**. This reduces the contributions by the back muscles when testing the arm's strength. Proceed to test the elbow flexors (**5C, 5E**) and extensors (**5D**). Testing of the biceps brachii and brachialis requires a fully supinated forearm, while the brachioradialis is best tested with a half-supinated forearm.

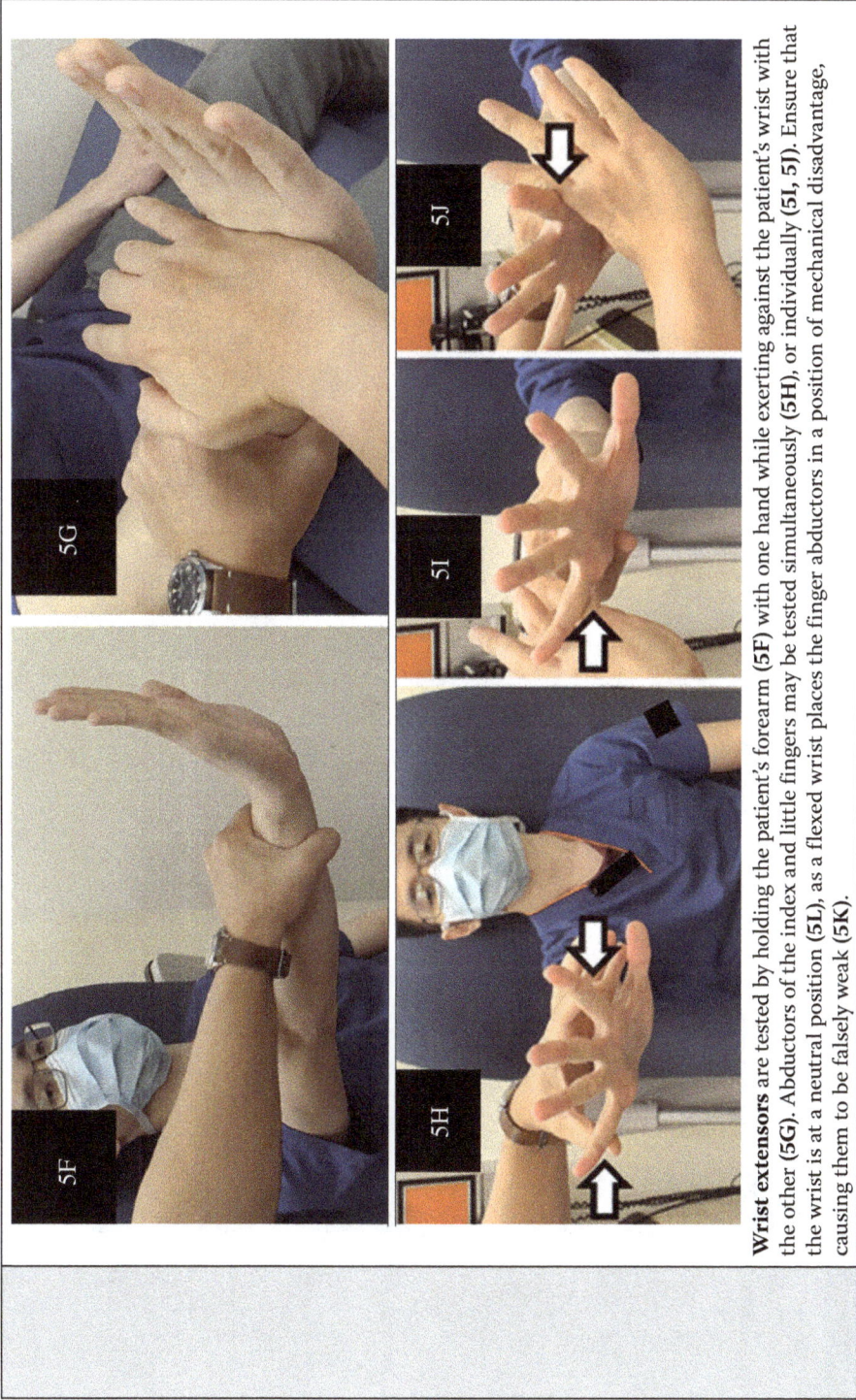

Wrist extensors are tested by holding the patient's forearm (**5F**) with one hand while exerting against the patient's wrist with the other (**5G**). Abductors of the index and little fingers may be tested simultaneously (**5H**), or individually (**5I, 5J**). Ensure that the wrist is at a neutral position (**5L**), as a flexed wrist places the finger abductors in a position of mechanical disadvantage, causing them to be falsely weak (**5K**).

(Continued)

(Continued)

Examination Steps

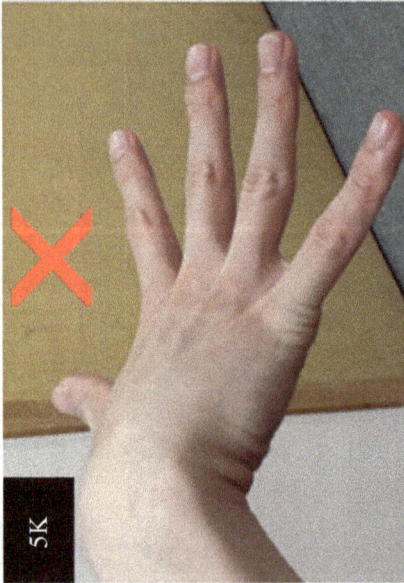

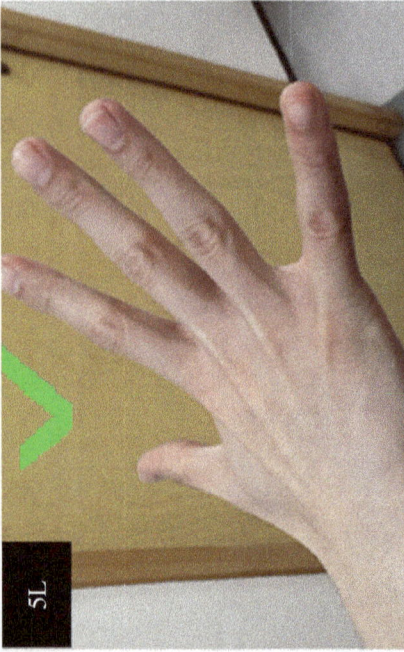

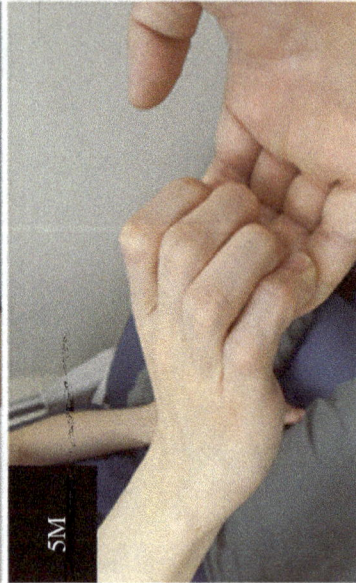

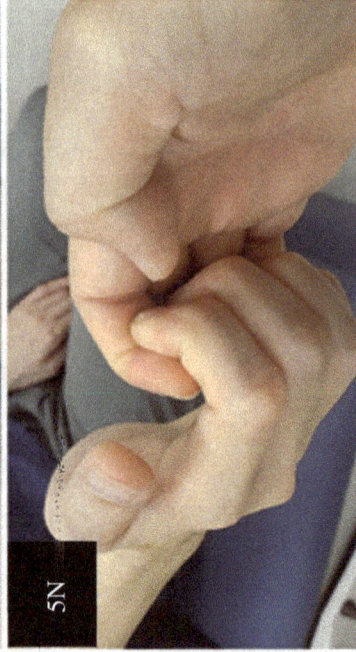

When testing the finger abductors and flexors, ensure that the wrist is at the neutral position (**5L**), as a flexed wrist places the finger abductors and flexors in a position of mechanical disadvantage, causing them to be falsely weak (**5K**). Testing of finger flexion is shown in **5M** and **5N**.

Sensory testing	6	

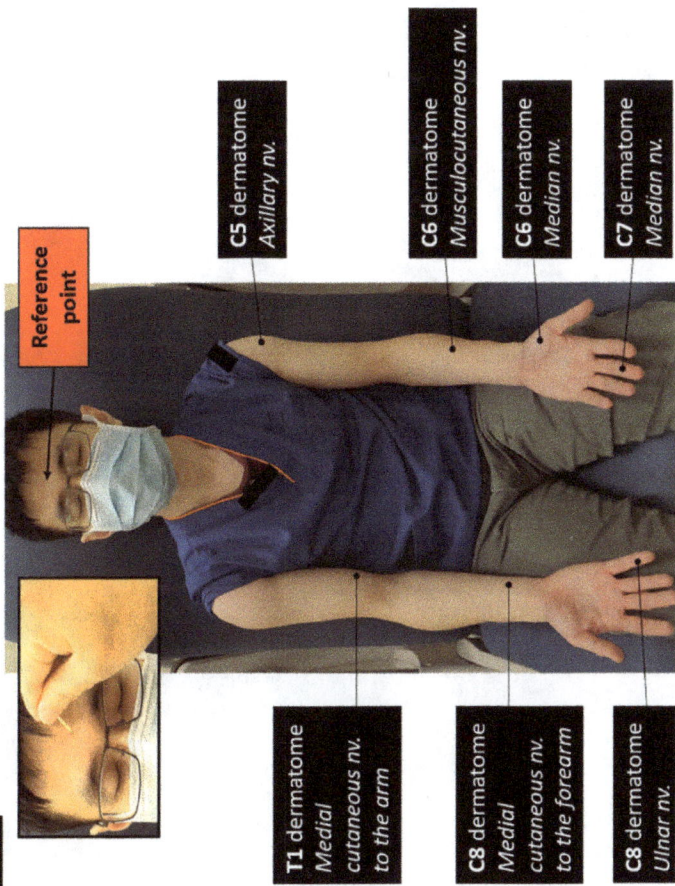

Reference point

C5 dermatome
Axillary nv.

C6 dermatome
Musculocutaneous nv.

C6 dermatome
Median nv.

C7 dermatome
Median nv.

T1 dermatome
Medial cutaneous nv. to the arm

C8 dermatome
Medial cutaneous nv. to the forearm

C8 dermatome
Ulnar nv.

Using an appropriate device, begin at the **reference point – the forehead.**

Illustrated here are the regions of interest, together with the nerves and dermatomes serving that area. A **Neurotip** or a **toothpick** should be used when assessing pain perception, while a **cotton wisp** is appropriate when assessing fine touch.

Sensory testing of the forearm is extremely important but often omitted. The patterns of sensory deficits over the forearms and the hands have significant localizing value when assessing a patient with hand numbness. In median neuropathy, for example, the sensation over the forearm is often spared, regardless of the proximity of the lesion, as the median nerve has no sensory branches supplying the forearm. This is unlike a C6 radiculopathy, in which sensory deficits over the forearm is expected. A similar concept applies to the ulnar nerve and the C8 root as well.

(Continued)

(Continued)

Examination Steps

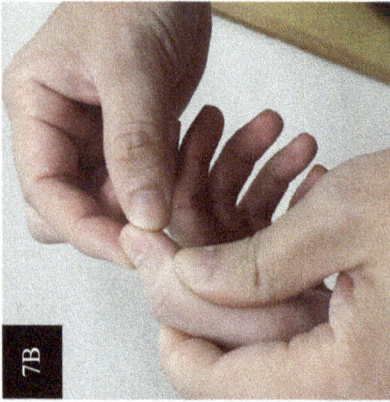

7A

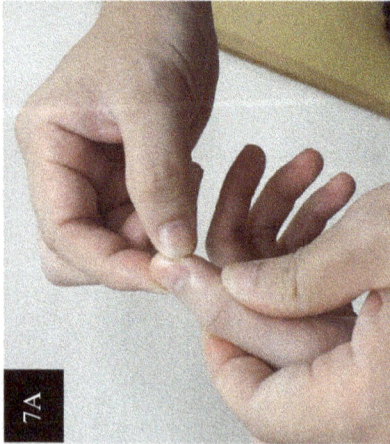

7B

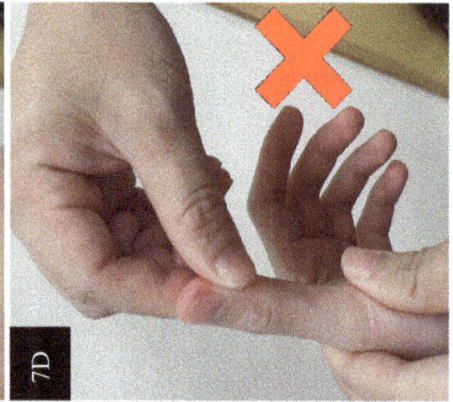

7C

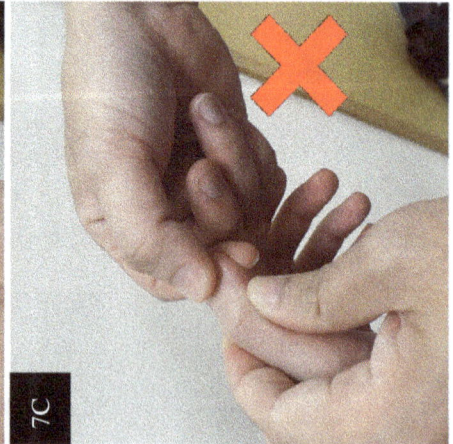

7D

When testing **proprioception** of the thumb, begin by gently holding the interphalangeal joint and the distal phalanx as shown (7A), and move the latter about the interphalangeal joint in **small and slow deflections** (7B). Avoid holding the distal phalanx at the nail (7C) or moving the thumb in large deflections (7D).

Proprioception is a highly-sensitive sensory modality, able to pick up small deflections. As such, deflections must be kept reasonably **small**. Additionally, the speed of the deflections should be **slow**, so as to avoid confounding the assessment with kinesthesia (sensation of motion).

The patient should be allowed **three responses** when asked about the perceived deflection — "up", "down", or "don't know" (see **Chapter 2**).

Cerebellar function

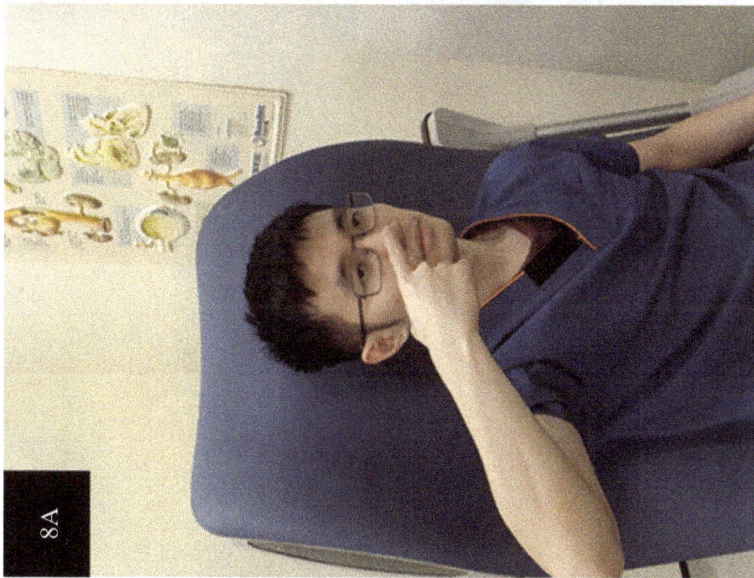

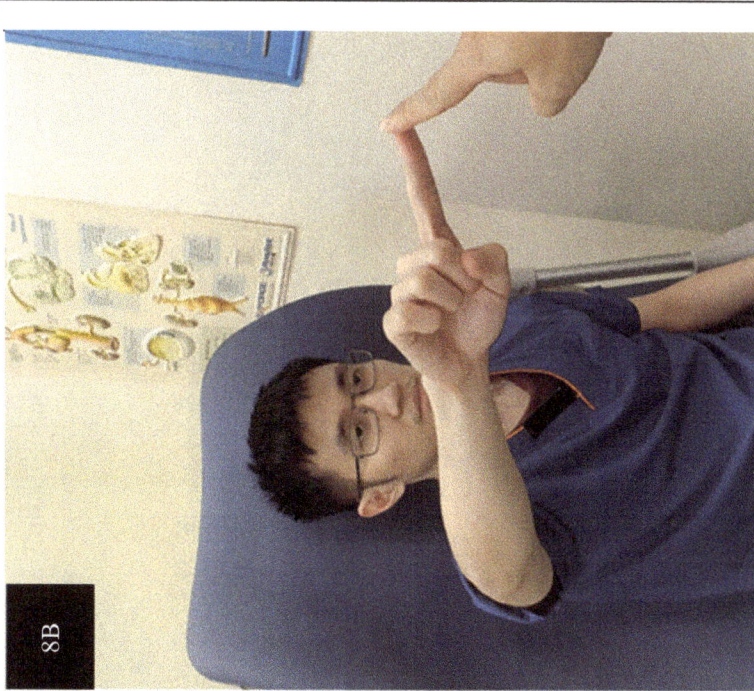

8A

8B

The **finger-nose test** for dysmetria is shown in **8A** and **8B**. Instruct the patient to alternately touch the **tip of his nose** and **your fingertip** with his **fingertip**. Dysmetria is present when the patient's fingertip over or undershoots the intended target.

(Continued)

(Continued)

Examination Steps

9

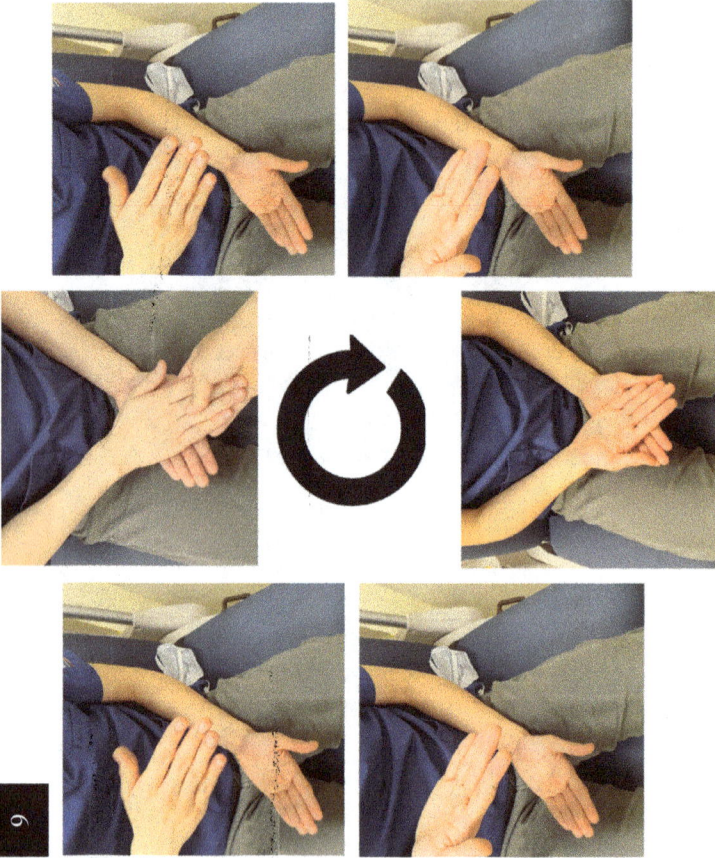

Dysdiadochokinesia, the inability to rapidly and precisely perform alternating movements, is tested by having the patient rapidly supinate and pronate the forearms whilst lightly tapping the bottom hand. Testing for right-sided dysdiadochokinesia is illustrated here (**9**).

Reference

1. Estanol BV, Marin OS. (1976) Mechanism of the inverted supinator reflex. A clinical and neurophysiological study. *J Neurol Neurosurg Psychiatry* **39**(9): 905–908. doi:10.1136/jnnp.39.9.905.

4

Examination of the Lower Limbs

A. Introduction

The neurological assessment of the upper limbs requires the same basic steps of most neurologic examinations, from inspecting the patient, to assessing for functional impairment. Generally, the flow of the examination follows the sequence below:

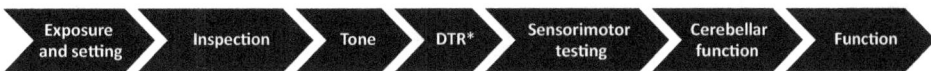

Exposure and setting > Inspection > Tone > DTR* > Sensorimotor testing > Cerebellar function > Function

*DTR: deep tendon reflex

This chapter aims to provide a step-by-step approach to the neurological examination of the upper limbs, aided by pictorial representations of a model (a kind volunteer and good colleague of mine). With the model's modesty and comfort in mind, he was kept attired in most of the pictures. In actual examinations and in clinical practice, however, the patient should be adequately exposed throughout. The deep tendon reflexes and their root levels, and the limb movements with their corresponding nerves and myotomes, are detailed in separate tables in **Chapter 2.**

Examination Steps		Description
Exposure, setting, and inspection	1	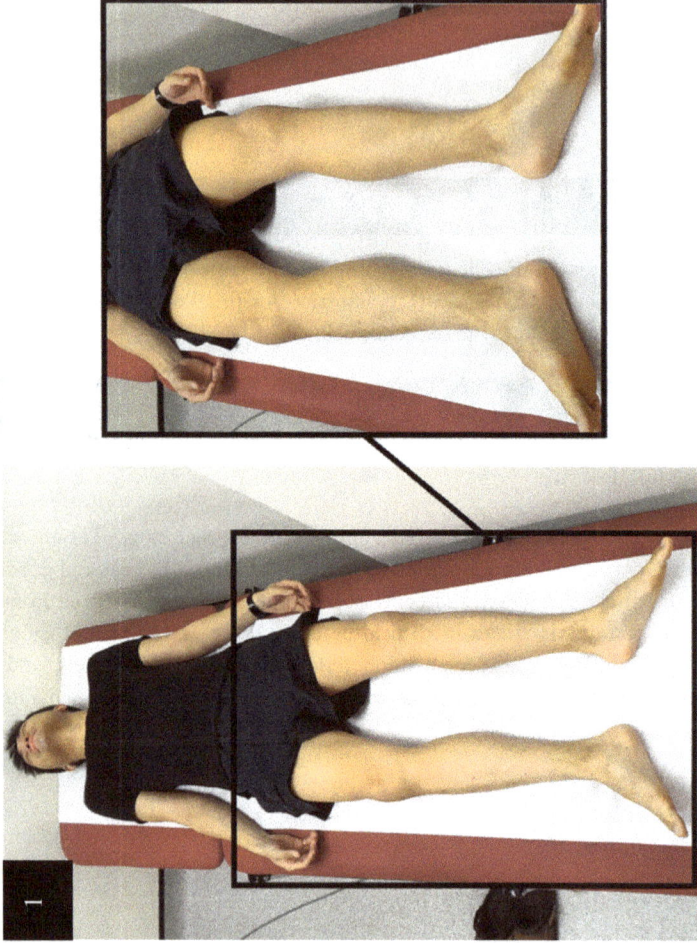 Expose the legs from the inguinal regions to the toes. However, the extent of exposure is ultimately dependent on the patient's comfort. In our attempt at preserving the model's modesty, we have left his inguinal region unexposed (1). Also, look around the room for **mobility aids**, which when present are indicative of underlying functional impairment.

Tone	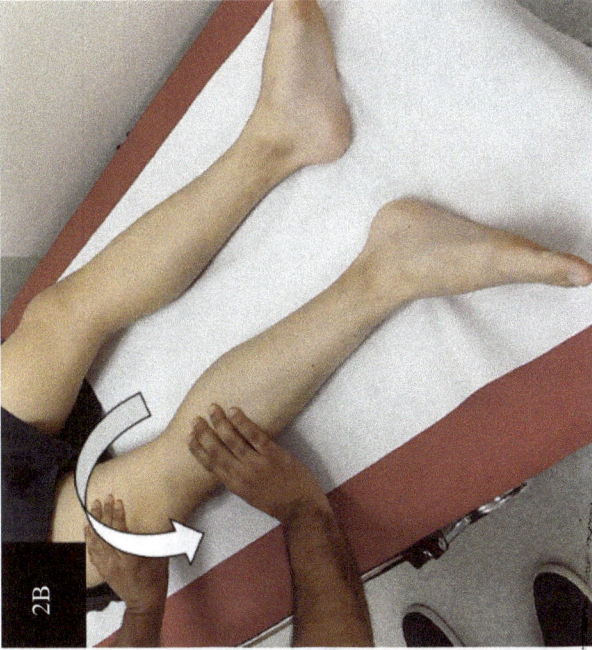 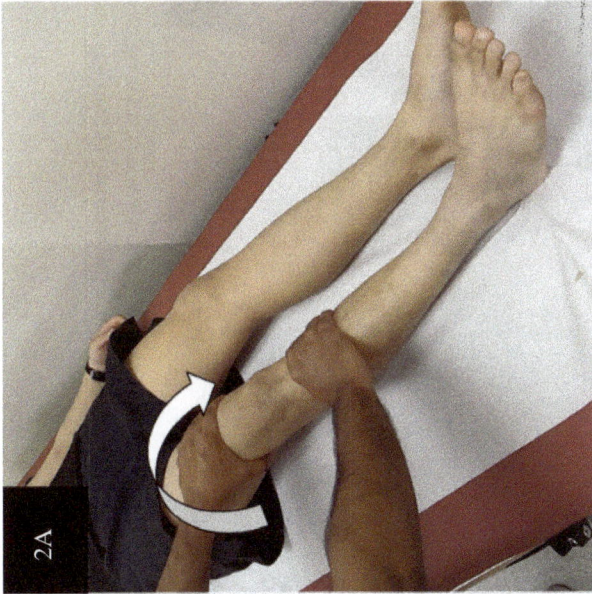

Assessment of the lower limbs' tone is as illustrated. Begin with the **leg roll** to assess the tone of the hip rotators (**2A, 2B**).

(*Continued*)

(Continued)

Examination Steps	Description
Tone	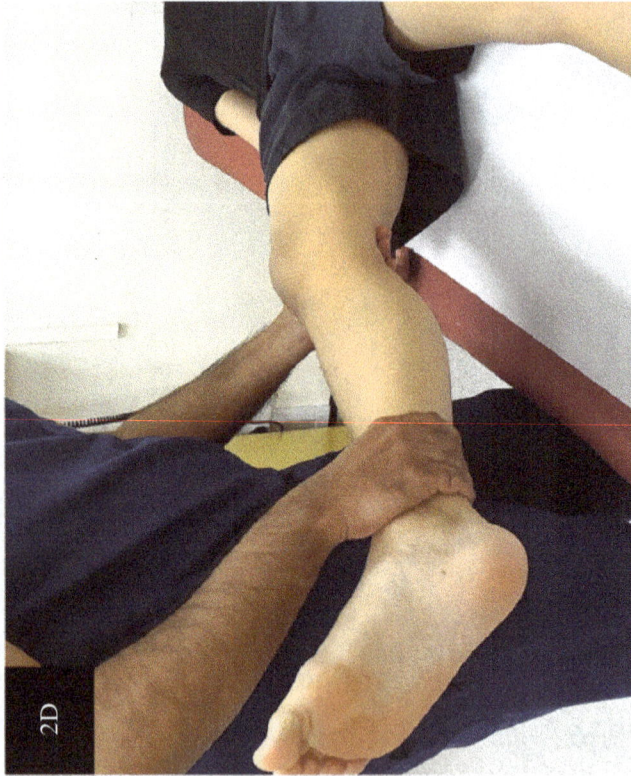 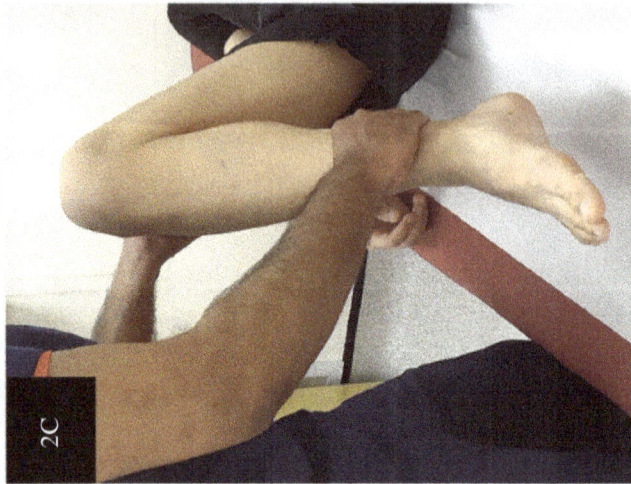 Next, **slowly flex and extend the knee** to assess for rigidity (**2C, 2D**). This also allows you to check the knee for any limitation in its range of motion and the presence of pain (e.g., osteoarthritis of the knees) before performing the leg-lift.

Next, perform the **leg-lift maneuvre** by briskly elevating the knee off the bed (**2E, 2F**) and observe the movement of the leg. In a normal leg, the heel will remain on the bed, while the foot of a hypertonic leg will be lifted off the bed.

The demonstration of ankle clonus is often performed immediately after the leg-lift maneuvre. This is incorrect, and will be discussed later in this chapter

Ensure that the limb is relaxed.

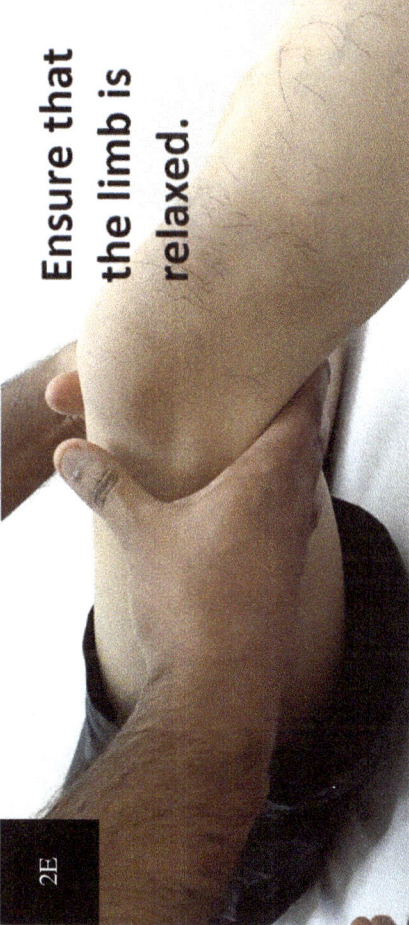

2E

Lift the leg briskly and observe the heel

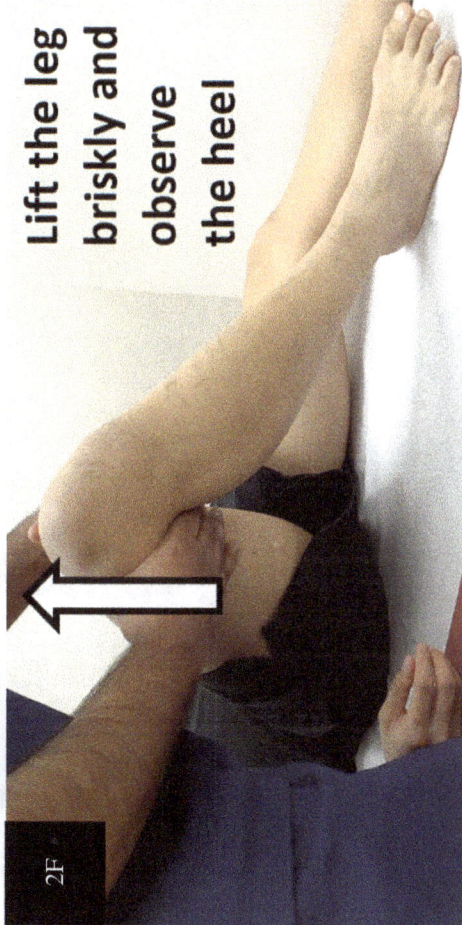

2F

(Continued)

(Continued)

Examination Steps	Description	
DTR	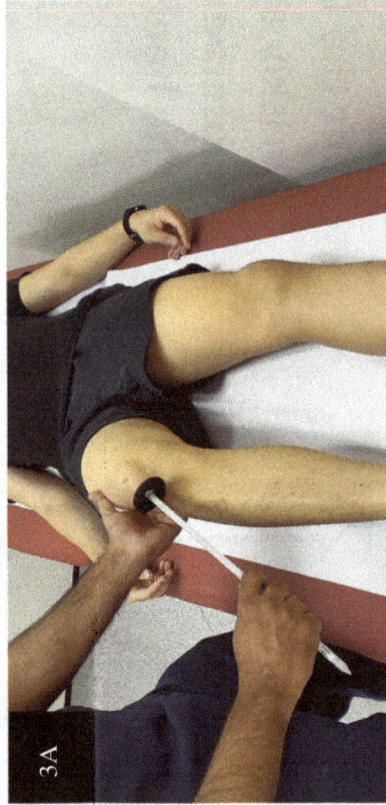 3A 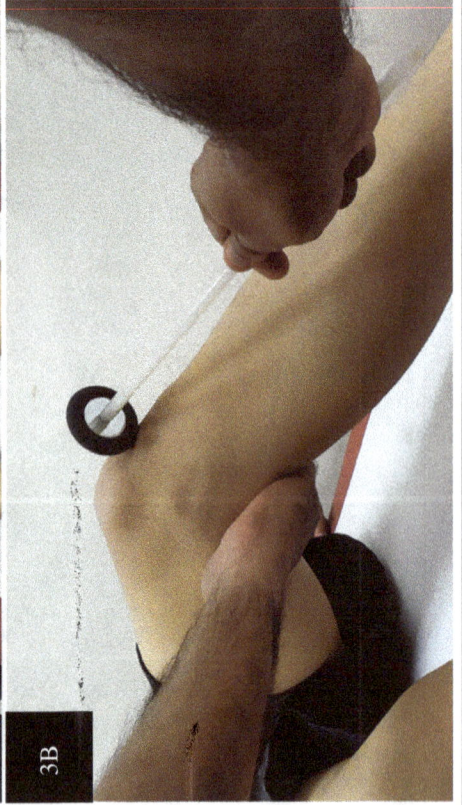 3B	The knee DTR (knee-jerk) is performed by striking the patellar tendon of a mildly-flexed knee with a tendon hammer, as shown in **3A** and **3B**.

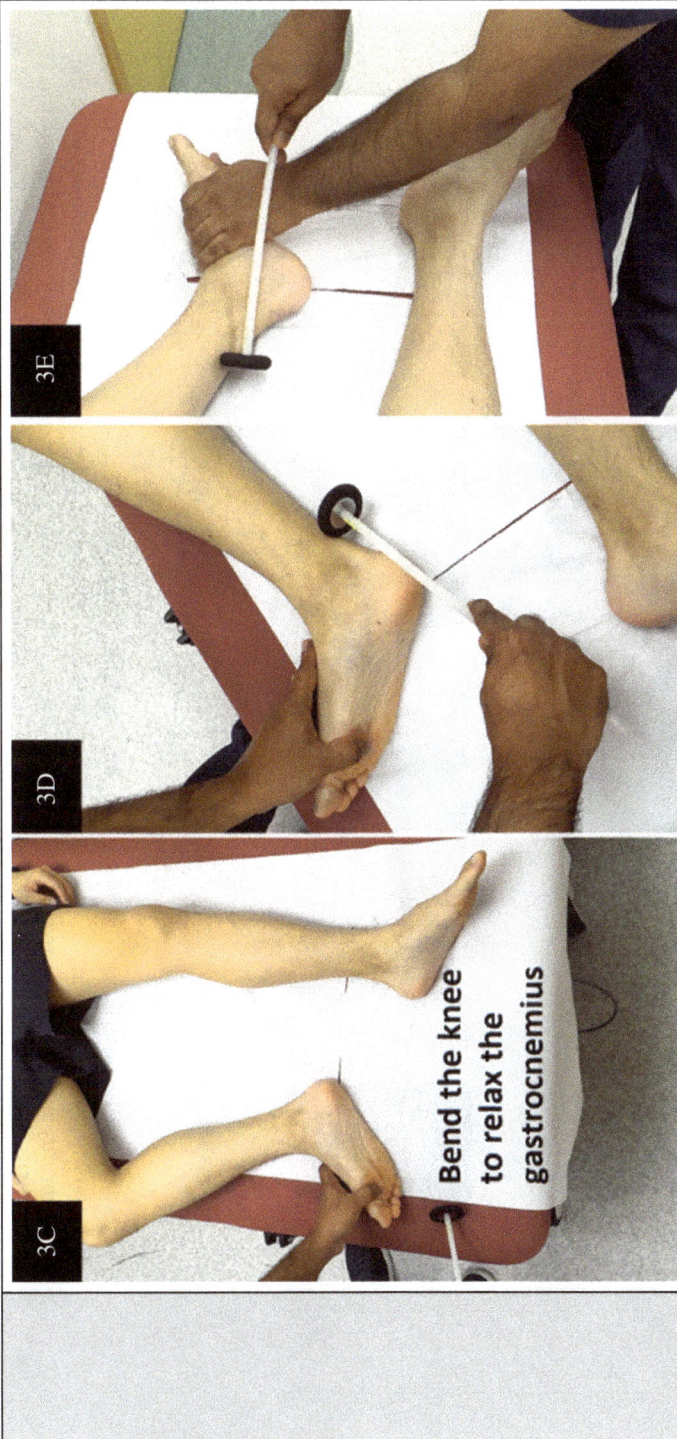

Bend the knee
to relax the
gastrocnemius

The ankle DTR (ankle-jerk) is performed by striking the Achilles tendon of a mildly-extended ankle with a tendon hammer, as shown in **3C**, **3D** and **3E**.

(Continued)

(Continued)

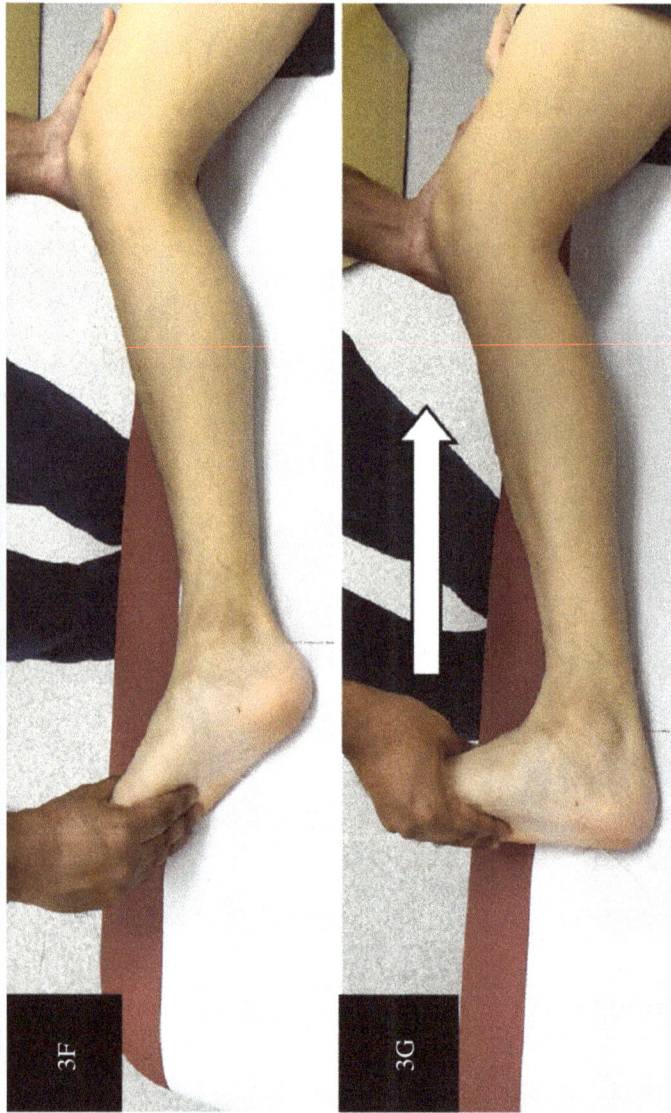

Examination Steps	Description
	 3F 3G The test for **ankle clonus** is often erroneously performed right after the leg-lift maneuvre. Ankle clonus describes the involuntary rhythmic contractions of the ankle flexors in patients with upper motor neuron (UMN) pathologies when the ankle is briskly and forcefully extended (**3F, 3G**). The knees are flexed slightly to relax the gastrocnemius. Although the number of beats required vary across literature, it is deemed present if three or more beats are observed (DTR score of 4), and described as sustained if the beats exceed five (DTR score of 5).

Plantar response	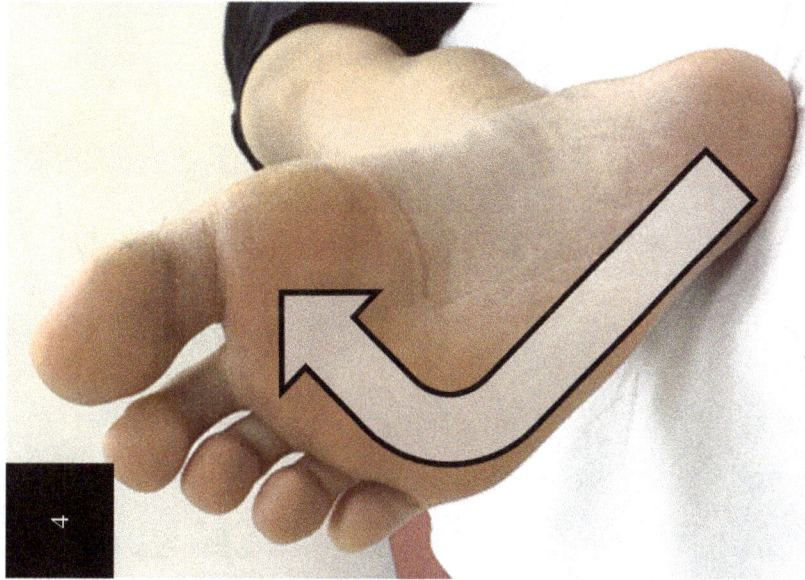

Plantar responses may be assessed using the **Babinski's test**. Using a blunt instrument (e.g., a small wooden stick), stroke slowly along the lateral plantar border towards the first metatarsophalangeal joint (**4**). The presence of an **extensor plantar response** (extension of the big toe), with or without fanning of the other toes, is suggestive of an UMN pathology, although it can be observed in healthy children below 2 years of age. There are many methods to elicit the plantar response (e.g., Chaddock sign, Oppenheimer sign, etc.), and their clinical implications are similar.

The Babinski's test and sign were originally described by Dr. Joseph Babinski in 1896 to portray the extension of the hallux, with or without fanning of the toes:

"On the paralysed side... excitation also results in flexion of the thigh on the pelvis, of the leg on the thigh, of the foot on the leg, but the toes, instead of flexing, execute a movement of extension upon the metatarsus"[2,3]

There are physicians who are pedantic with the use of "Babinski's sign" when describing plantar responses, deciding that the fanning of toes must be present. This departs from the original description. To avoid unnecessary confusion, we recommend using the term '**extensor plantar response**' rather than a 'positive Babinski's sign', when describing your findings. Regardless, the extensor response reflects dysfunction of the UMNs. A normal CST prevents sensory stimulation from spreading to the other cord levels. When the CST is diseased, painful stimulus to the lateral plantar surface (S1) spreads beyond the anterior horn cells at S1 to involve the neighbouring levels (L5, L4), resulting in extension of the hallux and ankle.[4]

(Continued)

(*Continued*)

Examination Steps	Description
Motor strength	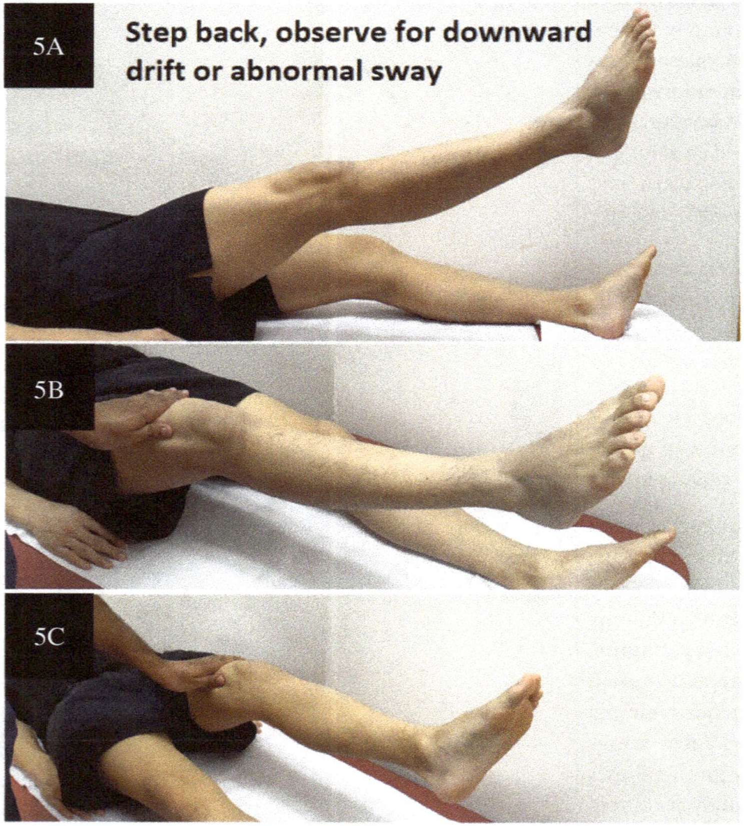 **Hip flexion** may be tested as illustrated (**5A–D**). The patient is instructed to elevate the leg at the hip (**5A**) before a downward force is applied at the thigh (**5B, 5C**). Step 5A also provides **an early opportunity to 'screen' for ataxia**. Before pressing down on the elevated leg, step back and observe for abnormal overshoot or sway of the leg, which when present may hint at the presence of ataxia (**5A**). This is a useful screening test during the undergraduate and postgraduate examinations, during which time is often limited.

5A **Step back, observe for downward drift or abnormal sway**

5B

5C

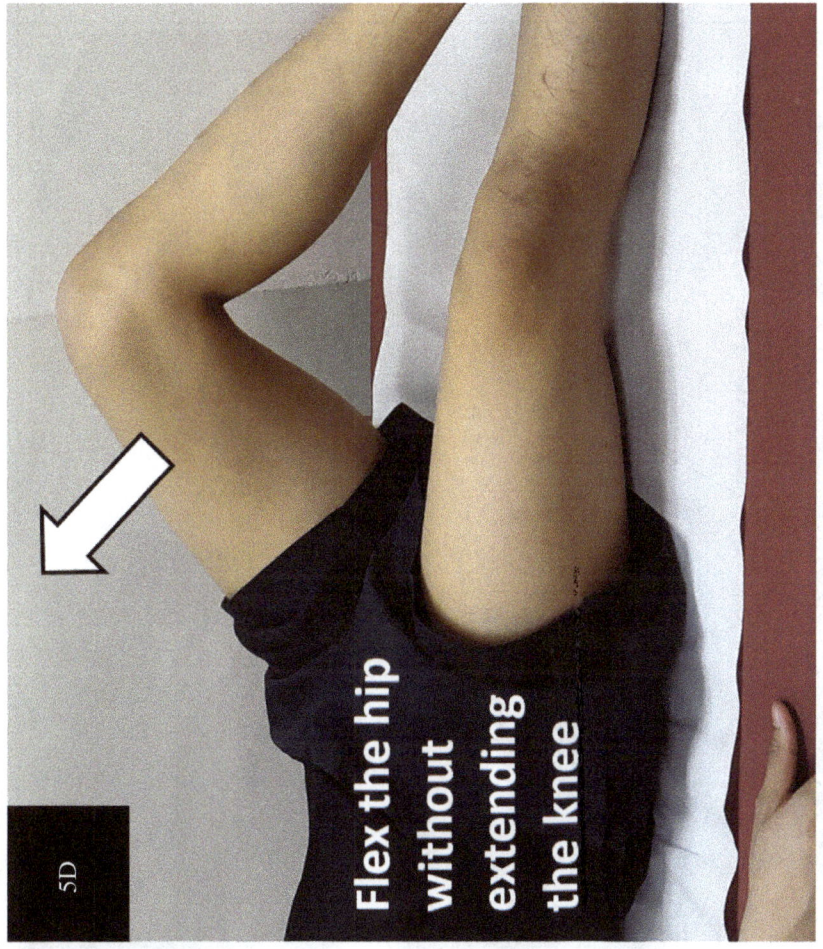

Assessment of the hip flexors may be confounded by weakness of the quadriceps (e.g., femoral nerve palsy) when performed using the method shown in **5A**. In that case, testing without maintaining an extended knee is more accurate and appropriate **(5D)**.

Flex the hip without extending the knee

5D

(Continued)

(Continued)

Examination Steps	Description
	Hip extension is best tested when lying prone (**5E**). In undergraduate and postgraduate examinations, frequent adjustments of the patient may be disruptive and time-consuming. As such, it is also acceptable to test the hip extensors by having the patient push against your hand while you exert an upward force at his/her knee or ankle (5F)

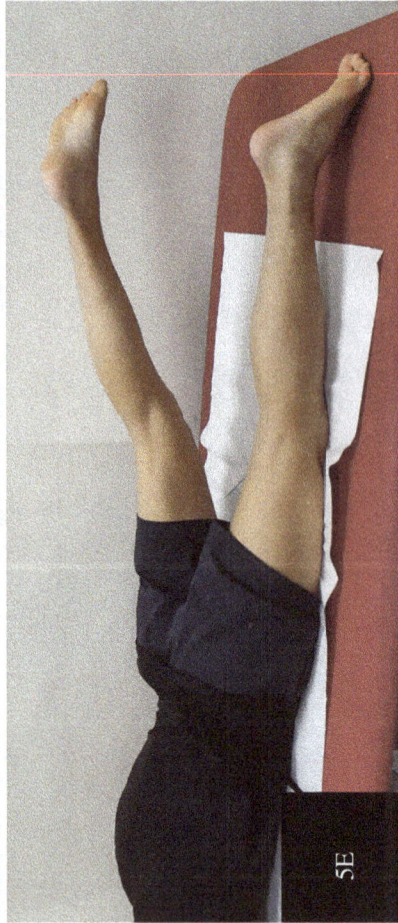

5E

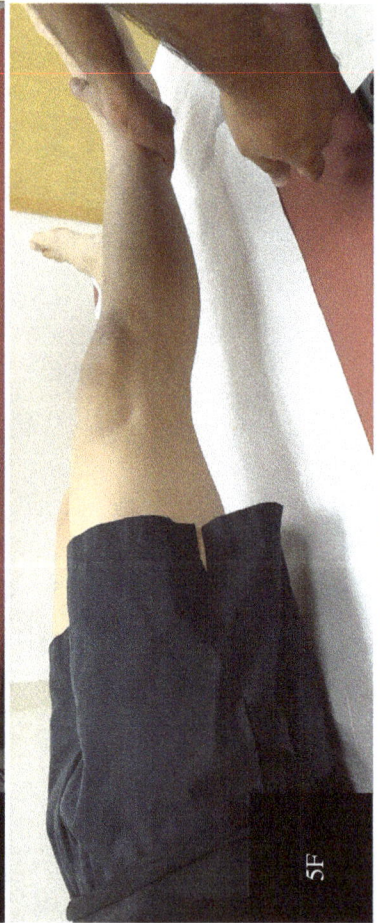

5F

Hip abduction should be performed when clinically necessary (e.g., patients with unilateral foot drop). Have the patient lie on his/her side when abducting the hip while you exert a downward force on the abducted leg **(5G, 5H)**. Be sensitive with your instructions to the patient. Avoid asking the patient to "spread their legs" as it can appear unprofessional and offensive to some.

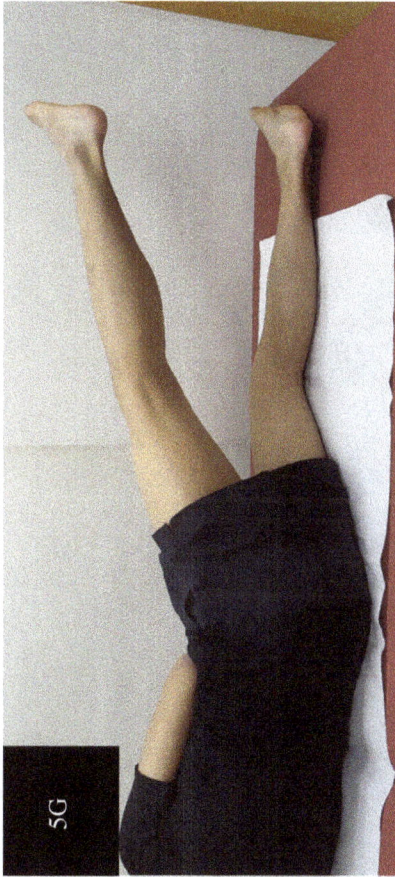

5G

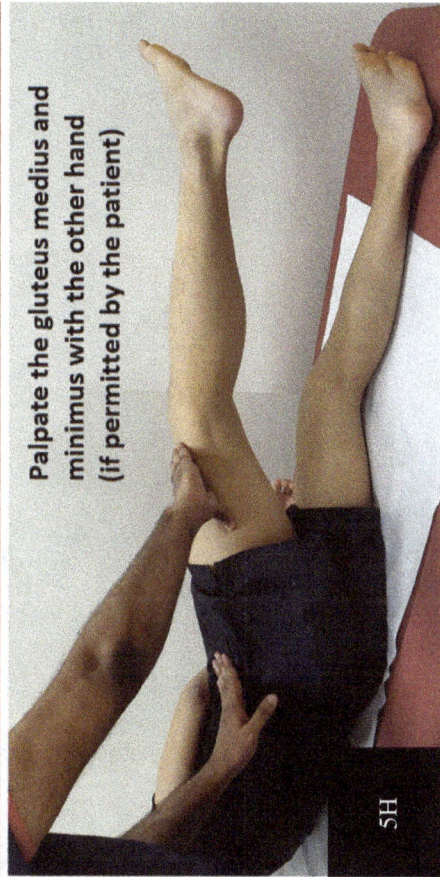

Palpate the gluteus medius and minimus with the other hand (if permitted by the patient)

5H

(Continued)

(Continued)

Examination Steps	Description

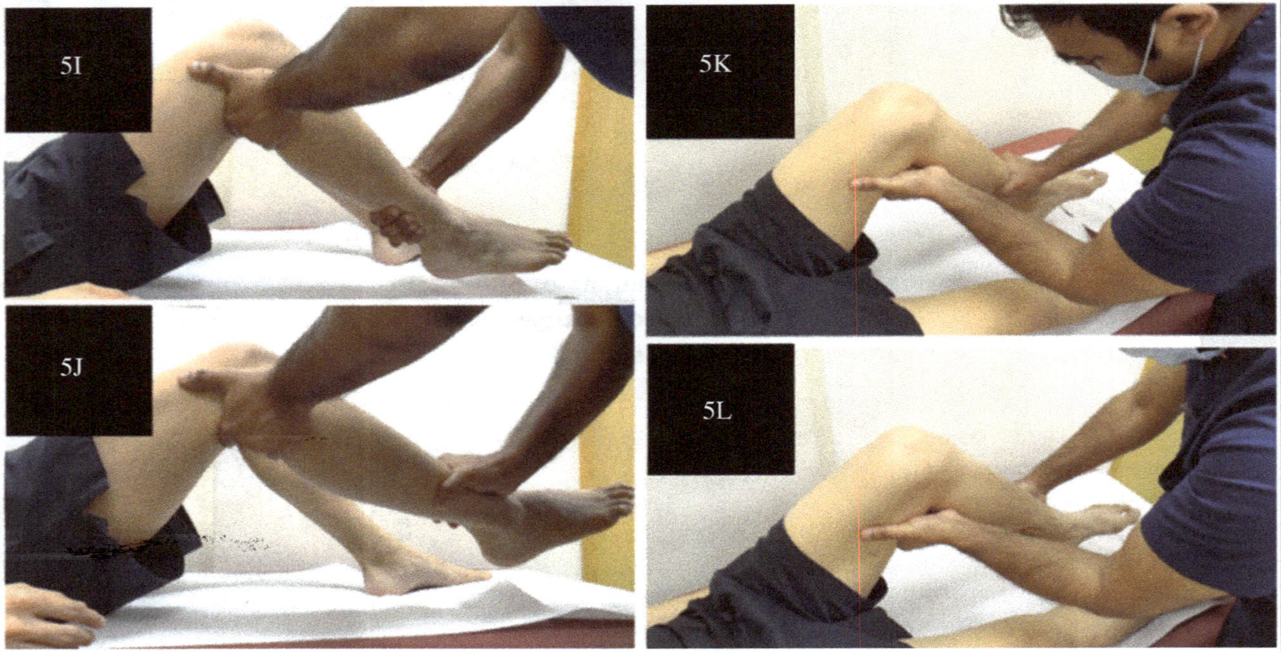

5I

5J

5K

5L

5I–5L demonstrate how the knee flexors and extensors should be examined. When testing, ensure that the heel is not in contact with the bed, as friction may confound your assessment.

The assessments of the **ankle flexors and extensors** are respectively shown in **5M** and **5N**. Stabilize the leg just proximal to the ankle with your left hand, and exert a strong, counteracting force with your right. The ankle extensors and flexors are strong muscles, and mild weakness may be missed when the force applied against the ankle is insufficient.

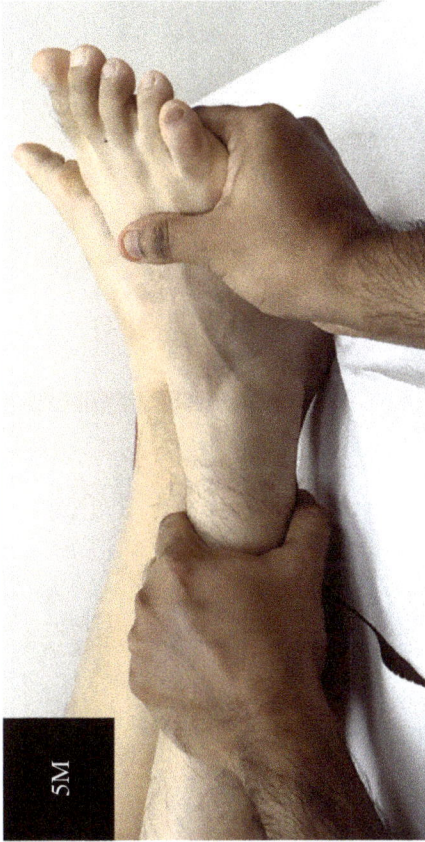

5M

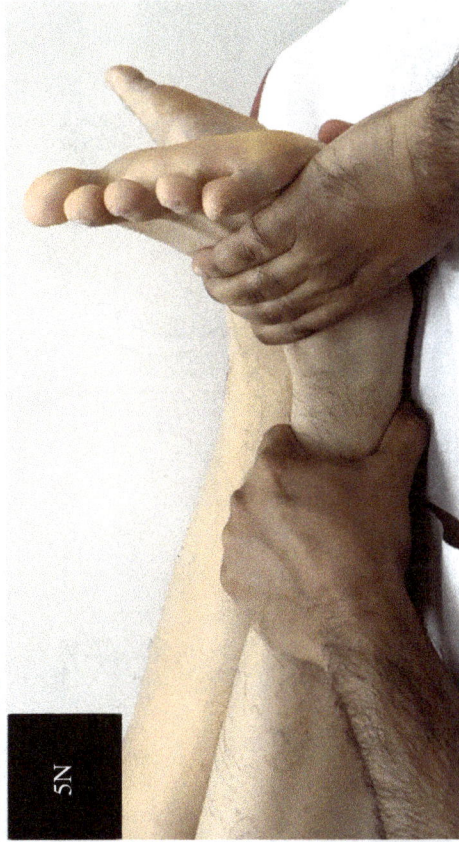

5N

(Continued)

(Continued)

Examination Steps	Description
	The testing of **ankle eversion (5O)** and **inversion (5P)** are shown here.

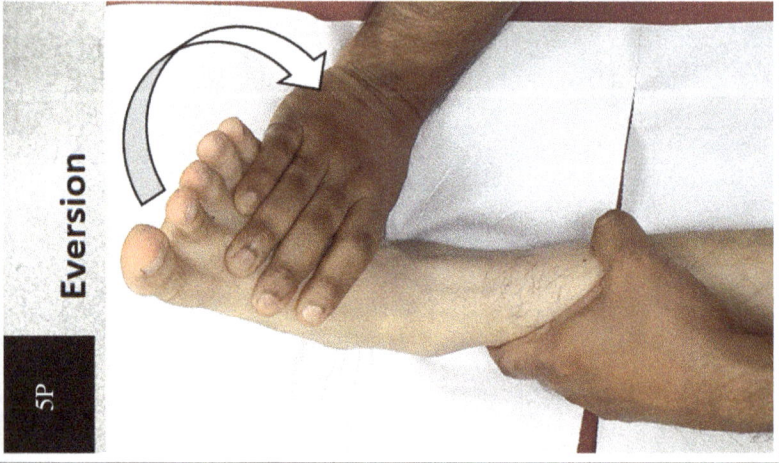

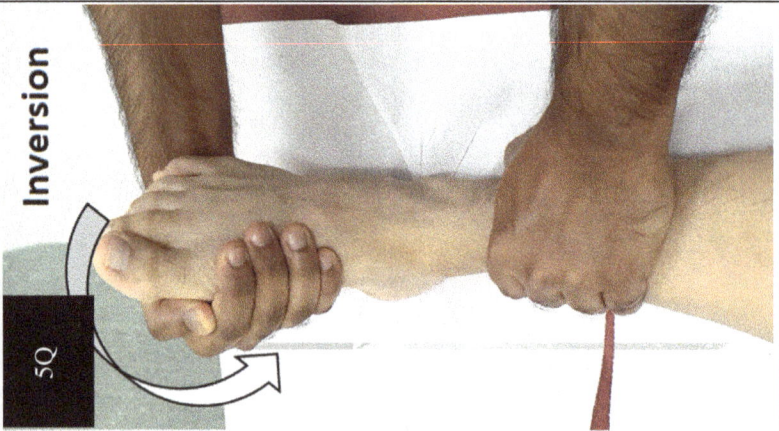

5P Eversion

5Q Inversion

| Sensory testing | 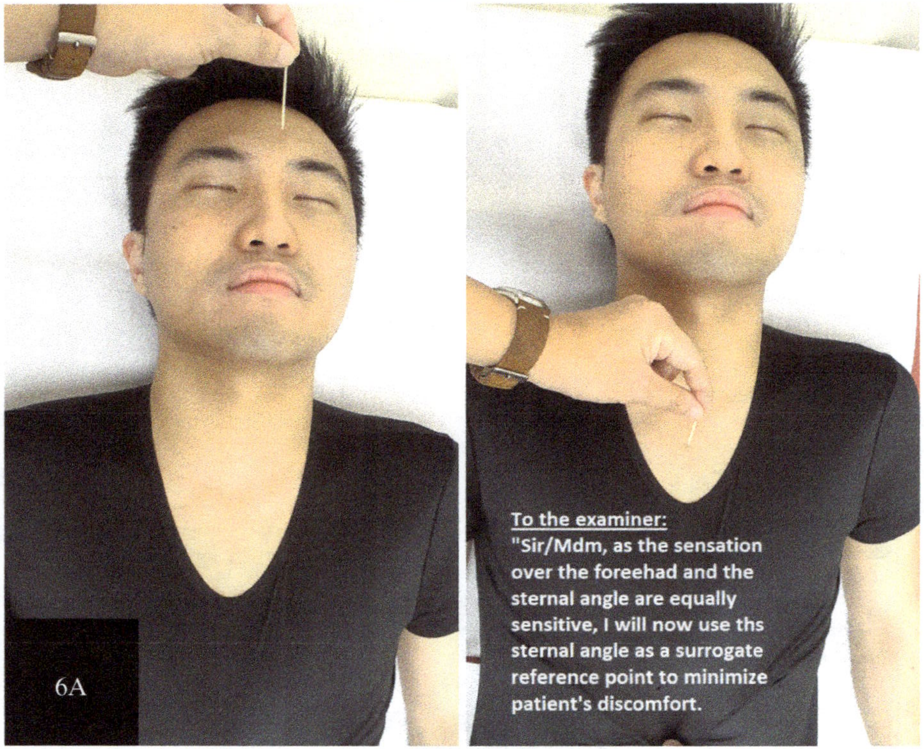 | When assessing sensation, the ideal **reference point** should be the **forehead**. To avoid having to touch the face repeatedly with a pin which has already touched the feet, the sternal angle is often used as the surrogate reference point, but only after it is tested to be as sensitive as the forehead (**6A**). |

To the examiner:
"Sir/Mdm, as the sensation over the foreehad and the sternal angle are equally sensitive, I will now use ths sternal angle as a surrogate reference point to minimize patient's discomfort.

6A

(*Continued*)

(Continued)

Examination Steps	Description
6B	Illustrated here are the regions of interest, together with their corresponding nerves and dermatomes **(6B)**. The anterior knee and the soles should be avoided, as these areas are naturally less sensitive than the forehead. Alternative regions which can be tested are the medial knee, and the lateral side of the foot.

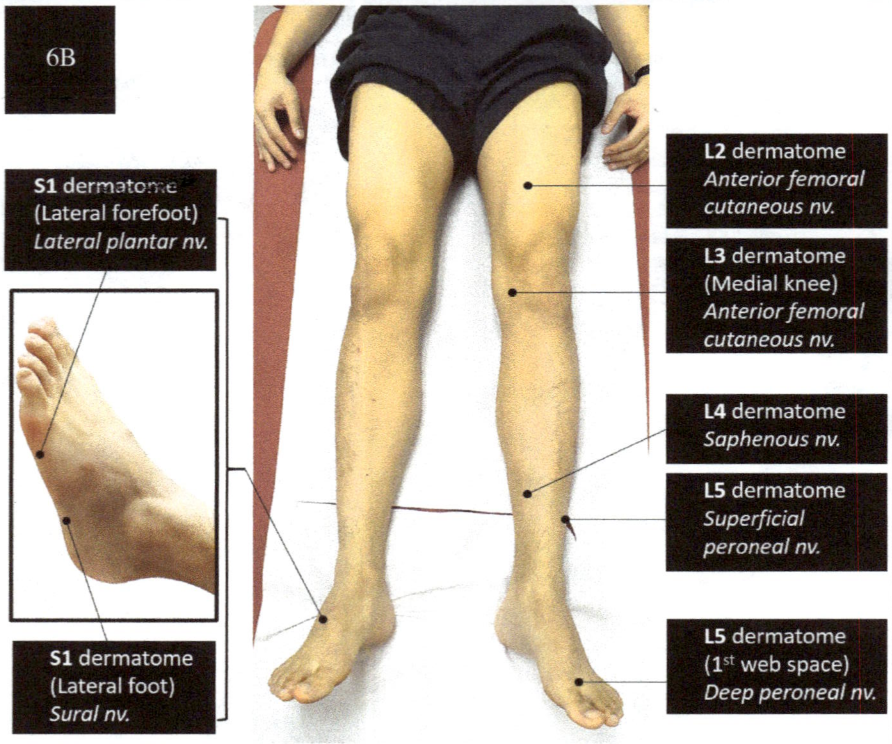

A Neurotip or a toothpick should be used when assessing pain perception, while a cotton wisp is appropriate when assessing fine touch. |

L2 dermatome
Anterior femoral cutaneous nv.

L3 dermatome
(Medial knee)
Anterior femoral cutaneous nv.

L4 dermatome
Saphenous nv.

L5 dermatome
Superficial peroneal nv.

L5 dermatome
(1st web space)
Deep peroneal nv.

S1 dermatome
(Lateral forefoot)
Lateral plantar nv.

S1 dermatome
(Lateral foot)
Sural nv.

When testing proprioception of the big toe, begin by gently holding the interphalangeal joint and the distal phalanx as shown, and move the latter **slowly** up or down about the interphalangeal joint in **small deflections (6C, 6D)**. Avoid holding the distal phalanx at the nail or moving the hallux in large deflections.

Proprioception is a highly-sensitive modality, able to pick up small deflections. As such, deflections must be kept reasonably **small**. Additionally, the speed of the deflections should be **slow**, so as to avoid confounding the assessment with kinesthesia (sensation of motion).

The patient should be allowed three responses when asked about the perceived deflection of his/her hallux — "up", "down", or "don't know" (see **Chapter 2**).

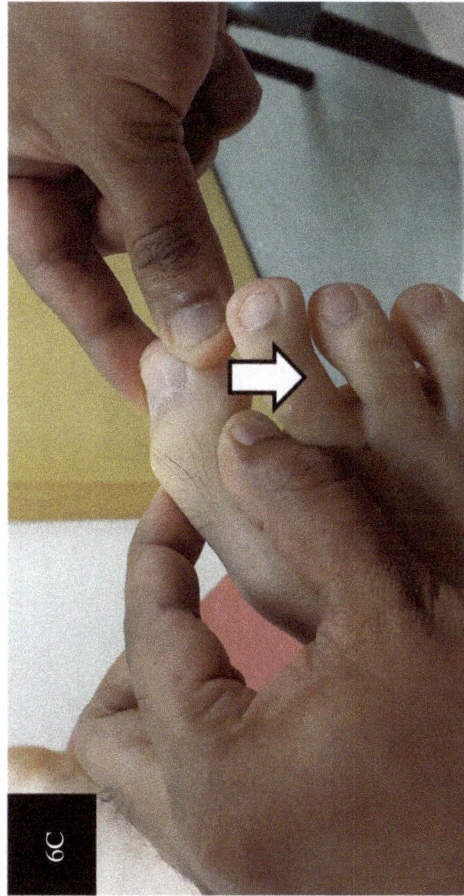

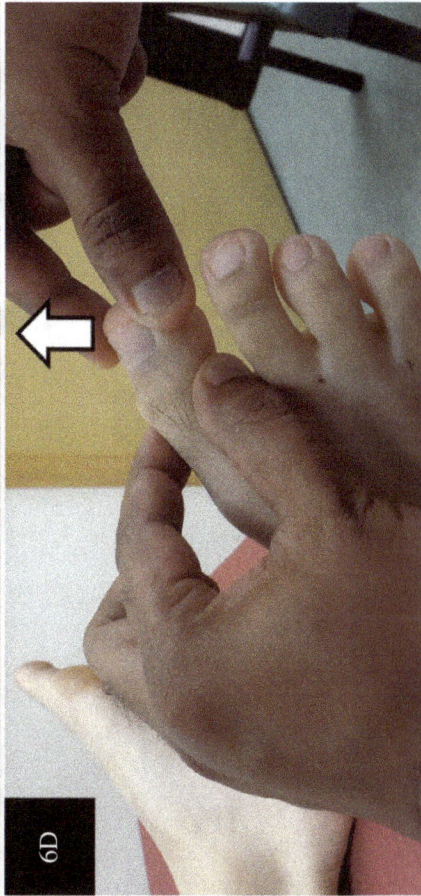

(Continued)

(Continued)

Examination Steps	Description
Heel-shin dysmetria	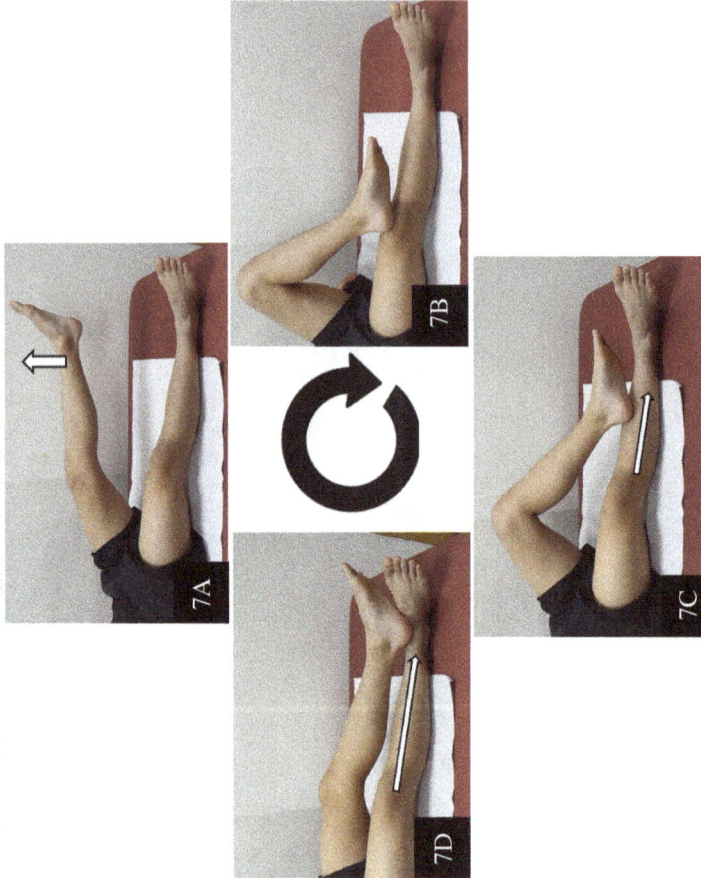

The heel-shin test (**7A–7D**). Instruct the patient to slide his/her heel down the bony prominence of the contralateral shin from the knee toward the ankle as rapidly and smoothly as possible. Abnormal cadence hints at ipsilateral cerebellar dysfunction, but may also be due to poor proprioception or abnormal motor control. There are multiple additions to this test, such as having the patient touch your finger with the big toe, before moving his/her heel to the knee. Such additions are acceptable. |

Romberg test	

8A

"Put your feet together."

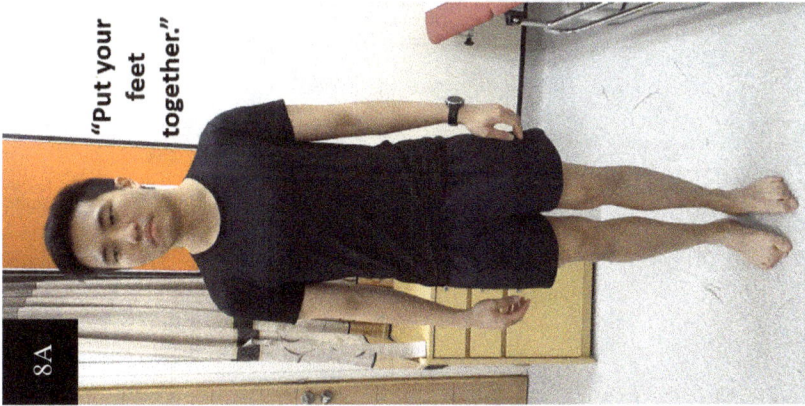

8B

"Close your eyes."

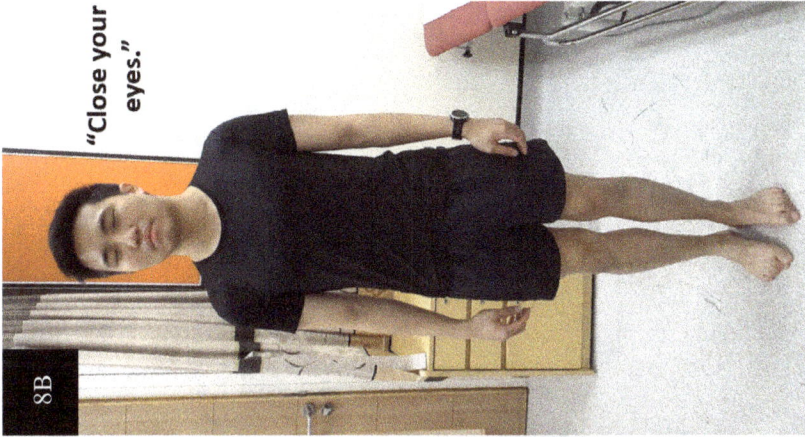

The **Romberg's test (8A, 8B)** is a test of disequilibrium. It compares the stability of a patient when standing with eyes wide open against that when with closed eyes. The test is considered positive (Romberg sign) when the patient **stands steadily with the eyes open**, but **sways or falls when the eyes are shut**. Thus, Romberg's test should not be performed on those who are already unsteady with open eyes (e.g., cerebellar ataxia). The original test/sign was described by **Dr. Moritz Romberg** in patients with tabes dorsalis:

"...ordered to close his eyes while in the erect posture, he at once commences to totter and swing from side to side; the insecurity of his gait also exhibits itself more in the dark."[5]

The need to place the feet close together was a later addition that is now accepted as part of the test.

A positive Romberg's test is suggestive of proprioceptive deficits. However, a positive test needs correlation with other sensory findings, and should not be interpreted in isolation.

(Continued)

(Continued)

Examination Steps	Description
Gait	

Begin the assessment by having the patient sit up, then stand up unsupported (**9A**). Observe for the following:

- Abnormal sway
- Abnormal posture (e.g., stooped, retrocollis, etc.)
- Abnormal position of the feet (e.g., broad based)

The Romberg's test may be performed here, just before assessing the patient's gait. Next, instruct the patient to walk a short distance, turn, and head back to the starting point (**9B**).

Regions		Comments
Base		Is the base broad, narrow, or normal?
Vertical axis		Abnormal posture of the neck and back.
Arms		Diminished arm-swing in Parkinson's disease, or excessive movement such as chorea, dystonia or tremors.
Walking straight	Initiation	Look for hesitation, or delays in the initiation of steps
	Cadence	Look for slowness in the cadence
	Stride length	Look for shortened stride length
	clearance	Look for high steppage gait, or dragging of the foot
	Progression	Observe for veering, freezing, festination or retropulsion
Turning		Observe for abnormalities in turning, such as freezing, turning in numbers and turning en masse.

References

1. Dohrmann GJ, Nowack WJ. (1972) The upgoing great toe. Optimal method of elicitation. *Lancet.* **1**(7799): 339–341.
2. Morrow JM, Reilly MM. (2011) The Babinski sign. *Br J Hosp Med* **72**(10): M157–M159.
3. Babinski J. (1896) Sur le reflexe cutane plantaire dans certaines affections du systeme nerveux central. *Comptes rendus des Seances et Memoires de la Societe de Biologie* 207–208.
4. Acharya AB, Jamil RT, Dewey JJ. (2021) *Babinski Reflex.* StatPearls Publishing, Treasure Island.
5. Pearce JMS. (1993) Romberg's Sign. *J Neurol Neurosurg Psychiatry* **56**(1): 51

5

Examination of the Cranial Nerves

A. Introduction

The cranial nerve assessment is an important part of the neurologic examination. For most trainees, the examination of the cranial nerves follows a sequential order, starting from the first to the twelfth cranial nerve. This guide provides a step-by-step approach in an order which we believe to be the "smoothest" during an undergraduate or post-graduate examination. However, there are many variations to the sequence, largely dependent on the clinical scenario. As we progress through this chapter, the cranial nerves will be interchangeably referred to by their roman numerals:

CN I	Olfactory nerve
CN II	Optic nerve
CN III	Oculomotor nerve
CN IV	Trochlear nerve
CN V	Trigeminal nerve • Ophthalmic division/nerve (V1) • Maxillary division/nerve (V2) • Mandibular division/nerve (V3)
CN VI	Abducens nerve
CN VII	Facial nerve
CN VIII	Vestibulocochlear nerve
CN IX	Glossopharyngeal nerve
CN X	Vagus nerve
CN XI	Accessory nerve
CN XII	Hypoglossal nerve
Abbreviations: CN, cranial nerve	

Examination Steps

Equipment

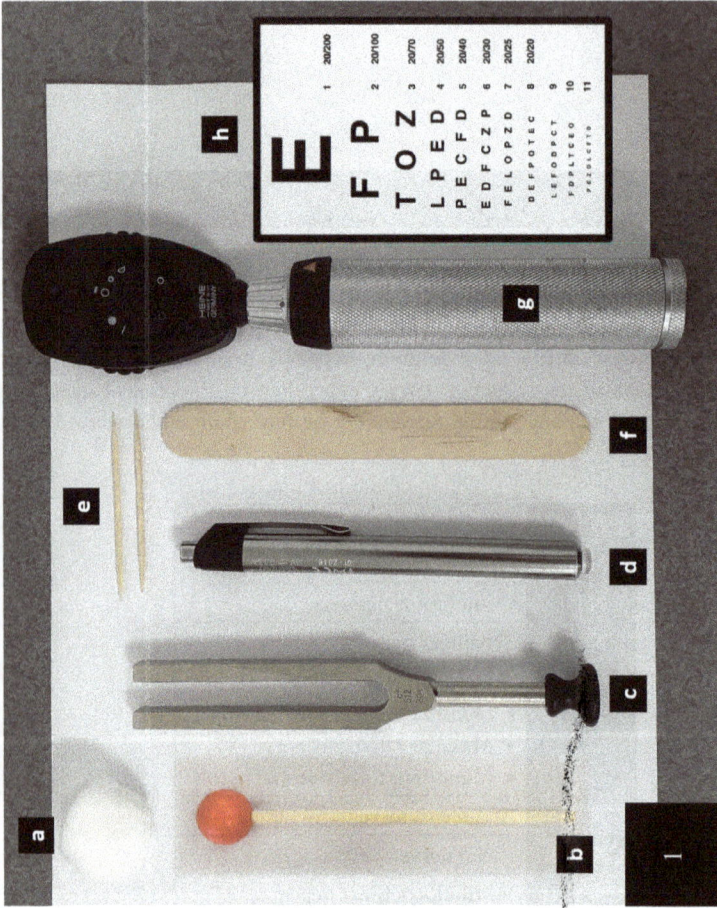

Before you start, prepare the appropriate equipment and devices needed to assess the cranial nerves (I): cotton ball (a), red hat pin fork (b), 512Hz tuning fork (c), pen torch or flash light (d), toothpick or neuro-tip (e), wooden tongue depressor/spatula (f), ophthalmoscope — optional (g), Snellen chart — regular size, or the mini version shown here (h).

Exposure, setting, and inspection	2A	The patient should be sitting up, with his/her face, neck, shoulders, and upper limbs exposed. The volunteer portrayed here in **2A**, however, opted to keep his shoulders covered.

When facing the patient, observe for:

- Facial dysmorphism
- Facial asymmetry
- Blepharoptosis
- Strabismus
- Abnormal posturing of the head and neck (e.g., torticollis)
- Atrophy of the anterior neck muscles
- Atrophy of the upper limbs

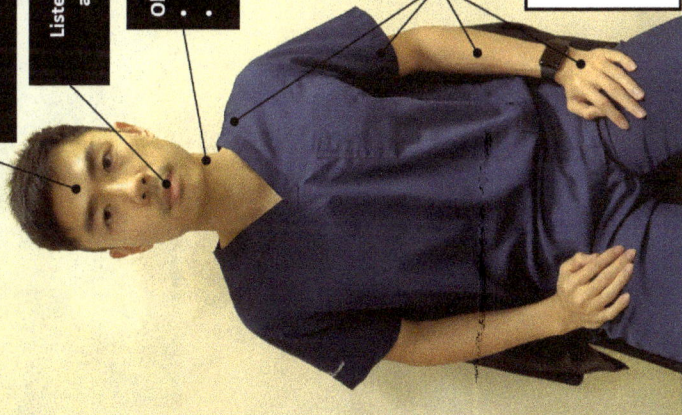

Observe the face for:
- Dysmorphic features
- Facial asymmetry
- Blepharoptosis
- Strabismus

Listen out for speech abnormalities

Observe the neck for:
- Muscle bulk
- Posture and position

Observe the shoulders, arms, forearms and hands for atrophy

Our volunteer opted to keep his shoulders covered. Under ideal conditions, however, the shoulders should be exposed to allow the trapezius and surrounding muscles to be inspected

(Continued)

(Continued)

Examination Steps

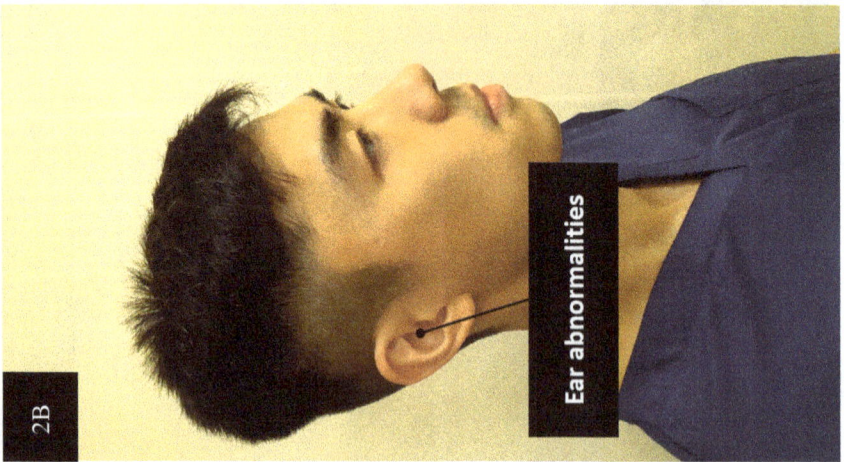

2B

Ear abnormalities

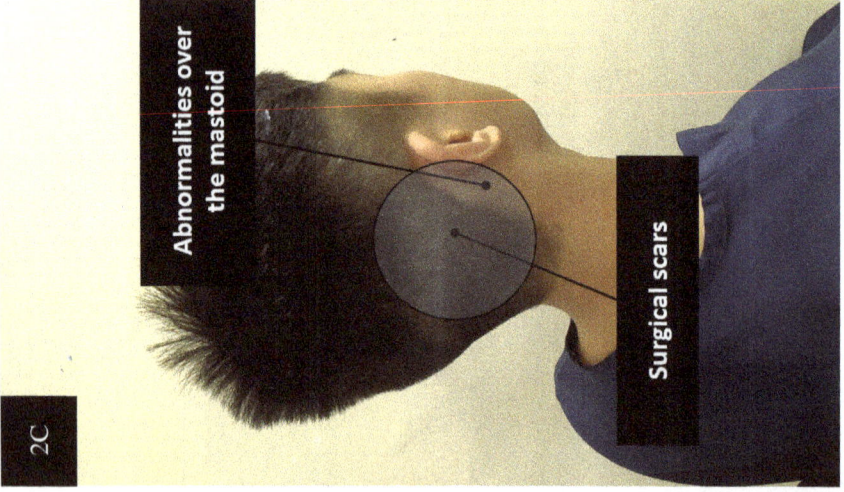

2C

Abnormalities over the mastoid

Surgical scars

Proceed to the patient's sides and observe for (**2B, 2C**):

- Ear abnormalities
  - ○ Otorrhea
  - ○ Vesicles
- Redness over the mastoid region
- Neurosurgical scars

Next, inspect the back for scars and deformities, and look for atrophy of the back muscles. Lastly, inspect the patient's surroundings.

| Sense of smell | 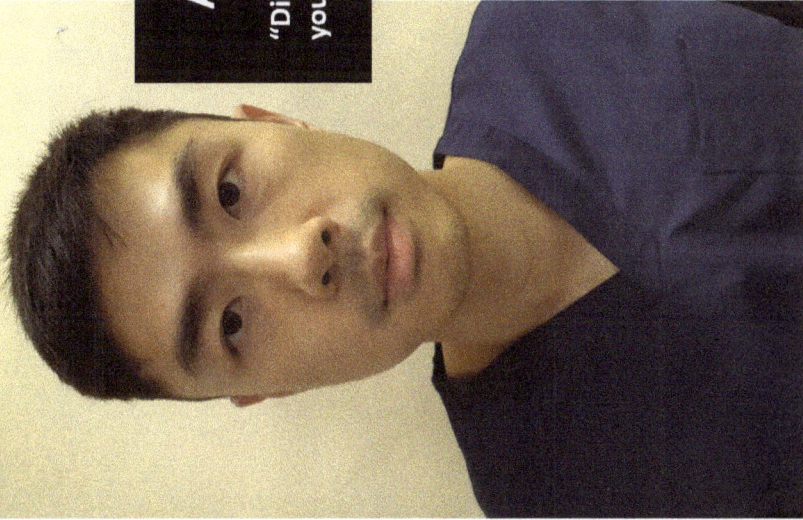

Ask the patient:

"Did you notice any change in your sense of smell or taste?" | The CN I transmits olfactory signals from the olfactory nerve endings in the upper part of the nasal mucosa to other areas within the central nervous system where they are processed and perceived as smell. Its function may be screened by **asking for changes in the patient's smell or taste,** the perception of the latter being closely linked to olfaction itself.[1]

Formal olfactory assessment may be performed later using available test batteries. However, these tests are time-consuming and exhaustive. |

(Continued)

(Continued)

Examination Steps

Visual acuity	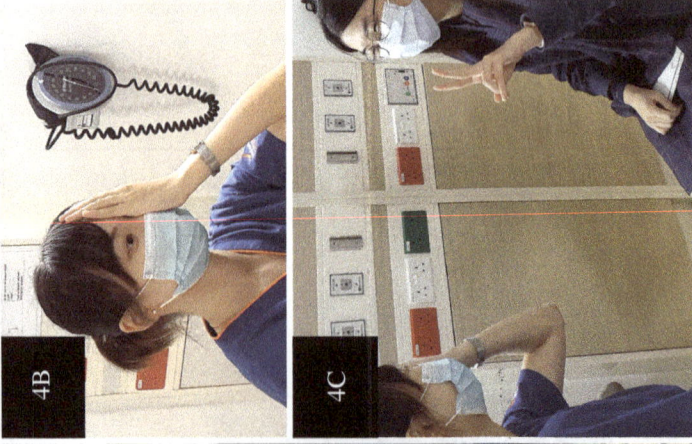 4A 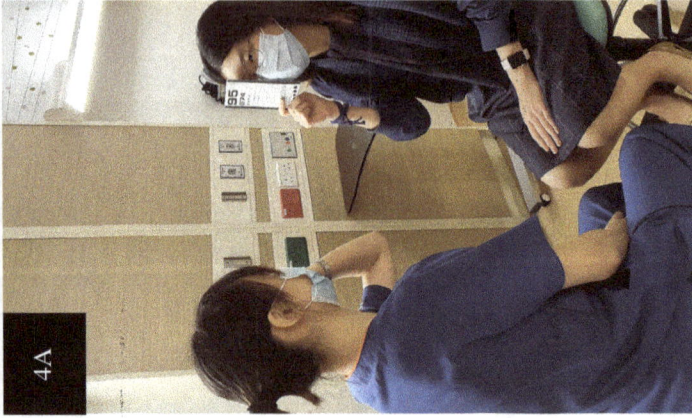 4B 4C CN II transmits sensory input from the retina to different parts of the brain responsible for conscious and unconscious processing of visual information. Visual acuity is tested using the **Snellen chart**. If spectacles or contact lenses are required, ensure that they are worn. A distance of **6 metres** is needed when using the Snellen chart. A **mini-Snellen chart (4A)** reduces the distance to **3 metres**, and may be used instead. Each eye should be individually tested **(4B)**. If the patient cannot read the topmost line, assess if he/she is able to count your fingers **(4C)**, detect your moving hand, or perceive light from a torch.

Pupillary light reflex	Testing of pupillary light reflexes must be done in a **dark room**. Illuminate both eyes from a distance, and observe the pupils for **anisocoria** (5A).

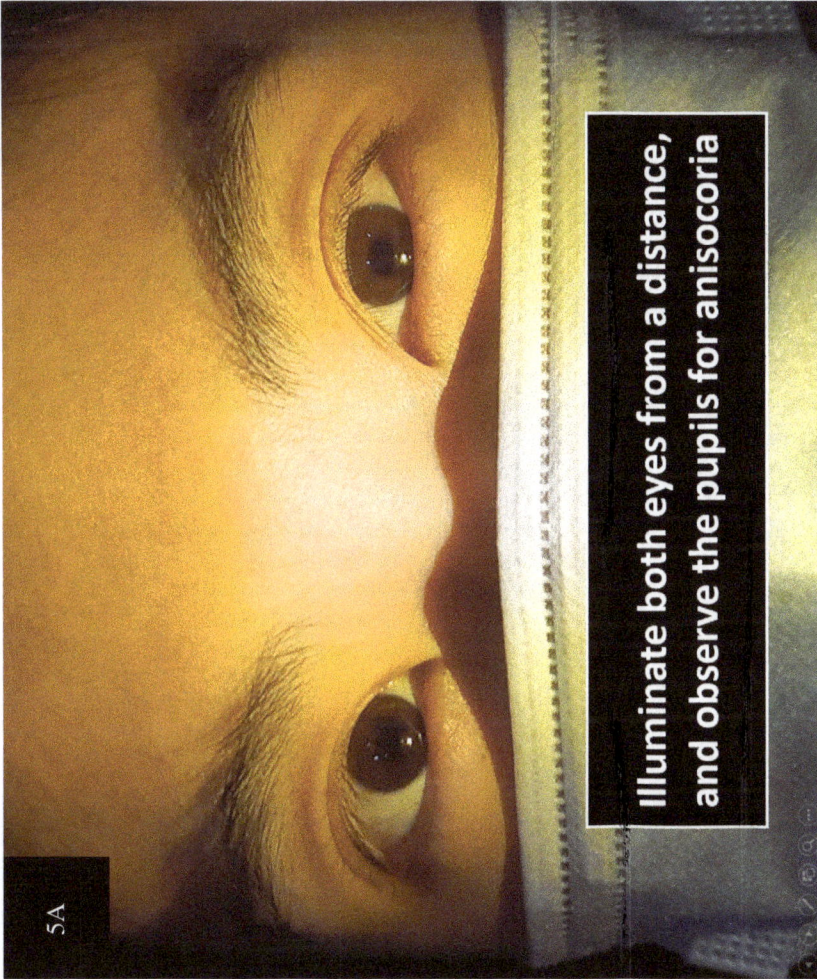

5A

Illuminate both eyes from a distance, and observe the pupils for anisocoria

(Continued)

(Continued)

Examination Steps

5B

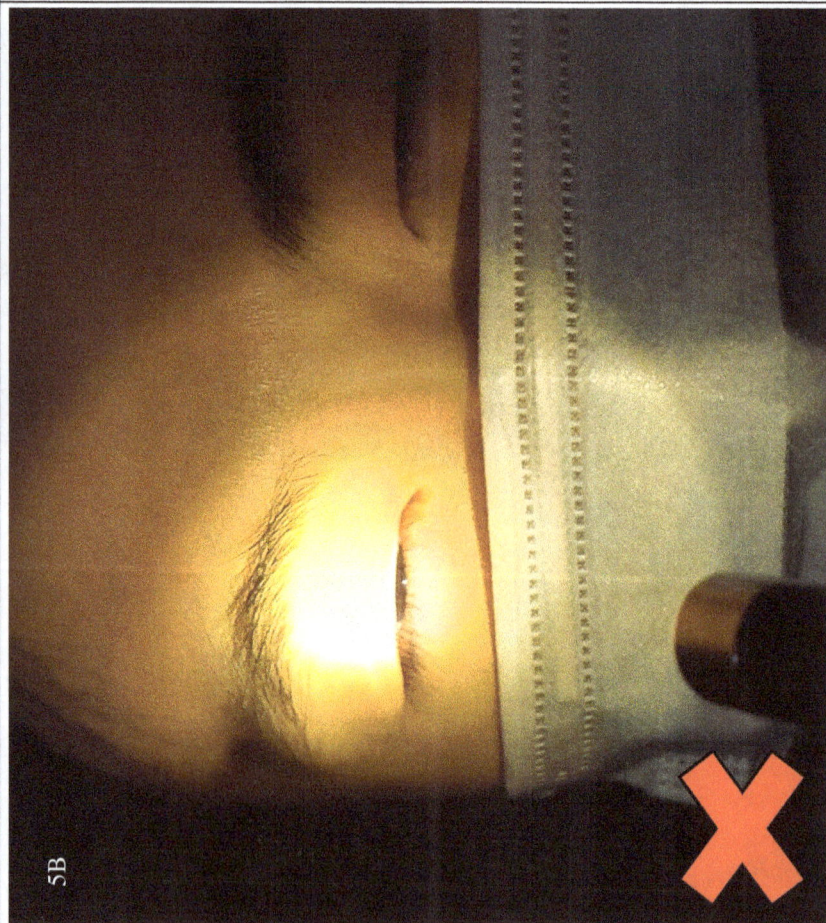

Next, test the direct light responses by shining the light at the eye. Because it is invariably uncomfortable to have a light shone directly at the eye (5B), we encourage **illuminating the pupil from a distance first (5C, 5E)**, before **bringing the torch closer to the pupil (5D, 5F)**. This reduces the patient's discomfort, and avoids causing the patient to blink **(5B)**.

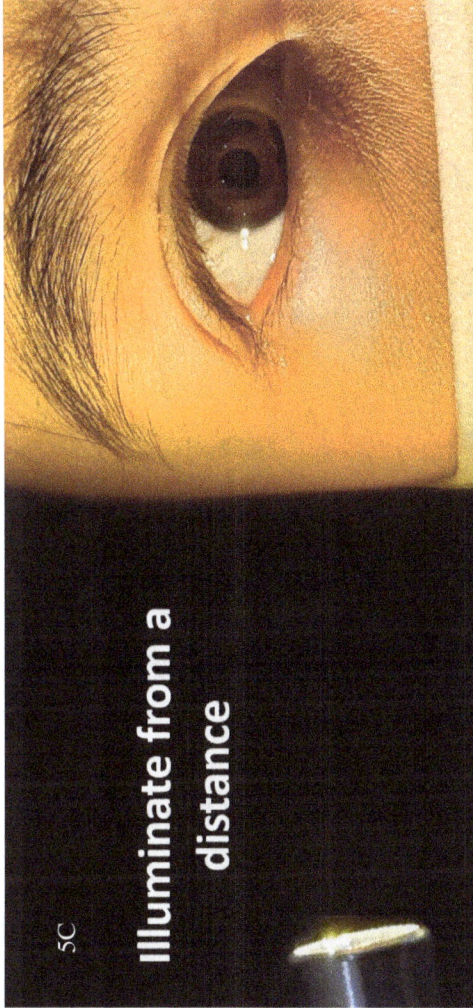

5C **Illuminate from a distance**

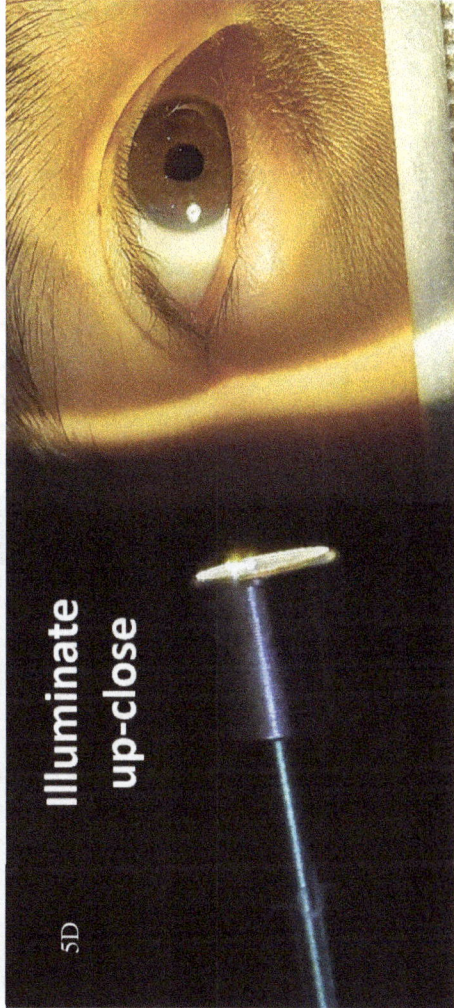

5D **Illuminate up-close**

(Continued)

(Continued)

Examination Steps

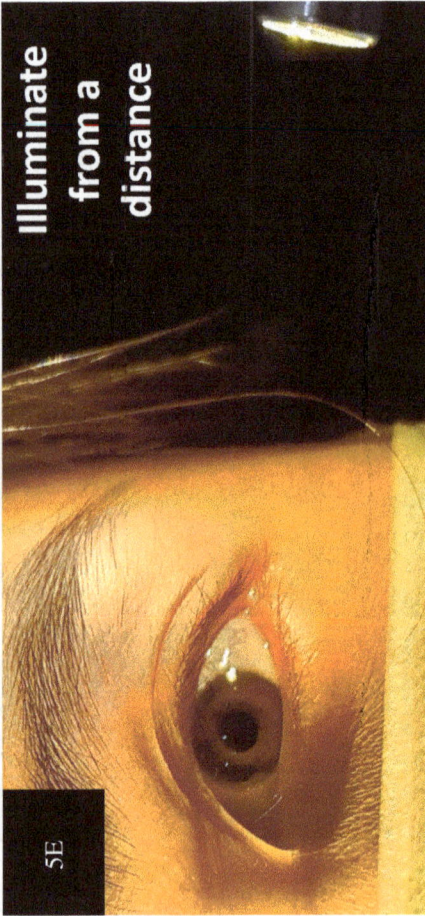

5E

Illuminate from a distance

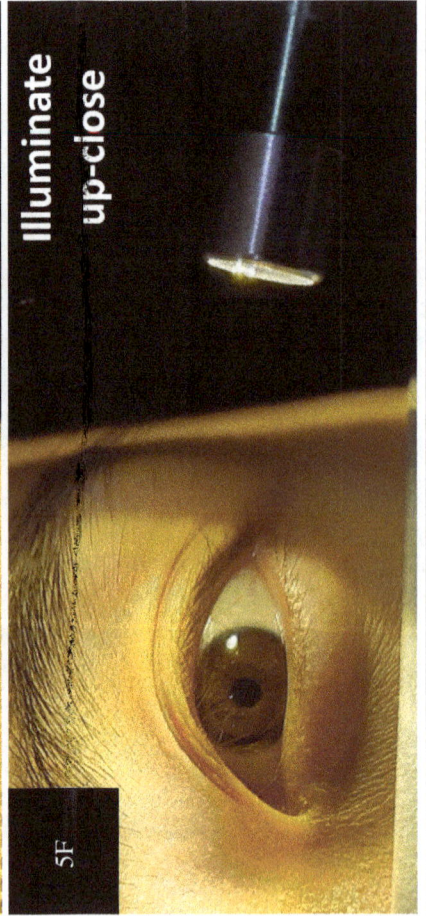

5F

Illuminate up-close

Illuminating the eye from a distance (5C, 5E) first before bringing the torch **closer to the eye (5D, 5F)** allows you to better appreciate the pupillary responses, whilst reducing the patient's discomfort.

Next, perform the **swinging torch test** as shown **(5G)**. The clinical interpretation and implications of **relative afferent pupillary defect (RAPD)** are discussed later in this chapter.

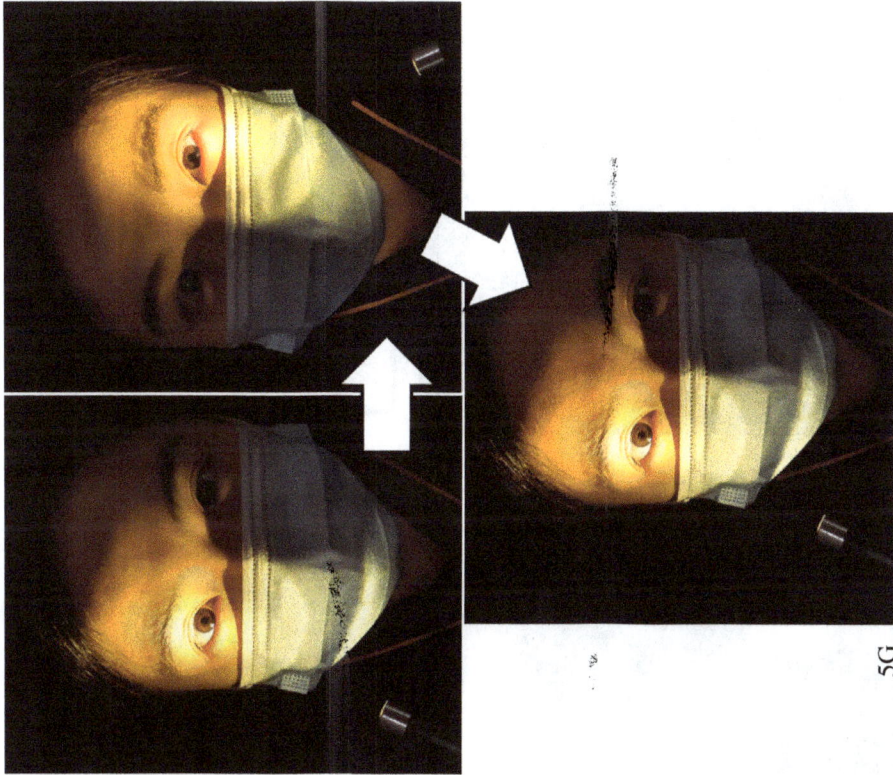

5G

(Continued)

(Continued)

	Examination Steps	
Visual fields	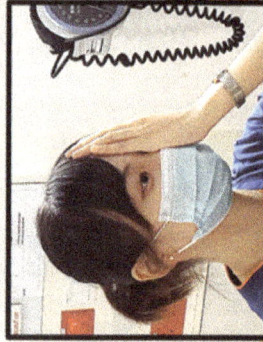 6A "I'm going to test your field of vision. I need you to use your left hand to cover your left eye, and I'm going to mirror you." "I will be bringing a red hat pin from the outside in. Inform me immediately when you see the pin".	VFs are assessed using the **confrontation testing technique**, during which the patient's VF is tested against yours. Begin by explaining to the patient what you are about to do **(6A)**.

Ensuring that your eyes are level with the patient's, continue to test each eye individually. Mirroring the patient by covering your opposing eye, instruct the patient to fixate on your uncovered eye (**6B**).

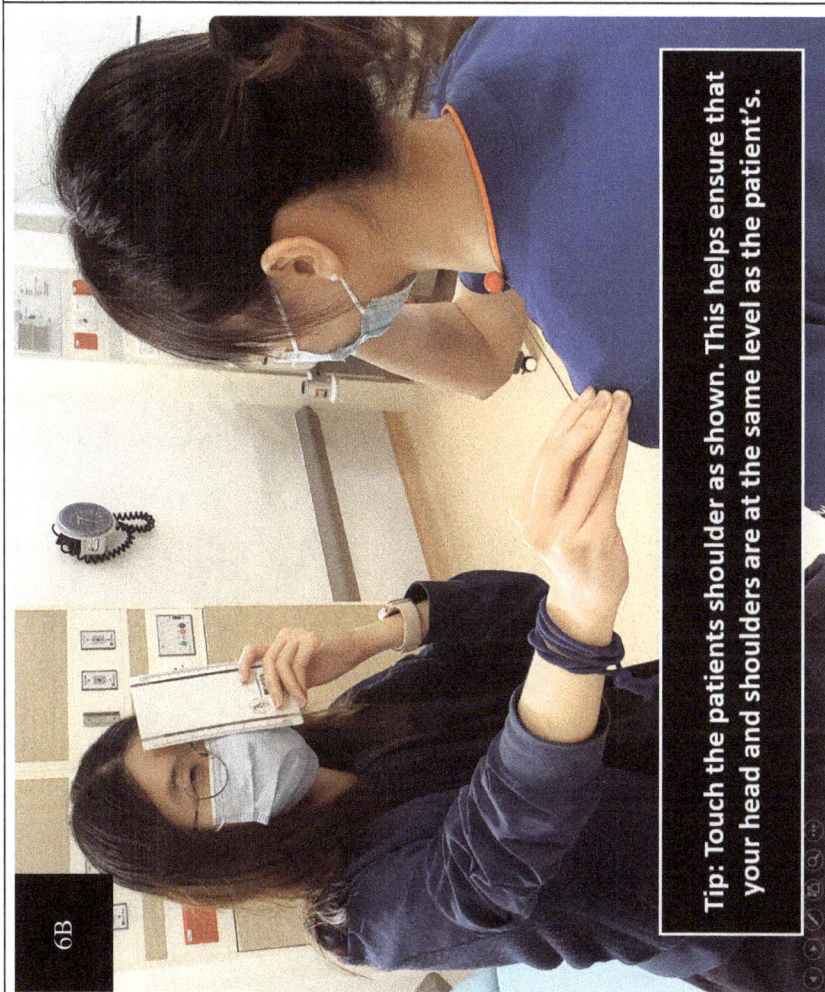

6B

Tip: Touch the patients shoulder as shown. This helps ensure that your head and shoulders are at the same level as the patient's.

(Continued)

(Continued)

Examination Steps

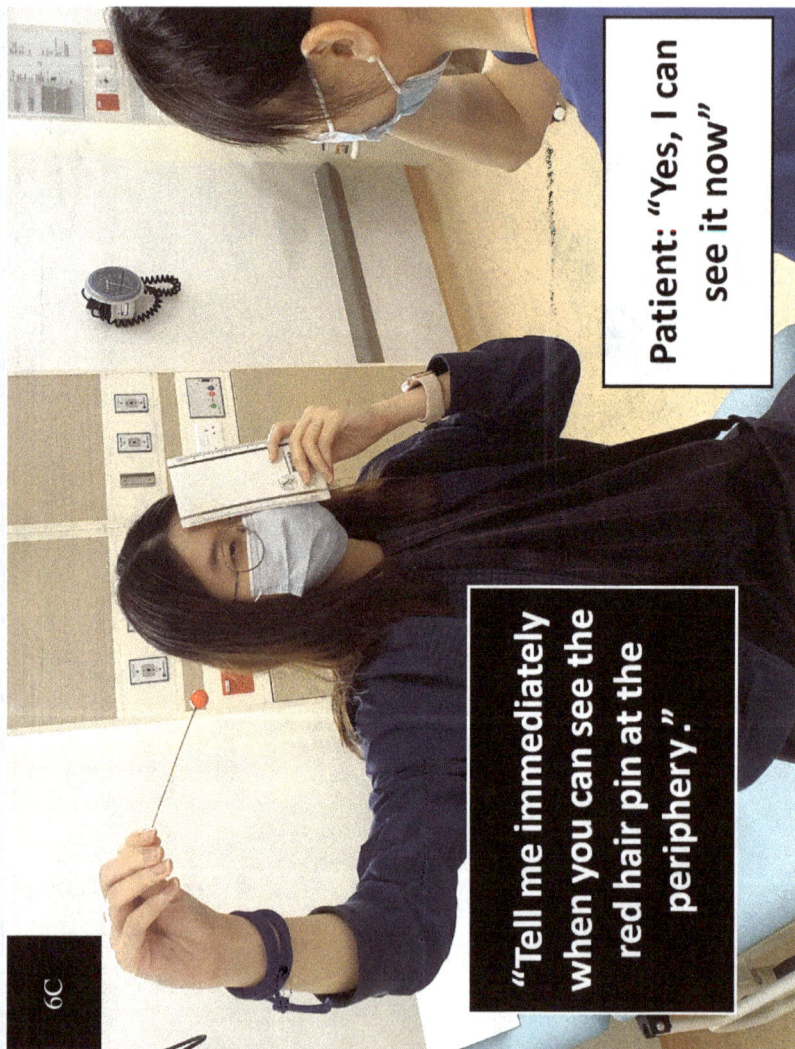

6C

"Tell me immediately when you can see the red hair pin at the periphery."

Patient: "Yes, I can see it now"

Next, present an object (e.g., a red hat pin) at the periphery and proceed to move it inwards as shown, until the object obscures the patient's uncovered eye (**6C**). Test all four quadrants and repeat the above on the other eye.

It is common for students and trainees to stop the test at the peripheries of the VF. Doing so merely samples 4 points along the peripheral limits of the patient's visual field, and may miss deficits which are situated nearer to the centre (e.g. scotomas).

6D and **6E** demonstrate how testing of the indicated VFs are performed.

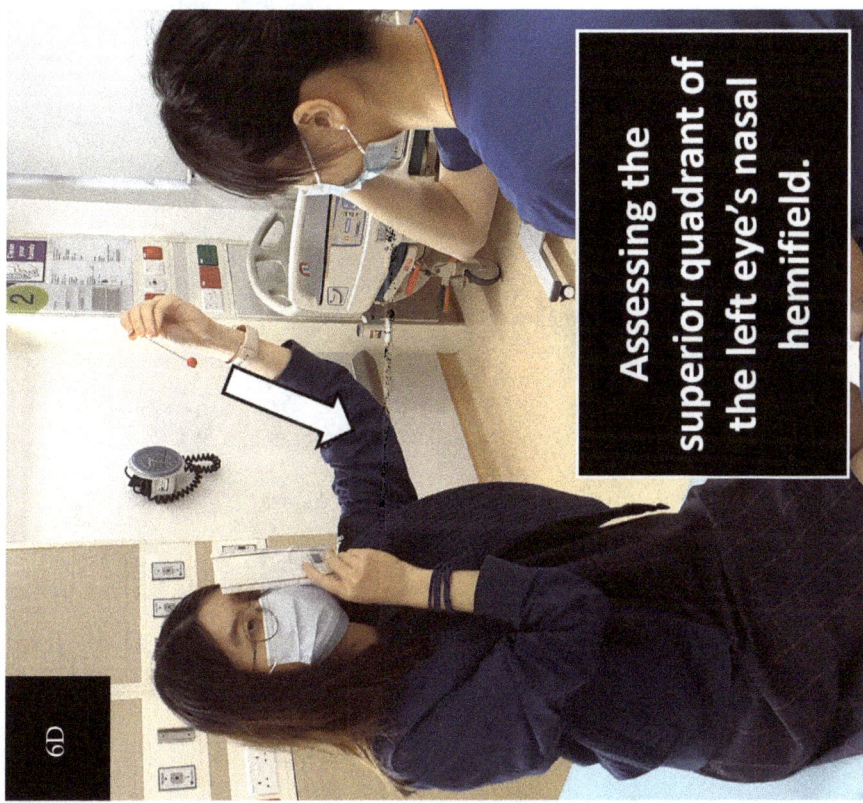

6D

Assessing the superior quadrant of the left eye's nasal hemifield.

(Continued)

(Continued)

Examination Steps

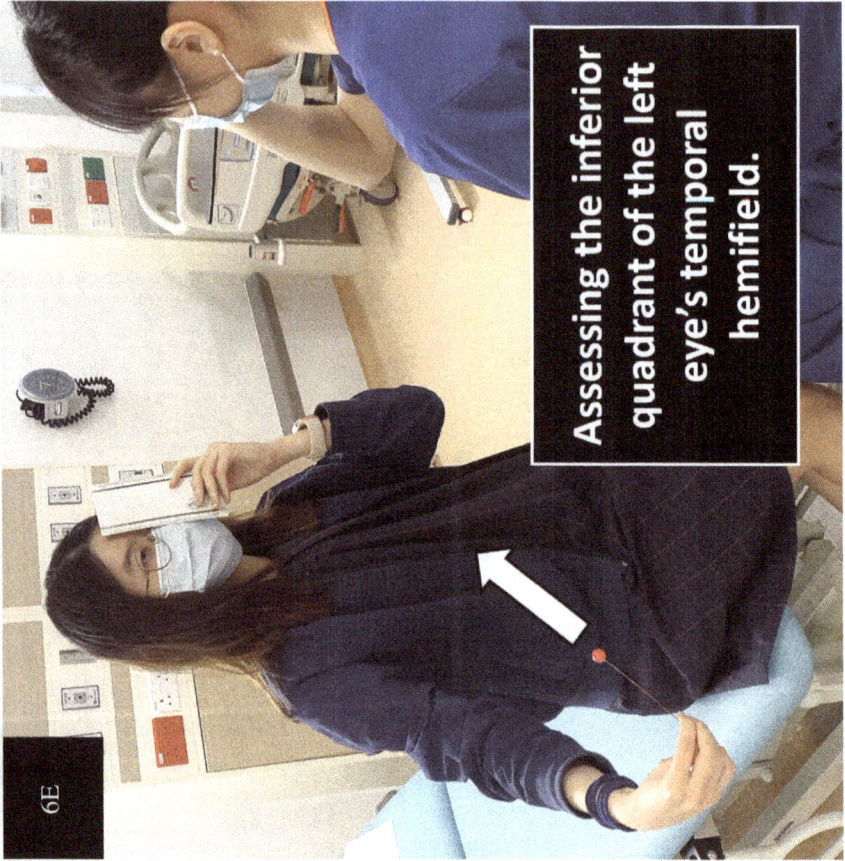

6E

Assessing the inferior quadrant of the left eye's temporal hemifield.

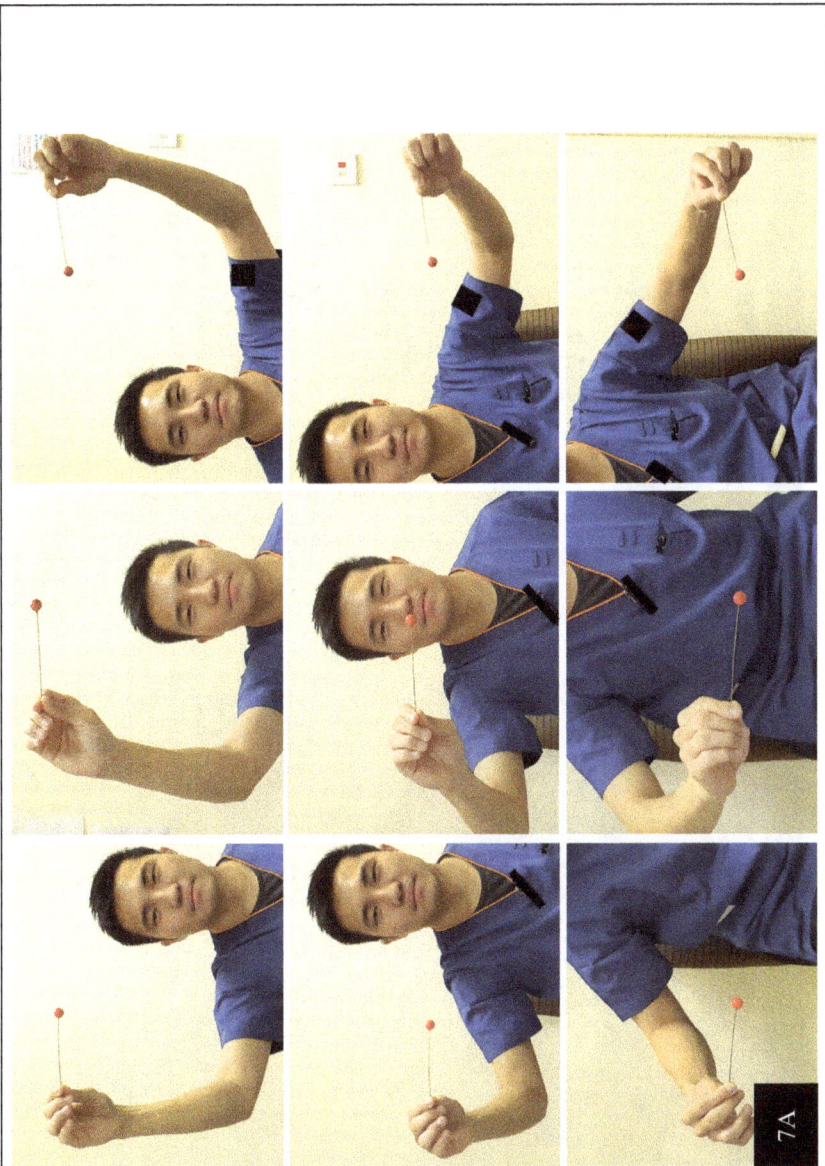

Extraocular movements

(Continued)

(Continued)

Examination Steps

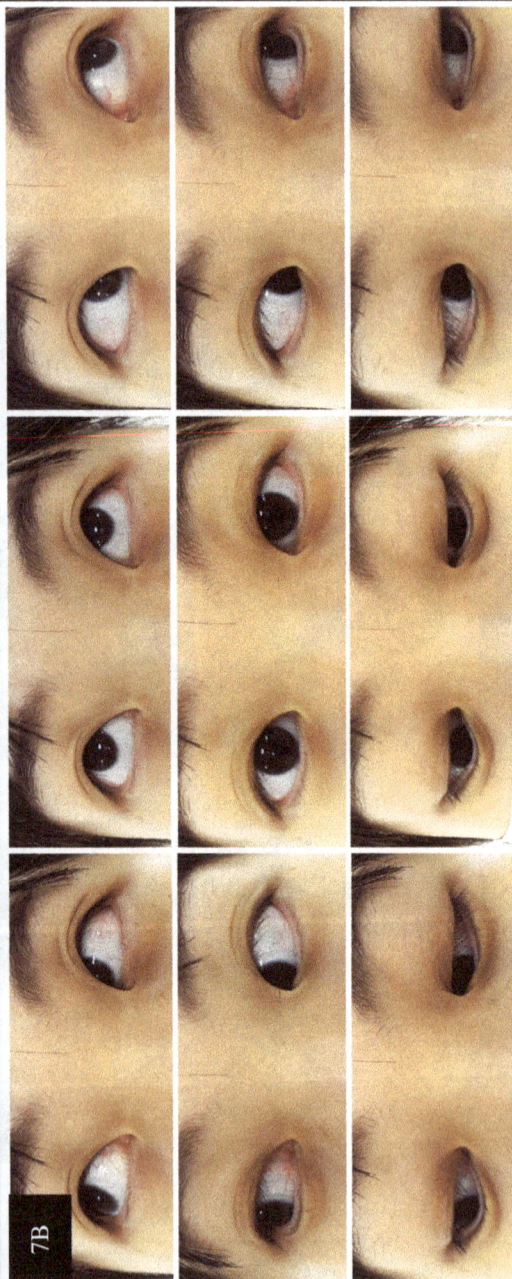

7B

When testing **slow pursuit**, instruct the patient fixate his/her eyes on a red hat pin or an equivalent object. Beginning at the eyes' primary position, move the pin slowly to the positions illustrated in 7A and 7B, **making sure to pause** at the horizonal and vertical extremes whilst observing for the presence of nystagmus.

Instruct the patient to look at the red ball, and then back at you nose quickly.

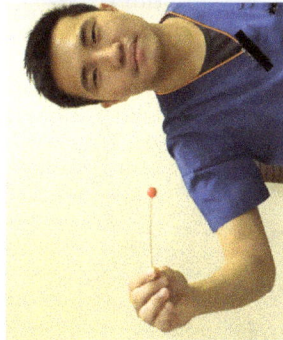

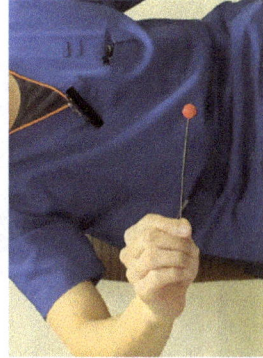

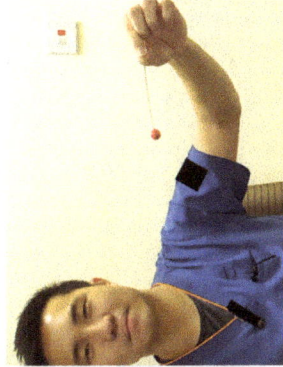

7C

Extraocular movements

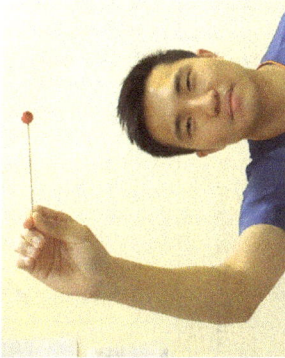

(Continued)

(Continued)

Examination Steps

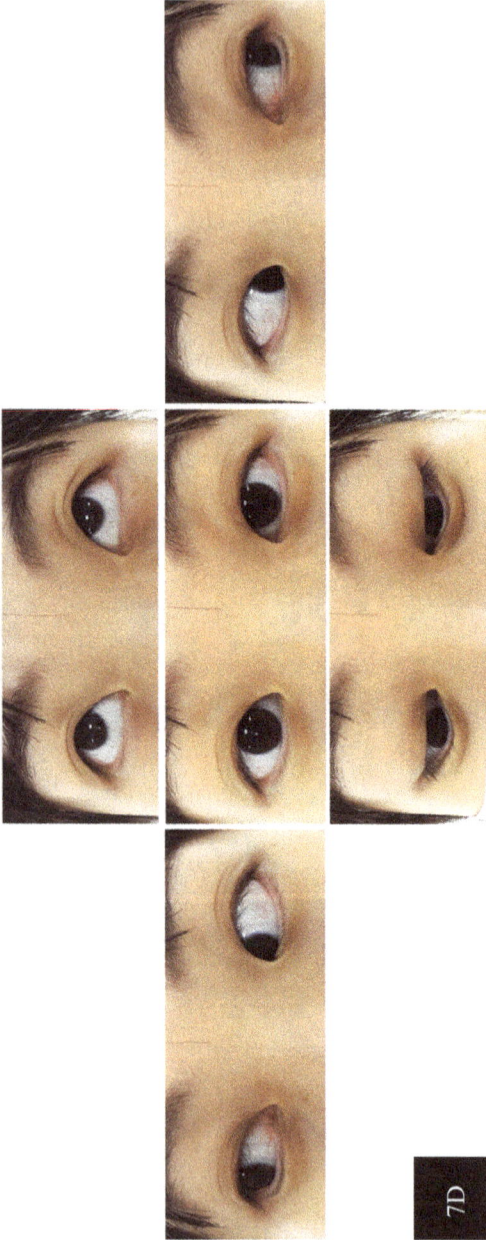

7D

When testing voluntary **saccades**, instruct the patient to shift his/her gaze to and fro between the object and your nose, as shown in **7C** and **7D**. Both vertical and horizontal saccades must be assessed. The testing of extraocular movements is discussed in greater detail **Chapters 8, 9 and 10.**

Motor assessment		I prefer to examine the motor domains of the remaining cranial nerves together (CN V, CN VII, CN IX, CN X, CN XI, CN XII), rather than assessing them sequentially according to their numerical order. This avoids having to repeatedly shuttle between the patient and your examination kit, thus minimising disruption to the examination process. This is by no means dogmatic, and I encourage the reader to modify the sequence appropriately to better suit your examination needs and style.

Instructions	CN	Tasks
Look up, frown, or wrinkle your forehead (**8A**)	VII	Observe for **facial asymmetry**
Squeeze your eyes shut, burry your lashes (**8B**)		
Puff up your cheeks, or blow a kiss (**8E**)		
Smile! (**8F**)		
Grimace, or show your lower teeth (**8G, 8H**)		Observe for **platysmal asymmetry**
Clench your jaw strongly (**8I, 8J**)	V	Palpate the **masseters** and the **temporalis** muscles
Open your mouth (**8K**)		Observe the tongue for **atrophy** and **fasciculations**
Say "ahhh"! (**8M, 8N**)	IX X	Inspect for asymmetric **palatal** elevation and deviation of the **uvula.**
Stick out your tongue (**8L**)	XII	Observe for deviation of the tongue
Push your tongue against your cheeks (**8O, 8P**)		Assess the tongue's strength
Turn your head to the left, and then to the right (**8Q, 8R**)	XI	Palpate the **sternocleidomastoid** muscles
Shrug both shoulders (**8S to 8V**)		Push down against the shrugged shoulders to assess the power of the **trapezius** muscles

The examination of facial muscles is discussed in greater detail in **Chapter 14.**

(Continued)

(Continued)

Examination Steps

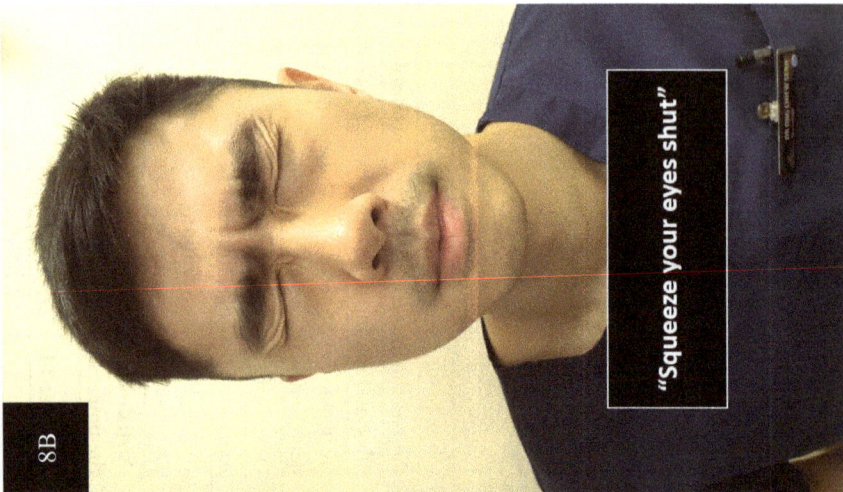

8A

"Look up, wrinkle your forehead"

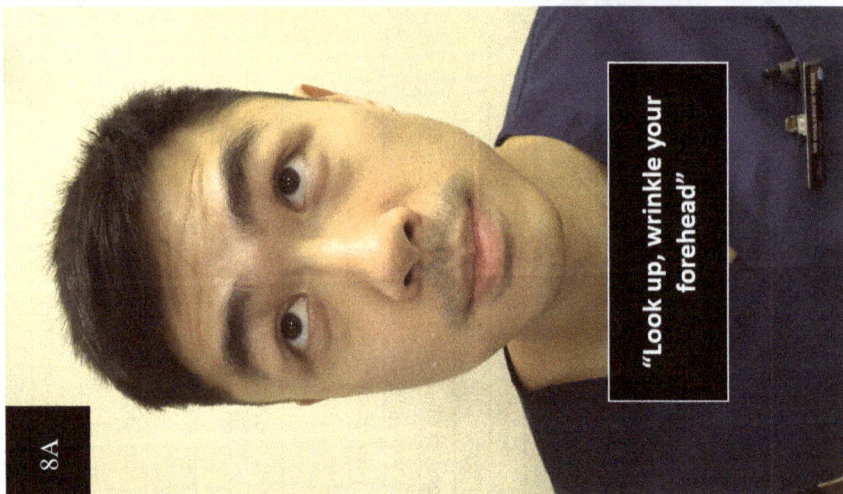

8B

"Squeeze your eyes shut"

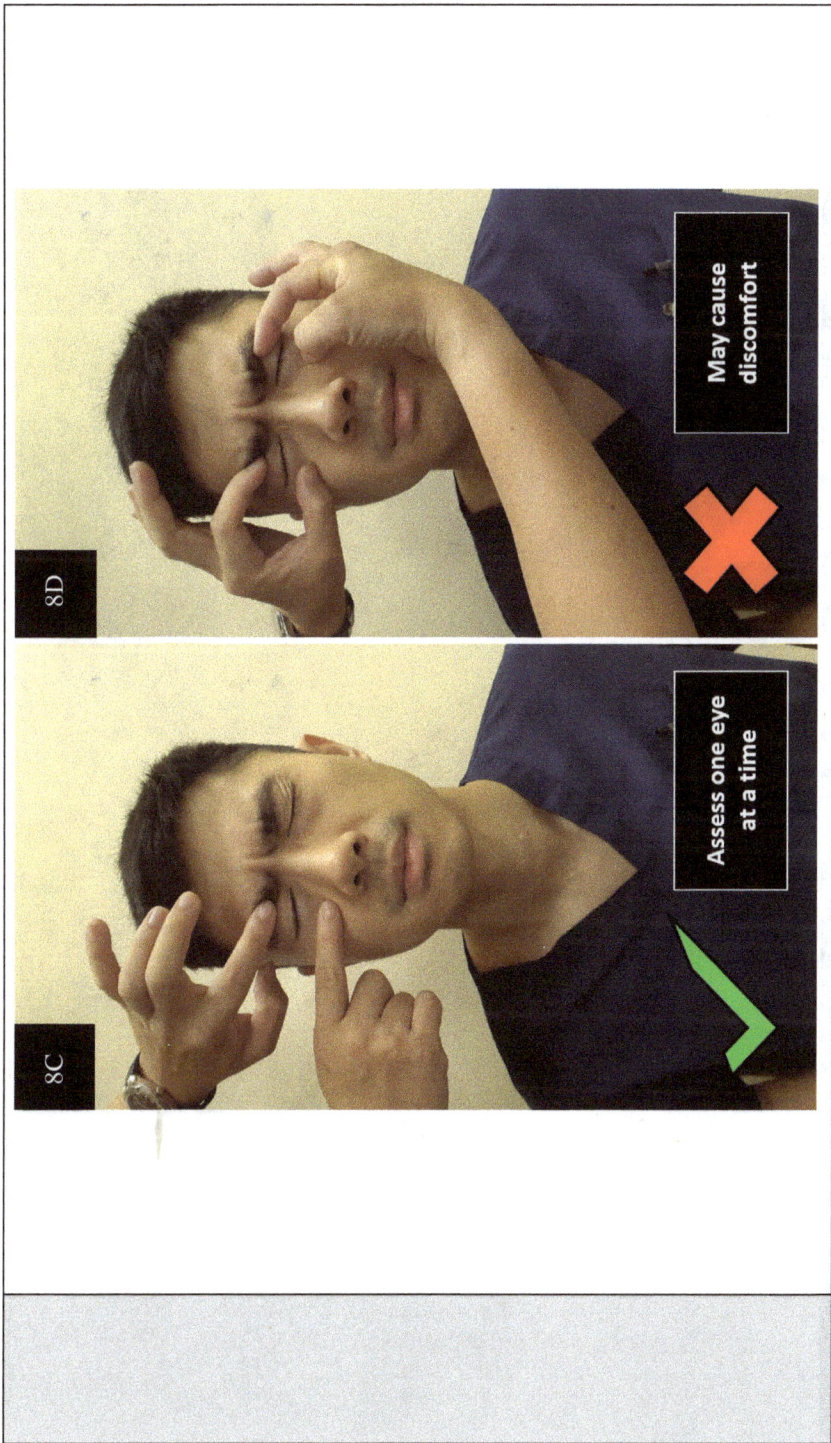

8C

Assess one eye
at a time

8D

May cause
discomfort

(Continued)

(Continued)

Examination Steps

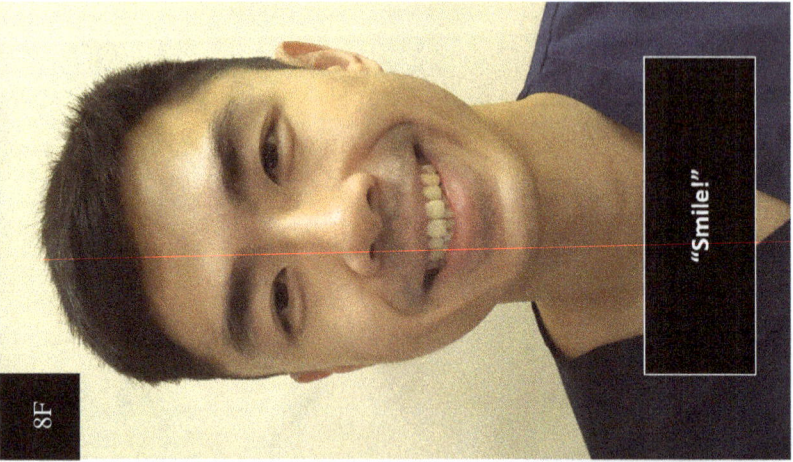

8F

"Smile!"

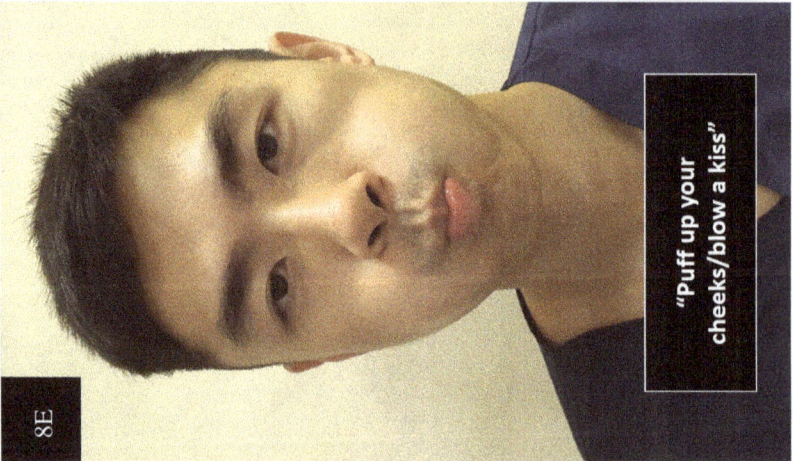

8E

"Puff up your cheeks/blow a kiss"

As the patient attempts to grimace, observe the platysma muscles (**8G, 8H**). Asymmetrical platysmal contraction due to unilateral weakness (the "**platysma sign**") may be seen in patients with unilateral facial palsy, regardless of it being due to an upper or lower motor neuron disorder.[2]

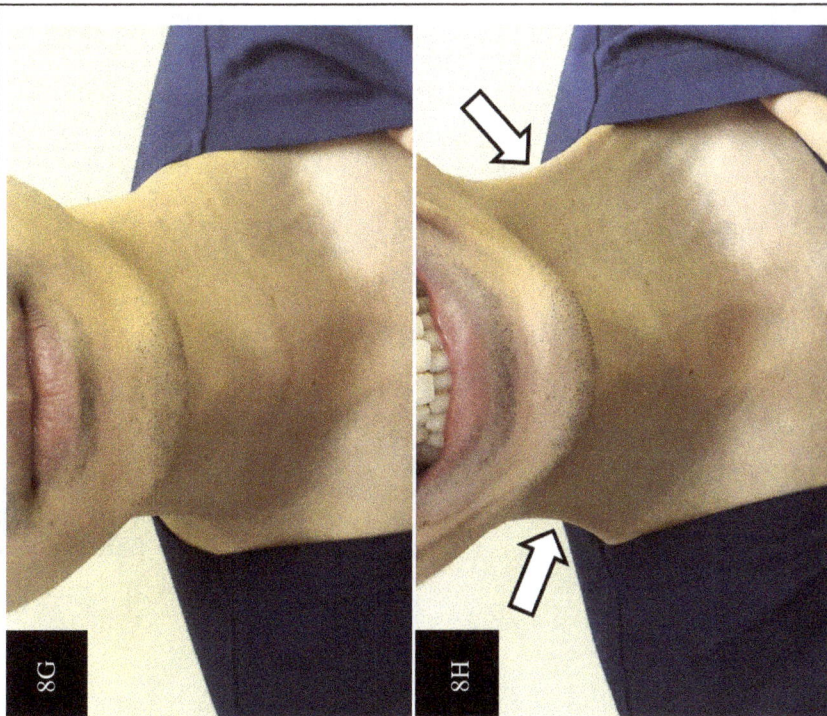

8G

8H

(Continued)

(Continued)

Examination Steps

8I

Palpate the temporalis muscle

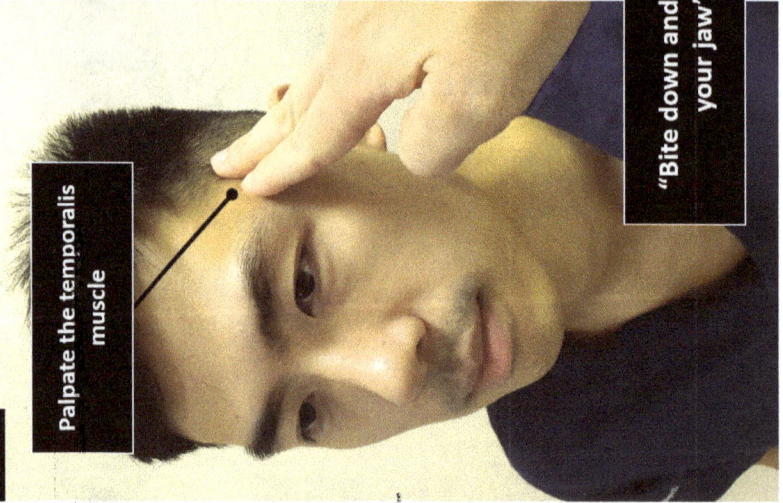

8J

Palpate the masseter muscle

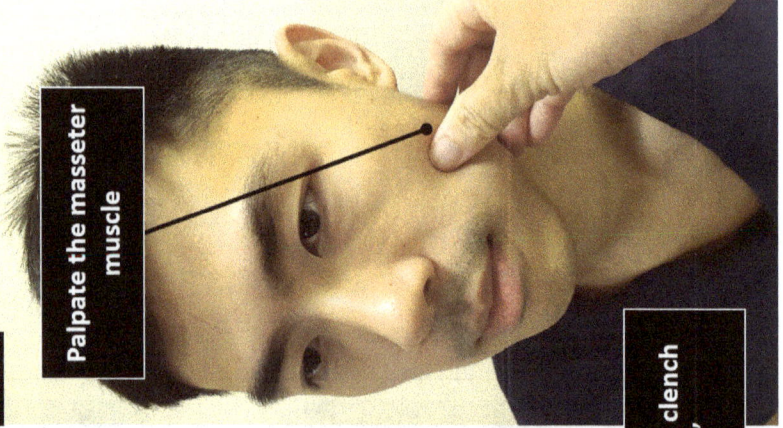

"Bite down and clench your jaw"

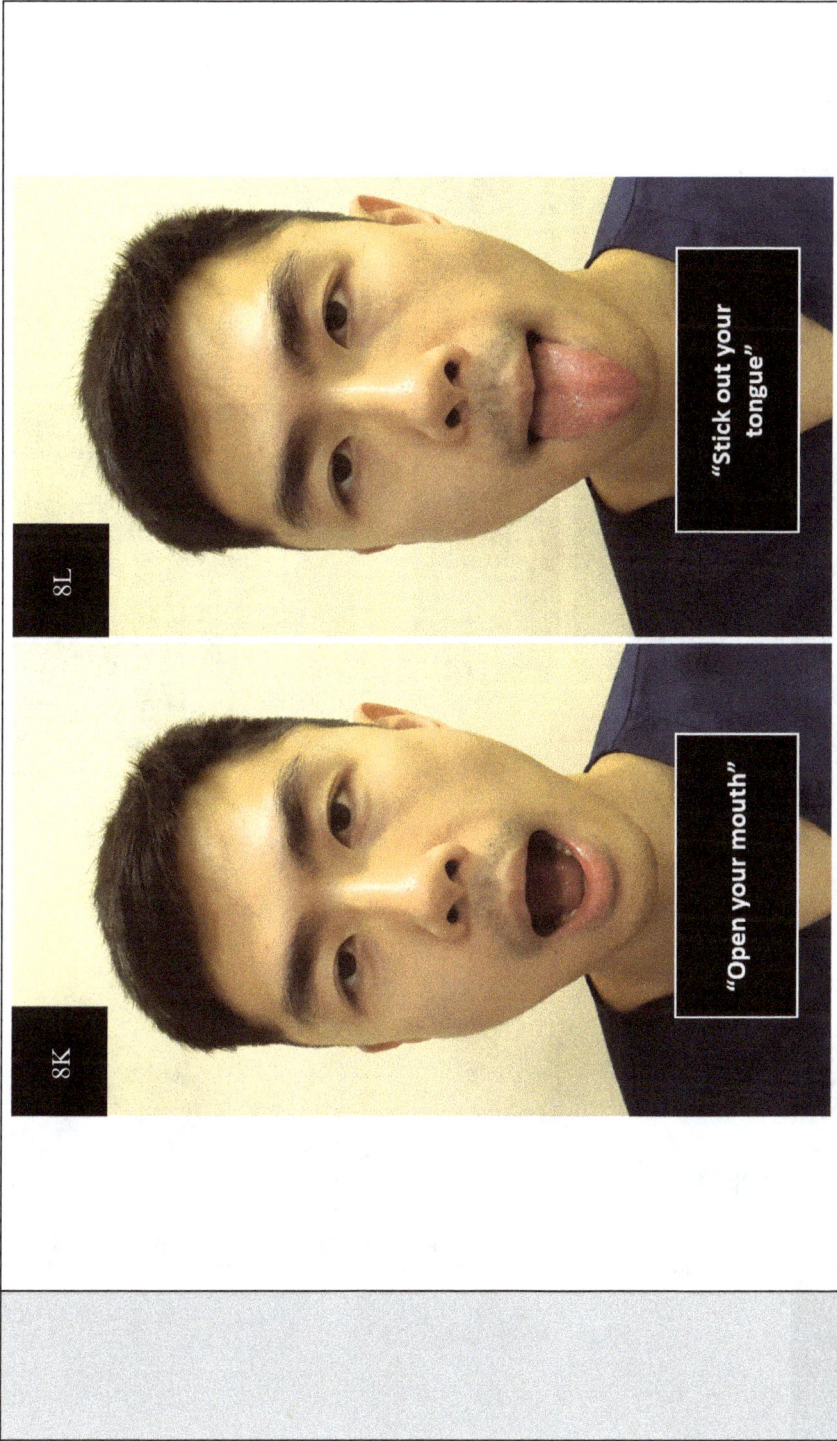

8L "Stick out your tongue"

8K "Open your mouth"

(Continued)

(Continued)

Examination Steps

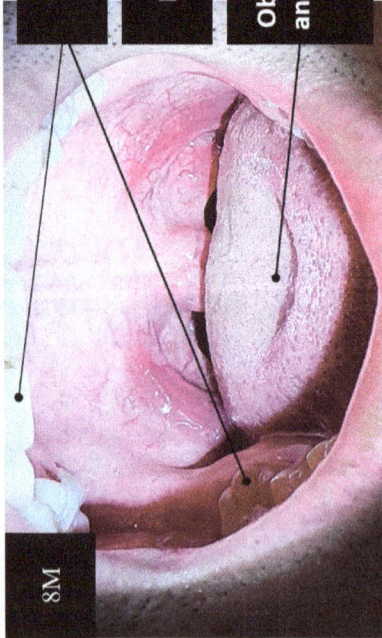

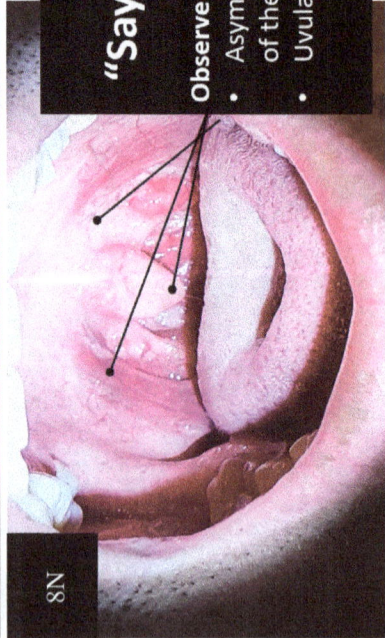

Dentition

Mucosal lesions

Observe for atrophy and fasciculations of the tongue

The innervation of the tongue is complex. Further reading will be required to better understand the tongue and to differentiate central from peripheral causes of unilateral tongue weakness. Regardless the cause, however, tongue deviation on protrusion indicates weakness of the **genioglossus muscle.**

"Say ahhhhh!"

Observe for:
- Asymmetrical elevation of the palate
- Uvular deviation

The genioglossus is an extrinsic muscle of the tongue. It protrudes and pushes the tongue towards the other side. Protrusion of the tongue along the midline (**8L**) requires both genioglossi to act together. Therefore, weakness on one side results in deviation of the tongue towards that side, as the normal genioglossus overpowers its weaker counterpart.

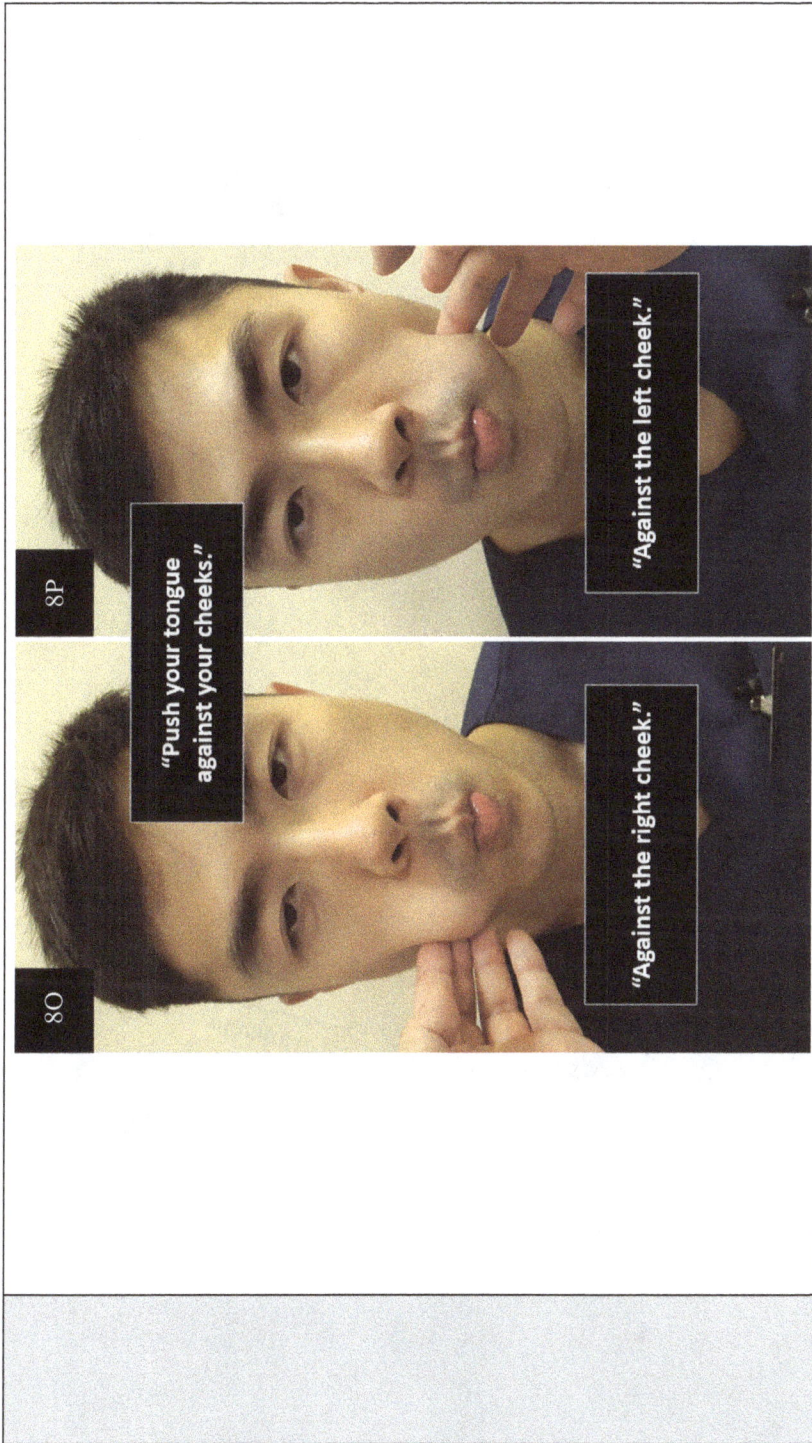

(Continued)

Examination Steps *(Continued)*

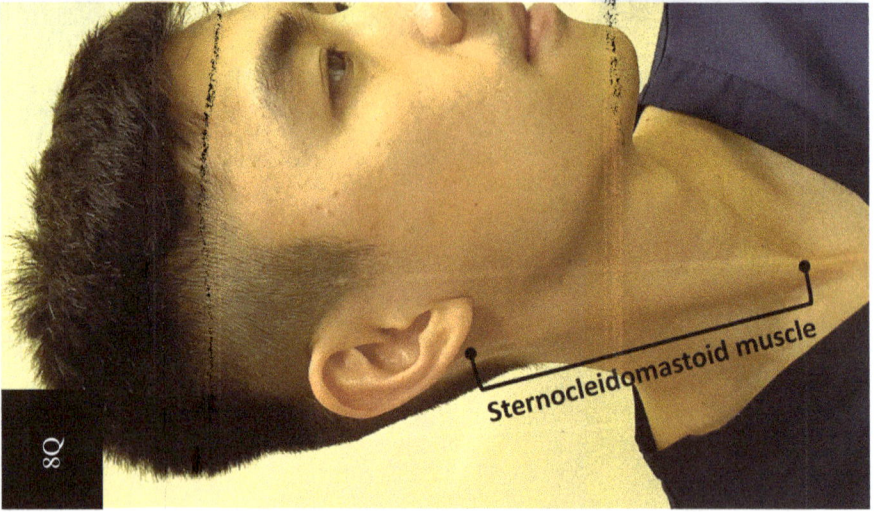

8Q

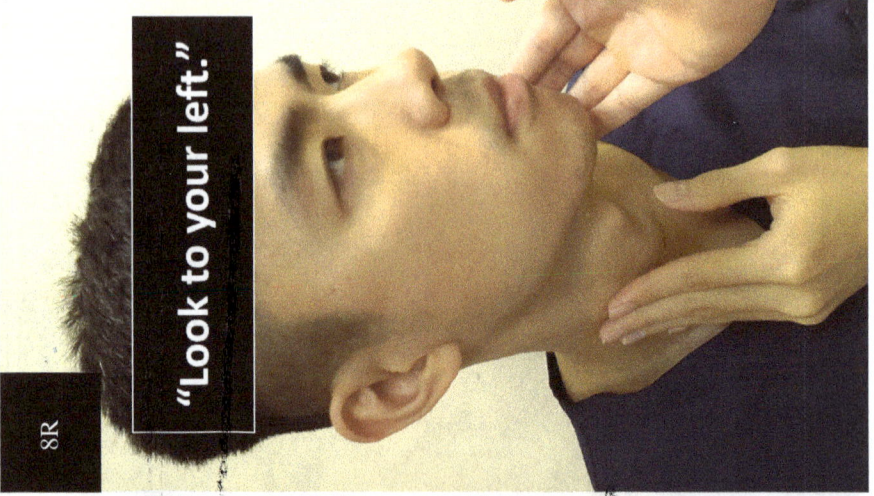

Sternocleidomastoid muscle

8R

"Look to your left."

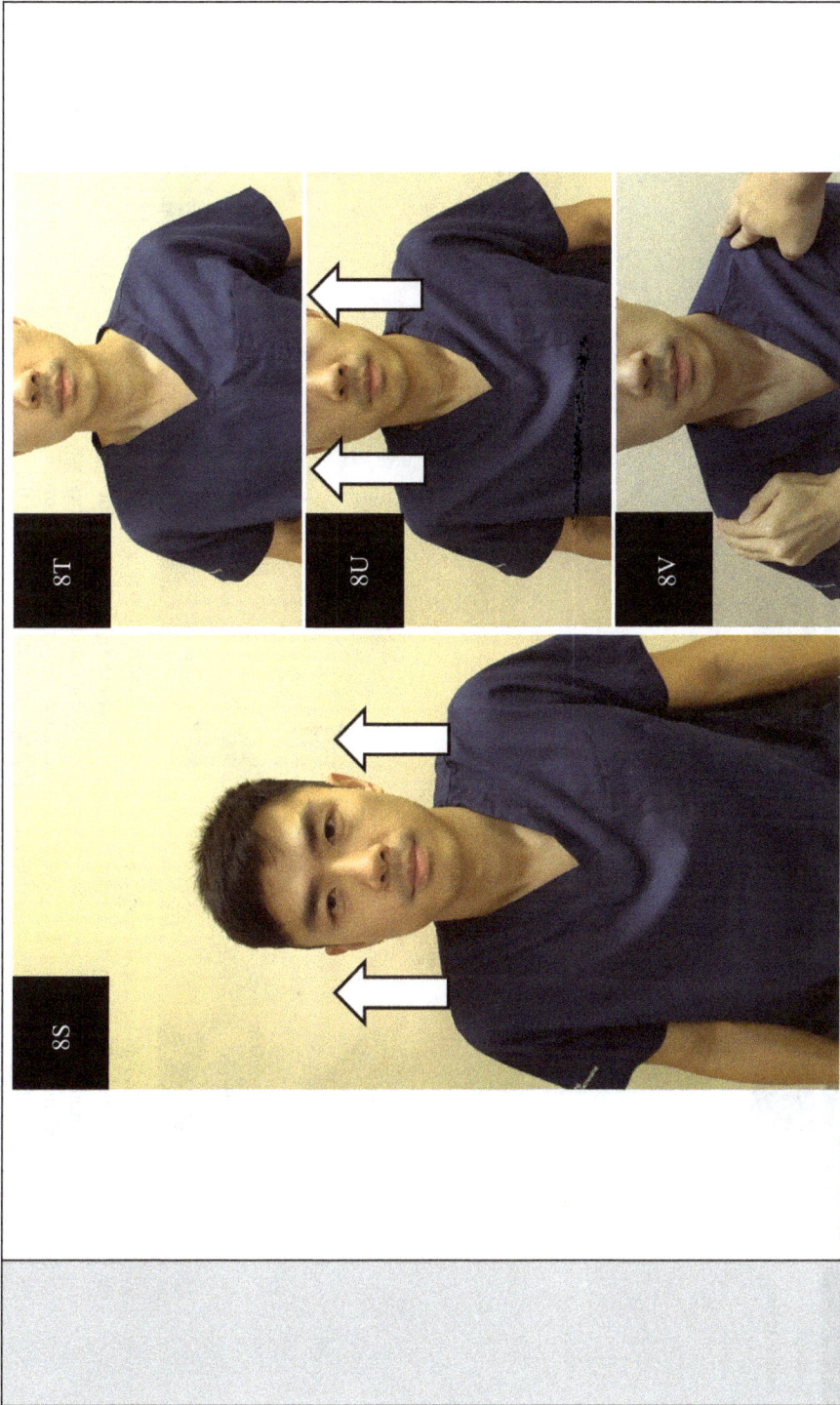

(Continued)

(Continued)

Examination Steps

Sensory assessment	

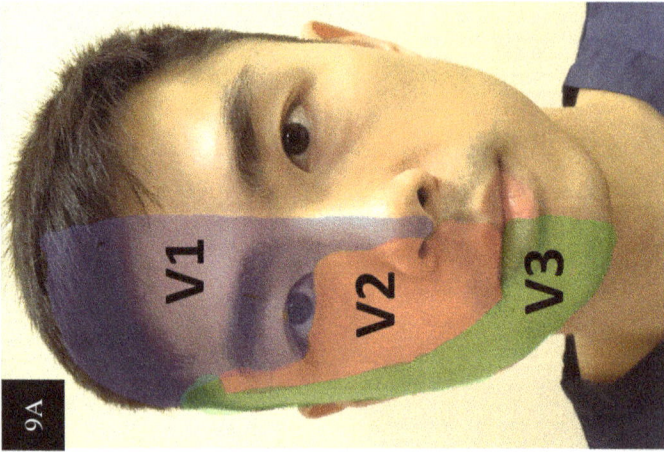

9A

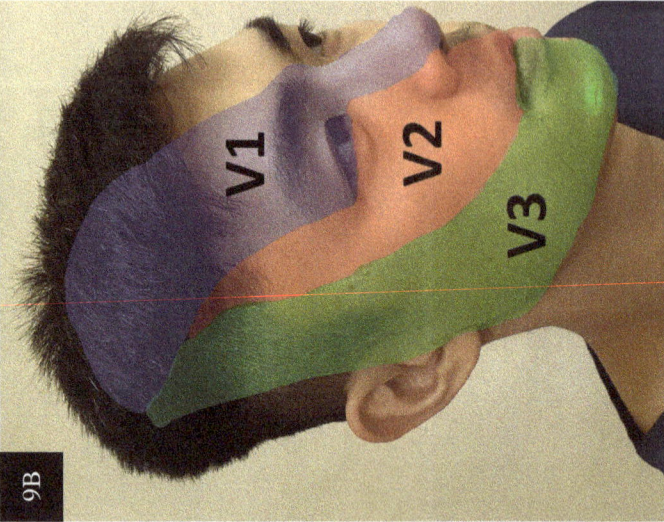

9B

Facial sensation should be tested using a wisp of cotton (**9A, 9B**). **Firstly**, a cotton wisp is more comfortable than a pin when used on the patient's face. **Secondly**, it assesses fine/light touch over the face, modalities processed by the pontine principal nucleus, where most trainees reflexively localize to when central causes of facial hypoesthesia are suspected. Alas, the trigeminal nuclear complex is extensive, occupying the entire brainstem and the superior cervical cord. The spinal nucleus receives nociceptive stimulus (e.g., pinprick). If a pin is used, sensory deficits cannot be attributed to lesions at the pons. As such, we recommend using a cotton wisp instead of a pin, except when diseases of the medulla oblongata are suspected (e.g., lateral medullary syndrome), for which pinprick will be preferred.

Hearing assessment	

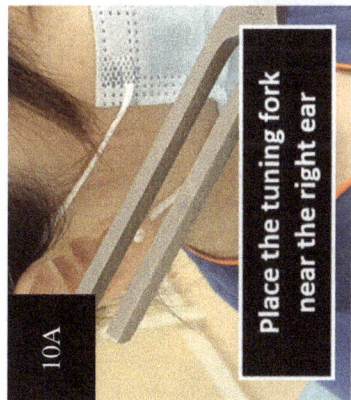

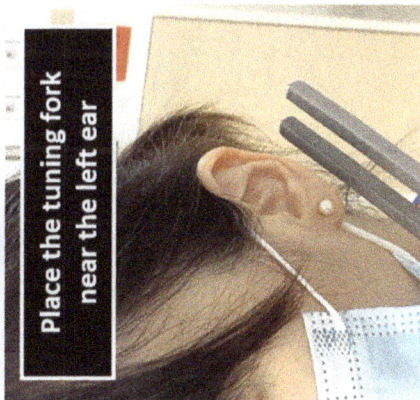

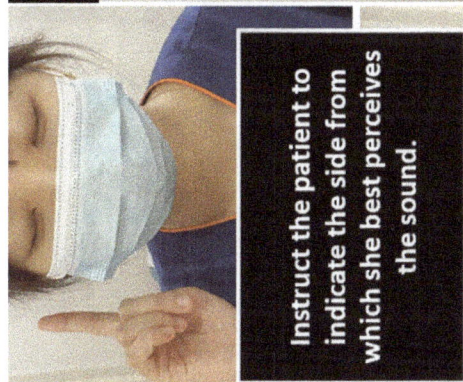

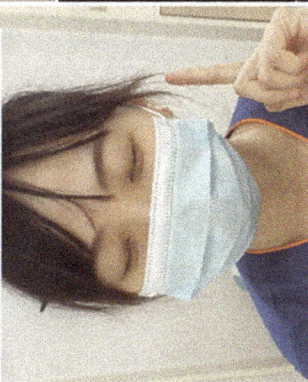

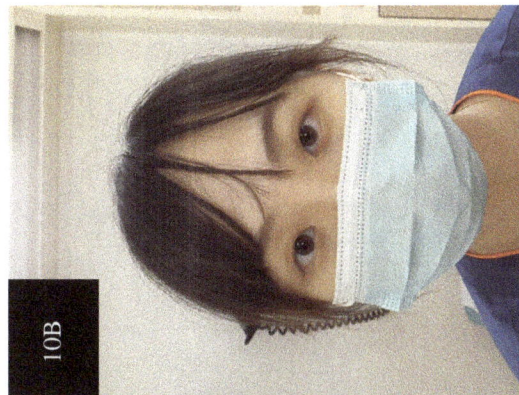

10A

Place the tuning fork near the right ear

Place the tuning fork near the left ear

Instruct the patient to indicate the side from which she best perceives the sound.

10B

Compare between the sides. Was it louder on one side?

Hearing may be screened with a 512 Hz tuning fork (**10A, 10B**). Instruct the patient to indicate with his/her hands the ear from which he hears the sound. To avoid confounding the assessment with unwanted noise, **do not speak to the patient during the test.** All pertinent instructions should be given prior to the test. **Weber** and **Rinne tests** are explained later in this chapter.

(*Continued*)

(Continued)

Examination Steps

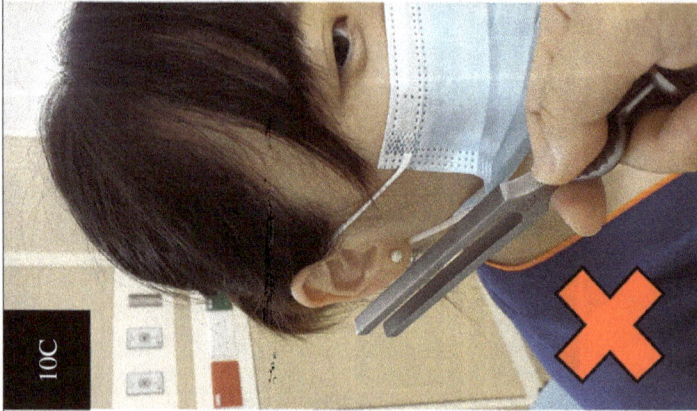

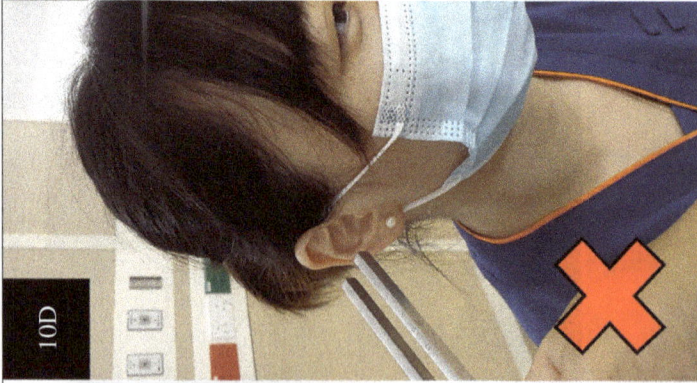

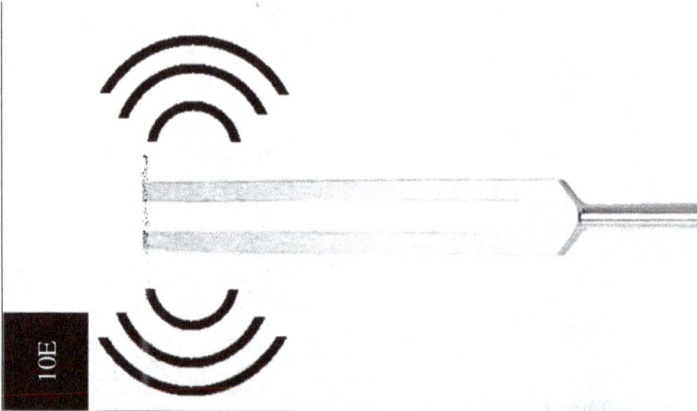

10C	10D	10E

Common mistakes when using the tuning fork are illustrated in **10C** and **10D**. Because sound is emitted from its sides (**10E**), the tuning fork should thus be held with its **sides toward the ear** (**10A**).

Additional examination	
	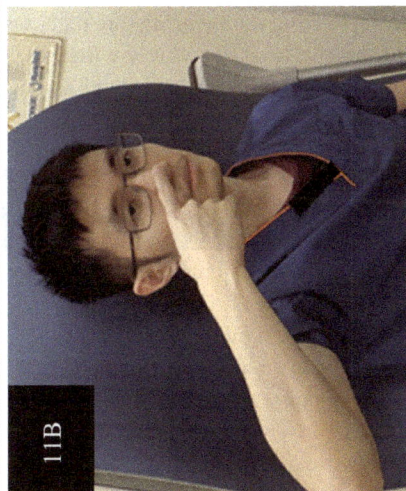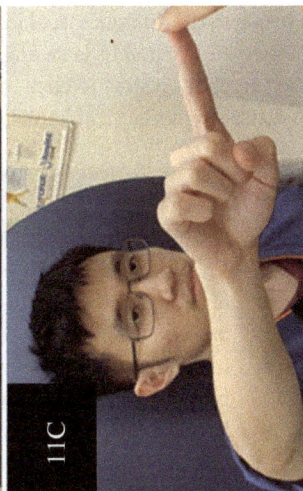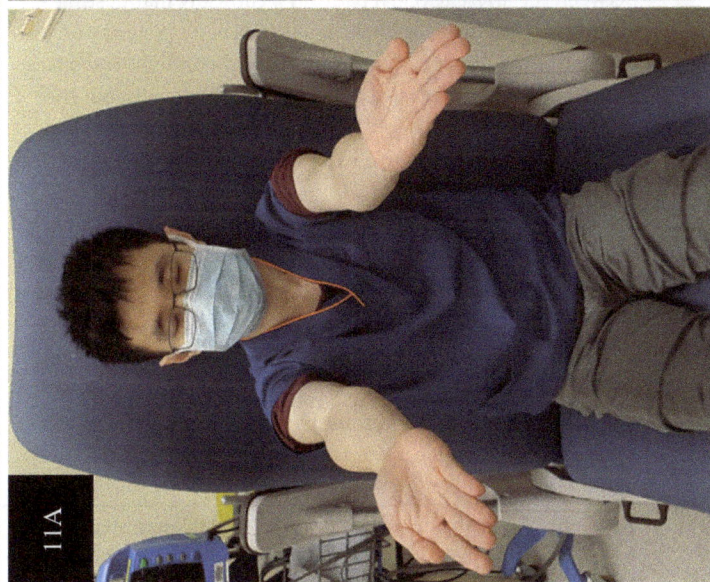 At the end of the examination, it is important to screen for long-tract deficits. Their presence localizes the lesion at the brainstem. In unilateral CN III palsy, for example, the presence of contralateral hemiparesis places the lesion along its fascicle at the midbrain, (Weber's syndrome) rather than a peripheral CN III palsy. Due to the artificial time limitations in professional examinations, testing for pronator drift (**11A**) and dysmetria (**11B** and **C**) will allow you to quickly screen for long-tract deficits.

B. Relative Afferent Pupillary Defect (Marcus Gunn Pupil)

Relative Afferent Pupillary Defect (RAPD) describes the clinical findings in patients with differential light perception between the afferent visual pathways. Using the swinging torchlight test, pupillary dilatation is observed when light is swung to that eye from the other eye (figures 5G and 5.1). Although RAPD is relatively easy to elicit, there are common misconceptions amongst medical students when discussing its clinical implications.

Common Misconceptions	Clarification
When direct light responses are present in both eyes, there's no need to perform the swinging torch test.	This misconception stems from the commonly-used description of a pupil with RAPD — defective direct light response with preserved consensual light response. While this description is somewhat true, some misunderstood it as saying that the presence of a/any direct light response immediately rules out RAPD, rendering the swinging torch test unnecessary. This is untrue. RAPD reflects the relative difference in light perception between the afferent visual pathways, clinically manifesting as differential "intensity" rather than the absolute presence or absence of the direct responses. As such, direct light responses of both eyes may be present when tested individually, but the differences in the "intensity" of the direct responses between both eyes in a patient with RAPD still requires elicitation by the swinging torch test.
The eye with RAPD is diseased eye. The other eye must be normal.	RAPD in one eye does not rule out disease in the other eye. It is here when the term "relative" becomes relevant, as it describes a relative difference in light perception between the afferent visual pathways. As such, RAPD can be present in patients with bilaterally diseased optic nerves, for example, if there is asymmetry of disease severity. In these patients, the eye with RAPD is more severely affected and thus perceiving less light than the other less-diseased eye, resulting in differential responses to light.
The lesion lies in the optic nerves or the retina.	Although classically described in cases of optic neuropathy and severe retinal disease, the lesion may lie anywhere along the afferent visual pathway. Cases of RAPD have been reported in patients with geniculate and retro-geniculate lesions.[3]

Normal

RAPD of the left eye

| Right Eye | Left Eye | Right Eye | Left Eye |

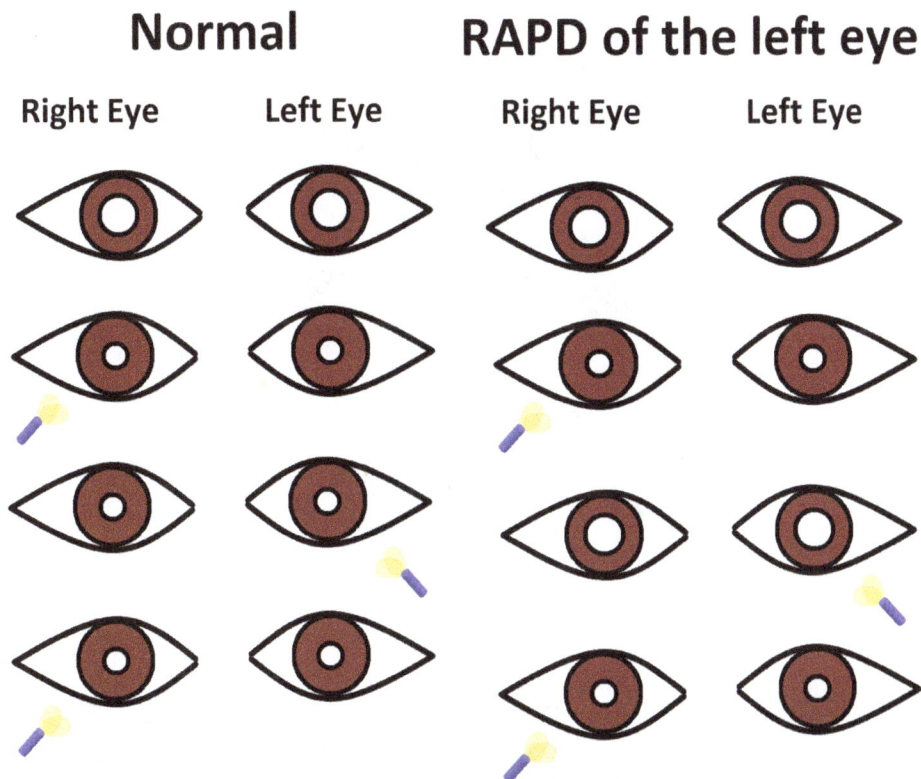

Figure 5.1.   Schematic drawing of the swinging torch test performed on a pair of normal eyes, and another pair with RAPD of the left eye.

C. The Weber and Rinne Tests

The **Weber** and **Rinne tests** are helpful in assessing the patient's hearing, and should only be performed in a quiet room. You will require a 512Hz tuning fork. Hold the stem, strike one side of the tines about 2/3 of its length from its base against a padded surface (e.g., a clothed elbow, or the fleshy parts of the palm). Avoid hitting the tuning fork against a hard surface as that may damage it and also introduce harmonic overtones.

The **Weber test** lateralises to the ear where the sound is perceived by the patient. After striking the tuning fork, place it against a bony region along the midline of the head (e.g., the forehead) for about 5 seconds (Figure 5.2). Thereafter, ask the patient from which ear is the sound best perceived.[4]

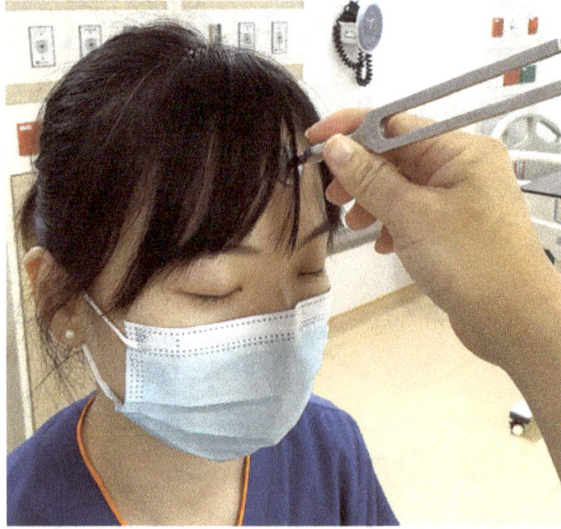

Figure 5.2.   Weber test.

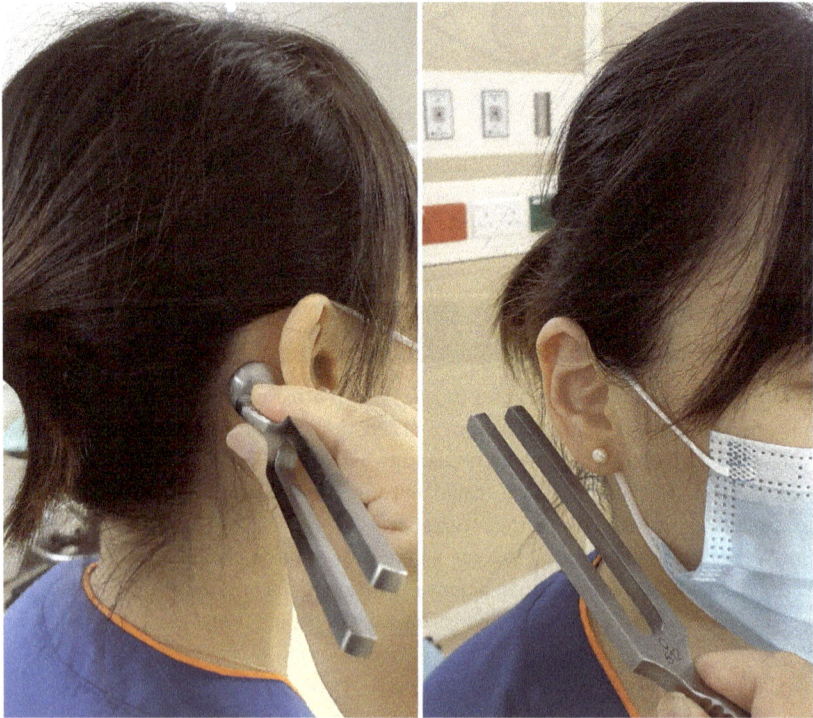

Figure 5.3.   Rinne test.

Interpretation of Weber Test	
Normal	The sound is perceived equally by both ears.
Conductive hearing loss	The sound is heard louder by the affected ear.
Sensorineural hearing loss	The sound is heard louder by the unaffected ear.

The **Rinne test** (Figure 5.3) compares the perception of the sound by **bone conduction (BC)** against **air conduction (AC)**. Begin at the ear where the Weber's test has lateralized to. Strike the tuning fork and place it against the mastoid process (tests BC). Instruct the patient inform you when the sound can no longer be perceived. Immediately move the tuning fork 2.5 to 4 cm in front of the external acoustic meatus (tests AC) and ask if the sound can be heard again.[4,5] If the patient is able to hear the sound, then sound perception by AC is deemed to be better than BC.

Interpretation of Rinne Test	
Normal	AC > BC (Rinne's positive)
Conductive hearing loss	BC > AC (Rinne's negative)
Sensorineural hearing loss	AC > BC (Rinne's false positive)

The Weber and Rinne tests are often used in combination, and their findings should be interpreted together.

Interpretation of Findings from Both Weber and Rinne Tests		
	Weber test lateralises to	Rinne test findings
Conductive hearing loss		
Normal ear	The symptomatic ear	AC > BC (positive)
Symptomatic ear		BC > AC (negative)
Sensorineural hearing loss		
Normal ear	The asymptomatic ear	AC > BC (positive)
Symptomatic ear		AC > BC (false positive)
		BC > AC (false negative, in patients with severe SNHL)

References

1. Spence C. (2015) Just how much of what we taste derives from the sense of smell? *Flavour* **4**: 30.
2. Wilhelm H, Wilhelm B, Petersen D, Schmidt U, Schiefer U. (1996) Relative afferent pupillary defects in patients with geniculate and retrogeniculate lesions. *Neuro-Opthalmology* **16**(4): 219–224.
3. Kong EL, Fowler JB. (2017) *Rinne Test*. [Updated 2020 Oct 27]. StatPearls Publishing, Treasure Island.
4. Butskiy O, Ng D, Hodgson M, Nunez DA. (2016) Rinne test: Does the tuning fork position affect the sound amplitude at the ear? *J Otolaryngol Head Neck Surg* **45**(1): 21.
5. Leon-Sarmiento FE, Prada LJ, Torres-Hillera M. (2002) The first sign of Babinski. *Neurology* **59**(7): 1067.

6

Approach to Brainstem Localisation

A. Introduction

The brainstem comprises of the **midbrain, pons**, and **medulla oblongata**, through which major tracts travel and in which the cranial nuclei reside. With many important structures tightly packed within the region, a small insult within the brainstem can have devastating clinical consequences. However, we can use this to our advantage. Like how the sailors of old interpret the constellations to navigate the uncharted seas, we can piece together the collection of neurologic deficits and pinpoint the likely location where the pathology dwells.

Brainstem neurolocalisation, as byzantine as it sounds, obeys a few basic rules that will certainly help you with your journey.

B. The Four Rules of Four

The **four rules of four** form the foundation of brainstem localisation. I found these rules easy to understand and simple to apply. Do take some time to familiarise yourself with them (see below).

	Rules	Description
#1	Four medially-located structures beginning with "M"	The four structures are: 1. Medial longitudinal fasciculus (MLF) 2. Motor tracts (corticospinal tracts, corticobulbar tracts) 3. Medial lemniscus 4. Motor nuclei (of the cranial nerves)
#2	Four laterally-located structures beginning with "S"	The four structures are: 1. Sympathetic tract 2. Spinothalamic tract 3. Spinocerebellar tracts 4. Sensory components of the trigeminal nerve
#3	Four cranial nerves above the pons, four at the pons, and four below the pons	• Above the pons: CN I to IV (CN III and IV are at the midbrain) • At the pons: CN V to VIII • Below the pons: CN IX to XII

(*Continued*)

(*Continued*)

Rules	Description
#4 Four medially-located motor nuclei Please note that we are **referring to the nuclei**, not the fascicles/nerves	They are: 1. CN III (midbrain) 2. CN IV (midbrain) 3. CN VI (pons) 4. CN XII (medulla oblongata)

We have to deal with three planes when navigating about a three-dimensional space (medio-lateral, cephalo-caudal and antero-posterior planes) (Figure 6.1). The four rules of four provide neurolocalisation clues in the medio-lateral and cephalo-caudal planes. **What about the antero-posterior plane?** Are there additional clues that give us clarity along the antero-posterior plane? Thankfully yes!

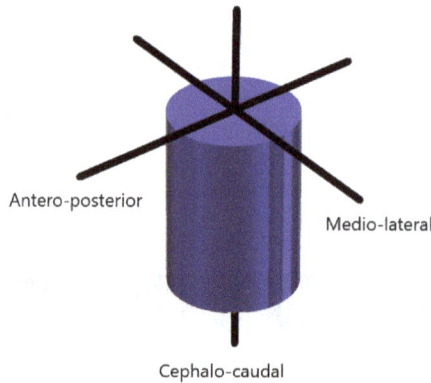

Figure 6.1.   Three-dimensional space in relation to its three planes.

- The **corticospinal tracts** run along the anterior portions of the brainstem (Figure 6.2):

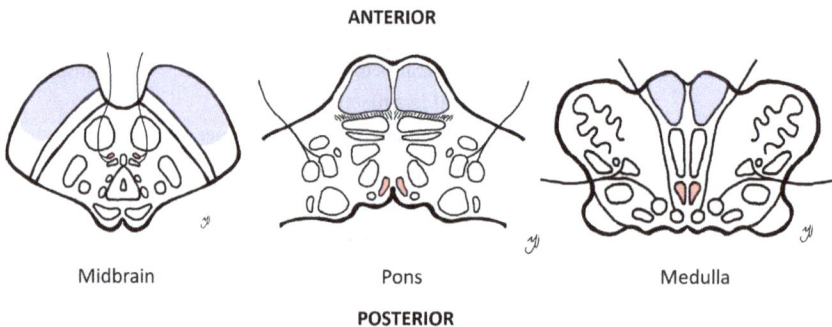

ANTERIOR

Midbrain   Pons   Medulla

POSTERIOR

Figure 6.2.   Schematic drawing of the brainstem along the axial plane (from the left: midbrain, pons, and medulla oblongata), showing the positions of the corticospinal tract (in blue) and the medial longitudinal fasciculus (in red).

- The **medial longitudinal fasciculus** runs along the posterior portions of the brainstem, except when within the midbrain (see below).

The involvement of these tracts can help us decide if the lesion is sited anteriorly or posteriorly within the brainstem.

> **WARNING!**
>
> These rules do not fit perfectly when applied on the midbrain.
> - The **motor tracts** run within the cerebral peduncle, extending from the medial to the lateral aspects of the midbrain, and thus are **not limited to the medial aspects** (rule #1).
> - Although the **medial longitudinal fasciculus** mostly lies in posterior aspect of the brainstem, it adopts a **relatively anterior course** as it traverses the midbrain.
> - The **cerebellar tracts** (superior cerebellar peduncle) lie medially within the midbrain, contradicting rule #2. A lesion at the medial midbrain can result in cerebellar deficits.
>
> As such, you should be cautious when applying the rules when the lesion is suspected to be at the midbrain. A degree of familiarity with midbrain anatomy will be helpful.

C. Practice!

Case A: A middle-aged gentleman with longstanding history of diabetes mellitus, hypertension, and hyperlipidaemia, presented acutely with binocular diplopia and left-sided weakness. He was drooling from the left side of his mouth and was unable to ambulate without assistance. An acute stroke was suspected. Examination revealed right blepharoptosis with the right eye adopting a "down-and-out" position. There was concomitant left hemiparesis.

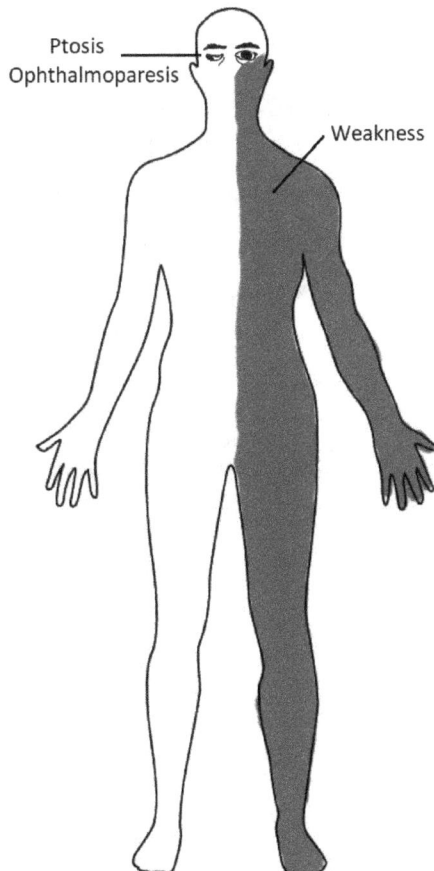

Discussion

The lesion likely involved the following structures:
- Right corticospinal tract (pre-decussation) → left hemiparesis
- Right oculomotor nerve → right blepharoptosis and ophthalmoparesis

Applying the four rules of four, the lesion is likely located:
- Medially:
  - Rule #1: corticospinal tract
- In the midbrain:
  - Rule #3: oculomotor nerve (fascicle)

With the knowledge that the corticospinal tract lies anteriorly, we are able to localise the lesion along the three planes:
- Antero-posterior plane: **Anterior**
- Medio-lateral plane: **Medial**
- Cephalo-caudal plane: **Midbrain**

As such, we now know that the stroke involves the left anteromedial region of the pons, resulting in symptoms and signs typical of **Weber's syndrome**.

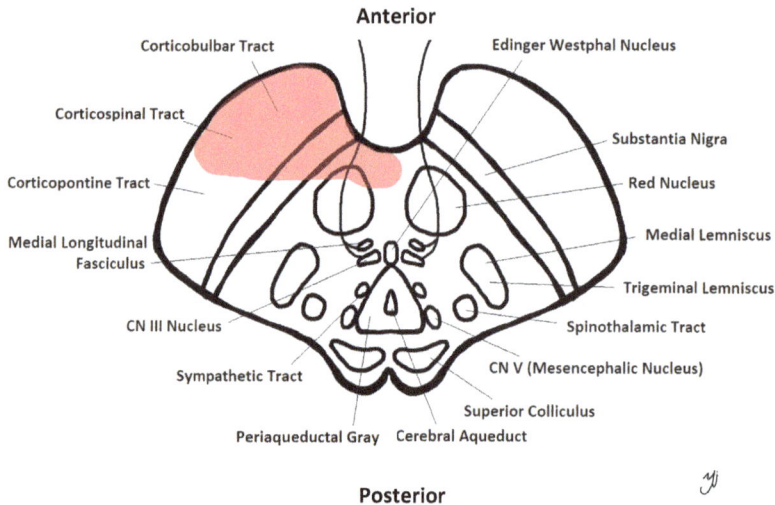

Case B: An elderly lady with a history of hypertension, presented acutely with binocular horizontal diplopia and right-sided weakness. An acute stroke was suspected. Examination revealed binocular horizontal diplopia that worsened on looking to the left, with impaired abduction of the left eye. There was accompanying left hemifacial weakness and right hemiparesis.

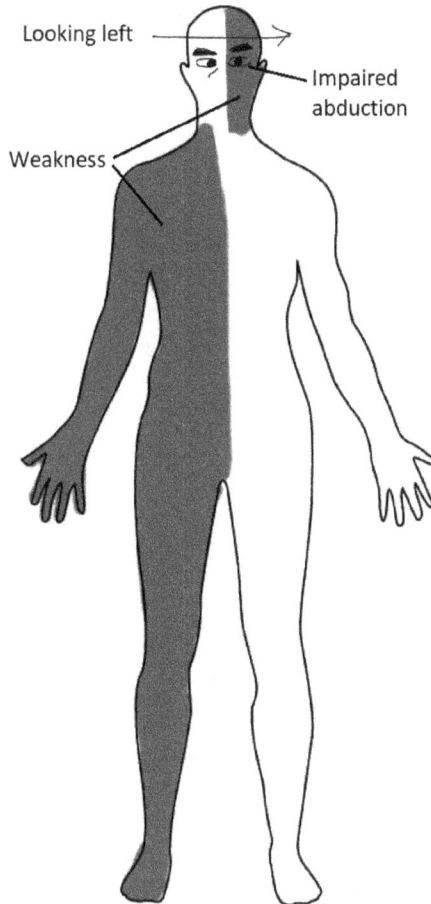

Discussion

The lesion likely involved the following structures:
- Left abducens nerve → abduction weakness of the left eye
- Left facial nerve or nucleus → left hemifacial weakness
- Left corticospinal tract (pre-decussation) → right hemiparesis

When we apply the four rules of four, the lesion is likely located:
- Medially:
  - Rule #1: corticospinal tract
- In the pons:
  - Rule #3: left facial and abducens nerve palsy

With the knowledge that the corticospinal tract lies anteriorly, we can localise the lesion along the three planes:
- Antero-posterior plane: **Anterior**
- Medio-lateral plane: **Medial**
- Cephalo-caudal plane: **Pons**

As such, the patient suffered a stroke at the left anteromedial region of the pons, resulting in symptoms and signs typical of **Millard-Gubler syndrome.**

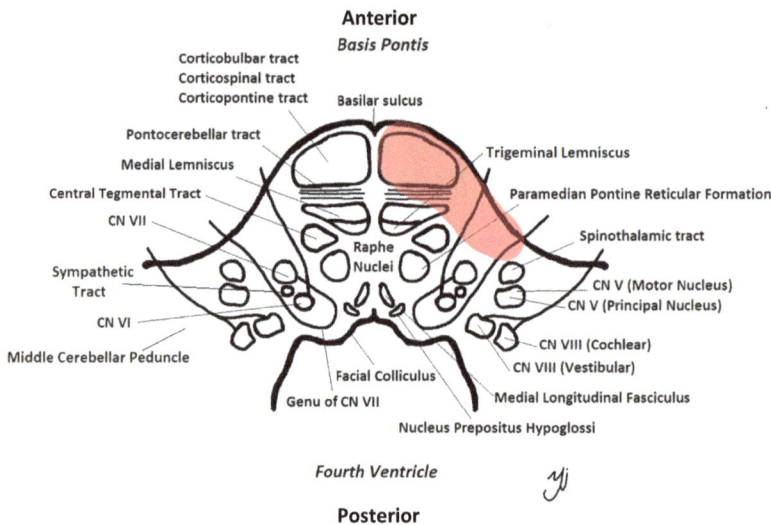

Case C: A middle-aged gentleman with vascular risk factors was admitted to your hospital for acute vertigo that was accompanied by severe vomiting. He complained of numbness over his right face and the left side of his body. He described difficulty swallowing and found his right arm clumsy. An acute stroke was suspected. Examination revealed the following signs:

- Right blepharoptosis with a miotic pupil
- Right facial hypoesthesia
- Impaired palatal elevation on the right
- Dysmetria of the right upper limb
- Hypoesthesia to pinprick of the left upper and lower limbs

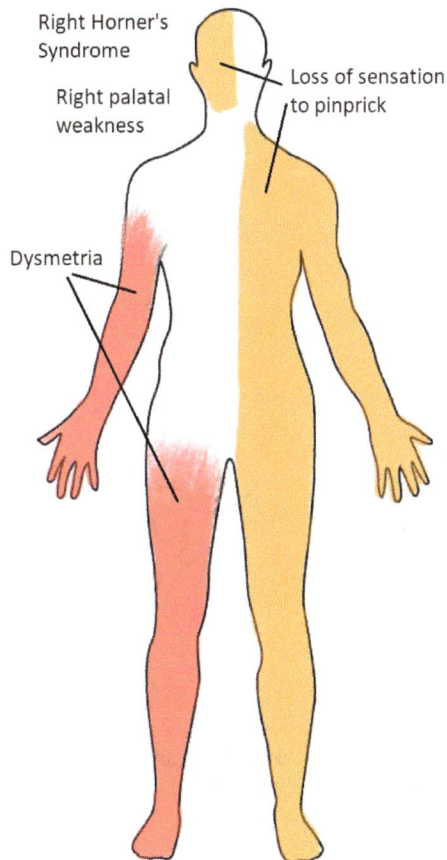

Discussion

The lesion likely involved the following structures:
- Right sympathetic pathway → right oculosympathetic failure
- Right spinal trigeminal nucleus and tract → right facial hypoesthesia
- Right nucleus ambiguus (with components of the glossopharyngeal and vagus nerves) → right palatal weakness
- Right spinocerebellar tracts → right dysmetria
- Right spinothalamic tract → left hemisensory deficits

When we apply the four rules of four, the lesion is likely located:
- Laterally:
  - Rule #2:
    - Spinothalamic tract
    - Sympathetic pathway
    - Spinal trigeminal nucleus and tract
    - Spinocerebellar tract
- In the medulla oblongata:
  - Rule #3: Palsy of the glossopharyngeal and vagus nerve

We can conclude that the lesion lies within the lateral aspect of the right hemi-medulla resulting in symptoms and signs typical of **Wallenberg syndrome**.

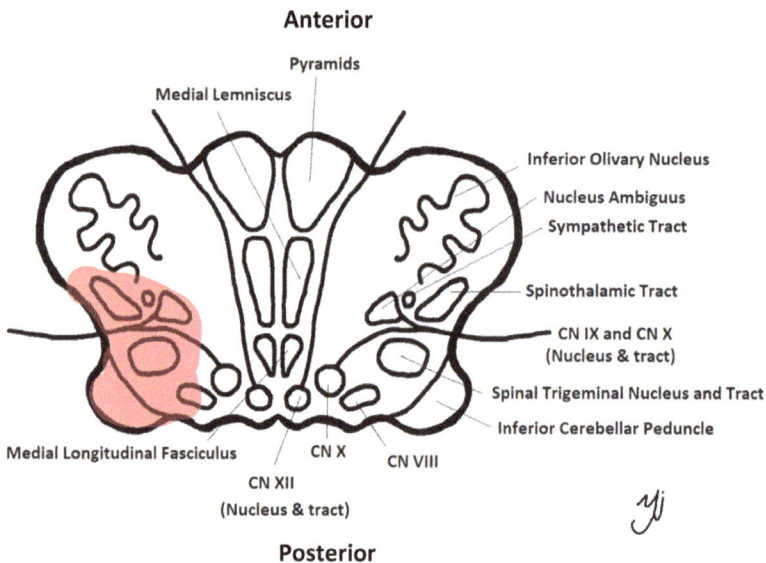

Case D: An elderly lady with diabetes mellitus and hypertension presented acutely with dysarthria. She experienced difficulty articulating her words, which was soon followed by weakness and numbness over her left. An acute stroke was suspected. Examination revealed the following signs:

- Tongue deviation to the right on protrusion
- Left hemiparesis
- Left-sided loss of fine touch, vibration sense, and proprioception

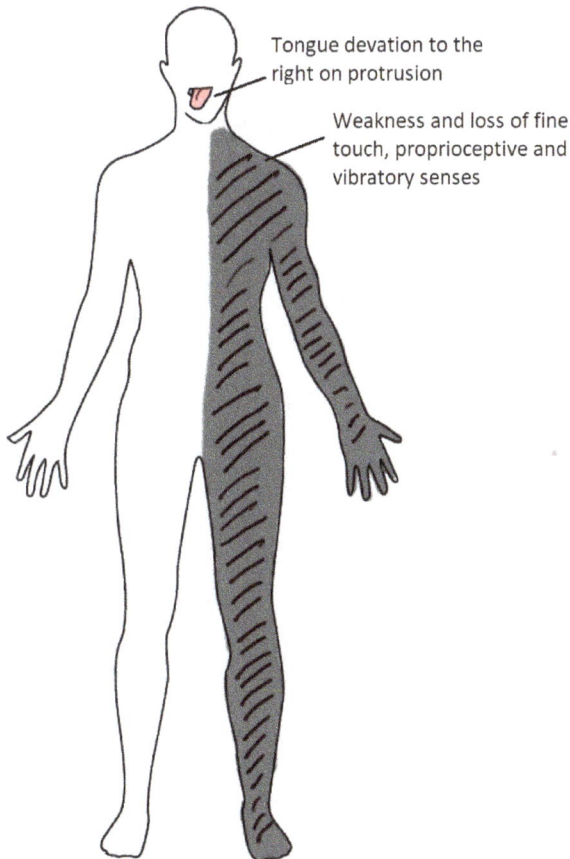

Tongue devation to the right on protrusion

Weakness and loss of fine touch, proprioceptive and vibratory senses

Discussion

The lesion likely involved the following structures:
- Right hypoglossal nucleus or nerve → tongue deviation to the right
- Right corticospinal tract (pre-decussation) → left hemiparesis
- Right Medial lemniscus → left sensory deficits to fine touch, vibratory and proprioceptive senses

When we apply the four rules of four, the lesion likely is likely located:
- Medially
  - Rule #1: Corticospinal tract, medial lemniscus
  - Rule #4: Hypoglossal nucleus or nerve
- In the medulla oblongata
  - Rule #3: Hypoglossal nucleus or nerve

We can conclude that the lesion lies within the medial aspect of the right hemi-medulla resulting in symptoms and signs typical of **Derjerine syndrome**.

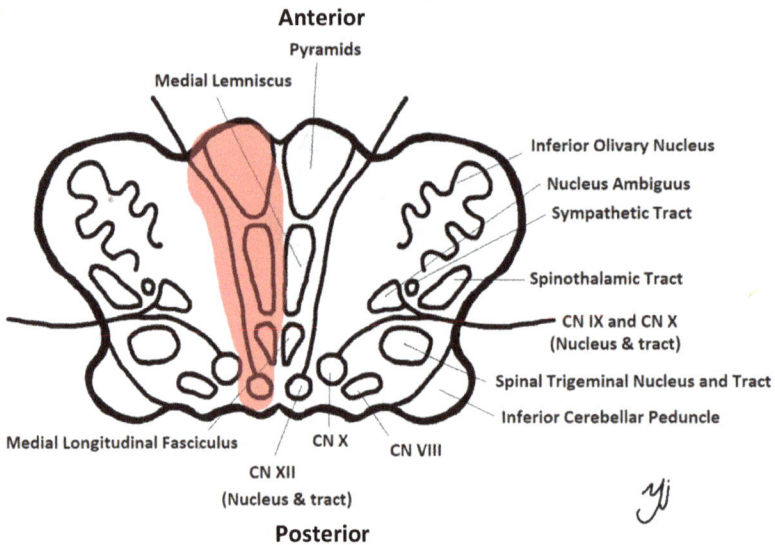

7

The Cranial Nerve Syndromes

A. Introduction

Familiarity with cranial nerve syndromes has significant neurolocalising value. This chapter will bring you through the classic cranial nerve syndromes that are important to recognise:

1. Cerebello-pontine angle syndrome
2. Jugular foramen syndrome
3. Cavernous sinus syndrome
4. Superior orbital fissure and orbital apex syndromes

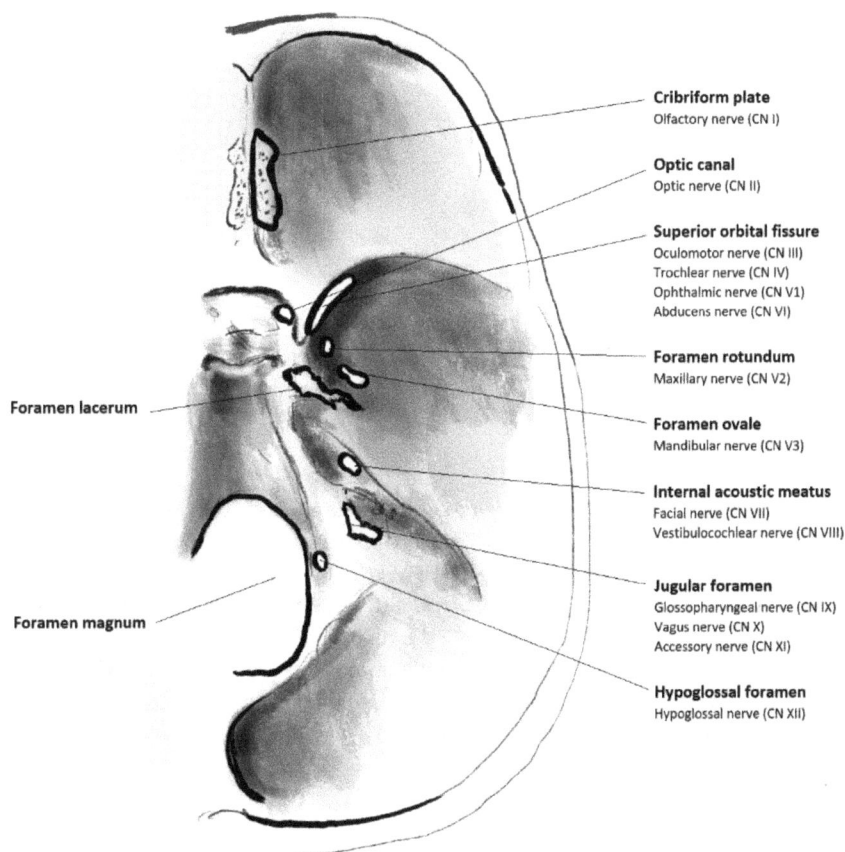

Cribriform plate
Olfactory nerve (CN I)

Optic canal
Optic nerve (CN II)

Superior orbital fissure
Oculomotor nerve (CN III)
Trochlear nerve (CN IV)
Ophthalmic nerve (CN V1)
Abducens nerve (CN VI)

Foramen rotundum
Maxillary nerve (CN V2)

Foramen ovale
Mandibular nerve (CN V3)

Internal acoustic meatus
Facial nerve (CN VII)
Vestibulocochlear nerve (CN VIII)

Jugular foramen
Glossopharyngeal nerve (CN IX)
Vagus nerve (CN X)
Accessory nerve (CN XI)

Hypoglossal foramen
Hypoglossal nerve (CN XII)

Foramen lacerum

Foramen magnum

Figure 7.1.   Cranial foramina at the base of the skull. Significant foramina are labelled together with their traversing cranial nerves.

B. Cerebello-pontine Angle (CPA) Syndrome

The CPA refers to the sharply angulated triangular space where the cerebellar folds over the pons (Figure 7.2). This space houses the cerebello-pontine cistern, a subarachnoid cistern filled with cerebrospinal fluid. The CPA contains two **cranial nerves (the facial and vestibulocochlear nerves)** and the **anterior inferior cerebellar artery (AICA)**. The trigeminal nerve passes over the superior aspect of the space and may be affected by diseases within the CPA.

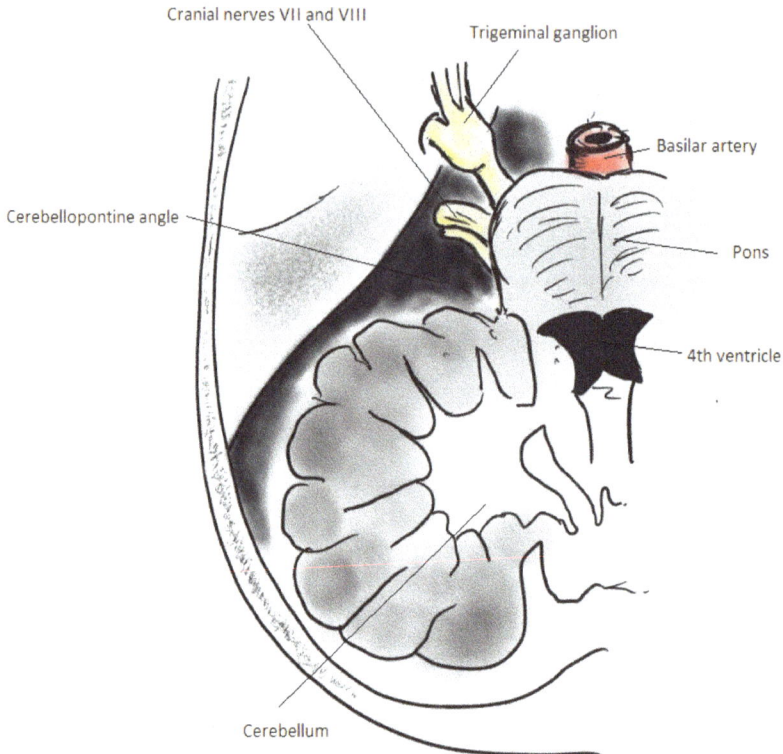

Figure 7.2.   Brainstem, axial view. The CPA is shown in relation to the neighbouring structures.

The commonest cause of CPA syndrome is a **tumour within that space,** compressing its contents and neighbouring structures. The CPA is the commonest site for neoplasms within the posterior cranial fossa and accounts for up to 10% of all intracranial tumours.[1] Vestibular schwannomas are benign neoplasms of the Schwann cells arising from the vestibular division of the vestibulocochlear nerve. They account for nearly 80% of tumours within the CPA.[2] Other tumours such as meningiomas, dermoid, and epidermoid cysts are comparatively rarer.[2]

The syndrome describes the constellation of signs and symptoms consequent from the structural distortion and compression within the CPA. The clinical features are:

Signs and Symptoms	Details
Ipsilateral sensorineural hearing loss and tinnitus	Compression of the vestibulocochlear nerve results in hearing loss. **Discrimination of speech** is often disproportionately worse than the hearing loss typical of a retro-cochlear localisation. As such, patients often complain of **difficulty following conversations**. Vertigo is an uncommon complaint in most patients with CPA syndrome due to the slow growth of the tumour.
Ipsilateral hemifacial weakness	Compression of the intracranial segment of the facial nerve results in ipsilateral hemifacial weakness. Facial nerve palsy usually occurs late in CPA syndrome from tumourous causes.[3]

Others Signs and Symptoms

Other accompanying symptoms and signs are dependent on the extent of the tumour's involvement within the brainstem and CPA.

- **Trigeminal nerve:**
  - Ipsilateral hemifacial sensory loss
  - Ipsilateral loss of corneal reflex
- **Cerebellum:**
  - Nystagmus
    - In addition to cerebellar nystagmus being present, Brun's nystagmus may be present with concomitant ipsilateral vestibular involvement. Brun's nystagmus is discussed in greater detail below.
  - Ataxia of the ipsilateral limbs
- **Abducens nerve**
  - Involvement of the abducens nerve is uncommon due to its antero-medial course within and upon exiting the pons, substantially distant from the CPA. However, abducens nerve palsy may still occur if the lesions are large and extensive enough.
  - Involvement of the abducens nerve weakens the ipsilateral lateral rectus muscle, resulting in horizontal binocular diplopia which worsens on gazing towards the side of the lesion.

Brun's Nystagmus

Brun's nystagmus is a rare and peculiar variant of bilateral nystagmus that is invariably mentioned in relation to CPA syndrome. Its presence reflects **concomitant ipsilateral cerebellar and vestibular dysfunction.**[4] Not only is the nystagmus bilateral, but the character of the nystagmus also varies depending on the gaze direction.

On looking **towards** the side of the lesion → **slow and large amplitude nystagmus.**[4]
- This is due to involvement of the cerebellar flocculus, an important neural integrator mediating the horizontal holding of gaze. Dysfunction of the flocculus results in inability to **maintain** eccentric horizontal gaze, resulting in high amplitude, coarse, and low frequency oscillatory nystagmus when the patient attempts to look towards the side of the lesion.

(Continued)

(Continued)

Brun's Nystagmus

On looking **away** from the side of the lesion → **fine, jerky, and small amplitude nystagmus (vestibular nystagmus).**[4]

- When looking away from the lesion, vestibular dysfunction results in slow-phase movement of the eyes back towards the centre, with a compensatory fast-phase movement away (corrective saccades).

Brun's nystagmus, when present, elegantly demonstrates the extent of the lesion's involvement and hints at its considerable size.[4] As such, a degree of familiarity with this sign will be helpful in your assessment of patients suspected to have CPA syndrome.

Case Example for the Examination Candidate

A 35-year-old gentleman presented with chronic and progressive right-sided hearing loss. He was increasingly unable to follow conversations and his friends observed that his face was asymmetrical just a week ago.

Examination of the patient revealed the following:
- Right sensorineural hearing loss
- Right hemifacial weakness
- Right facial hypoesthesia and diminished right corneal reflex

The patient's symptoms and signs are consistent with dysfunction of the right vestibulocochlear, trigeminal, and facial nerves, placing the lesion within the right CPA. Knowing that a vestibular schwannoma is the commonest cause of CPA syndrome, you may proceed to look for cutaneous features of neurofibromatosis type 2 especially when bilateral CPA syndrome is suspected, or for surgical scars from prior neurosurgical procedures.

Investigations you should offer include:
- Contrasted magnetic resonance imaging (MRI) of the brain
- Audiometric tests
- If neurofibromatosis 2 is suspected:
  - Gene testing for mutations of the "Merlin" gene (chromosome 22)
  - Slit lamp examination for posterior subcapsular lenticular opacities

C. Jugular Foramen Syndrome (JFS) — Vernet's Syndrome

The jugular foramen is a sizeable opening at the base of the skull through which the **glossopharyngeal, vagus and accessory nerves,** as well as the sigmoid and inferior petrosal sinuses run "(Figure 7.3 and 7.4). Diseases of the jugular foramen result in JFS.

JFS manifests clinically as signs and symptoms expected when the traversing cranial nerves are compromised and dysfunctional:

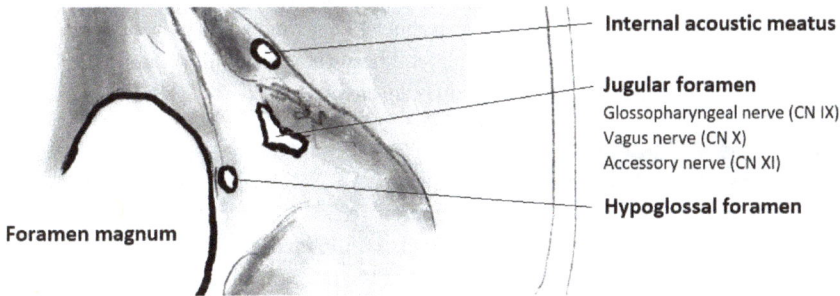

Figure 7.3.   A diagram of the skull base showing the jugular foramen in relation to its neighbouring structures.

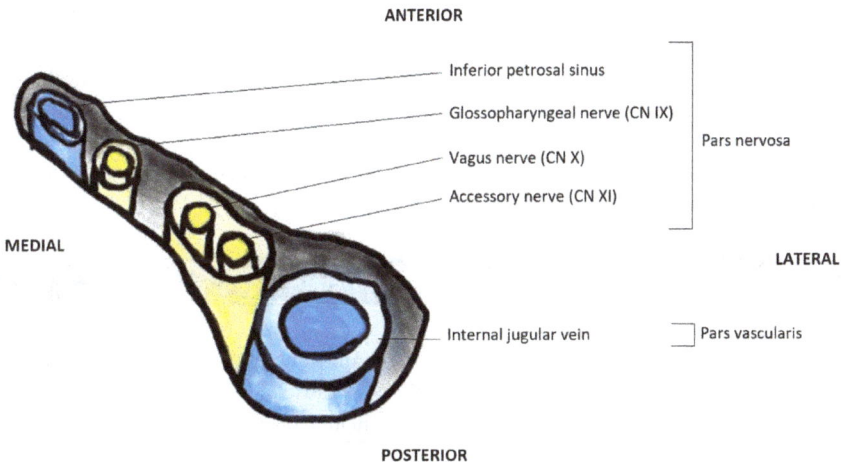

Figure 7.4.   A detailed drawing of the right-sided jugular foramen illustrating its nervous and vascular contents. Vagus and accessory nerves share a common dural sheath.

Signs and Symptoms	Details
Hoarseness of voice, nasal pitch **Impaired elevation of the ipsilateral soft palate** **Deviation of the uvula to the contralateral side**	These symptoms reflect **palsy of the vagus nerve.** The vagus nerve supplies muscles of the larynx and the soft palate. Weakness of the laryngeal muscles results in hoarseness. Weakness of the soft palate results in dysphagia, nasal pitch, and uvular deviation.

(Continued)

(Continued)

Signs and Symptoms	Details
Loss of somatic sensation and taste over the posterior third of the ipsilateral half of the tongue **Loss of gag reflex**	The **glossopharyngeal nerve** receives somatic and special sensory input from the posterior third of the tongue. It serves an important role as the afferent pathway of the pharyngeal/gag reflex.
Weakness of the trapezius and sternocleidomastoid muscles	The spinal **accessory nerve** supplies the ipsilateral sternocleidomastoid and trapezius muscles. Weakness of the sternocleidomastoid muscle causes weakness of contralateral head rotation, while weakness of the trapezius causes weakness of the ipsilateral shoulder shrug.
Others	
If the **venous sinuses are obstructed**, the resultant venous congestion, cerebral edema, and raised intracranial pressure may cause **headache, papilledema, and focal neurologic deficits**. Patients with concomitant involvement of the hypoglossal nerve from jugular foramen lesions such as glomus jugulare tumour and jugular venous thrombosis have also been documented (Collet-Sicard syndrome).[5,6]	
A rare condition associated with JFS is the **glossopharyngeal neuralgia syncope syndrome**. These patients complain of paroxysms of sharp stabbing pain over the affected half of the pharynx and posterior tongue. These attacks may be triggered by mastication or swallowing, and may be associated with syncope and cardiac arrhythmias in rare occasions.	

The causes of jugular foramen may be grouped into the following categories, of which the **neoplastic aetiologies are the commonest**[7]:

Aetiologies	Details
Tumours	• **Primary:** Paragangliomas • **Metastatic:** Metastasis by distant tumours to the skull base is a common (if not the commonest) cause of JFS. Cancers known to metastasize at the skull base include breast, lung, and prostate cancers.
Vascular disorders	• Aneurysms of the extracranial internal carotid artery or the vertebral artery[8] • Thrombosis of the internal jugular vein • Protruding jugular bulb • Jugular diverticulum
Infections	• Herpes virus[9] • Varicella Zoster[10]
Non-infectious inflammatory causes	• Giant cell arteritis, causing ischemic JFS[11] • Granulomatosis with polyangiitis • Sarcoidosis
Trauma	• Skull-base fractures

Case Example for the Examination Candidate

A 65 years-old gentleman presented with 3 months of progressive dysarthria, hoarseness of voice, and dysphagia. He is a chronic smoker and is currently undergoing treatment for his lung cancer.

Examination of the patient revealed the following:
- Cachexia
- Nasal and hoarse speech
- Diminished palatal elevation on the right, with deviation of the uvula towards the left
- Weak shrug of his right shoulder
- Weakness of the right sternocleidomastoid muscle

The patient's neurologic signs suggest dysfunction of the right-sided glossopharyngeal, vagus, and spinal accessory nerves, consistent with diagnosis of JFS. Knowing that a neoplastic aetiology is especially likely in view of his active lung malignancy, a contrasted MRI of the brain will be the next most appropriate investigation to evaluate for metastasis to the skull base.

D. Cavernous Sinus Syndrome (CSS)

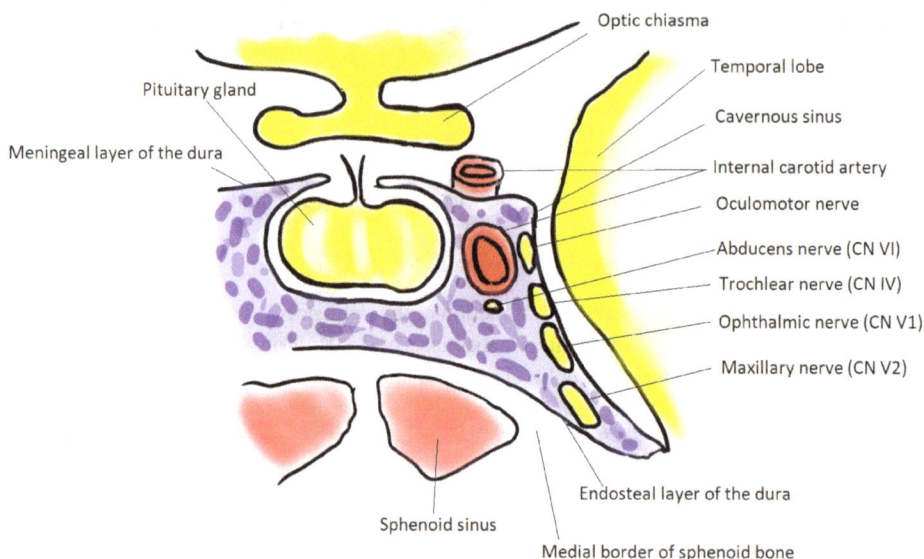

Figure 7.5.   Left cavernous sinus (coronal). This picture shows the vascular and nervous contents within the cavernous sinus. Sympathetic fibres traveling the internal carotid artery are not depicted.

The cavernous sinuses are major dural venous sinuses located just lateral to the sella turcica. It sits below the optic nerves and the optic chiasma, surrounds the pituitary gland, and is laterally bordered by the temporal uncus (Figure 7.5).

The cavernous sinus is well connected to the other intracranial venous structures, receiving blood from the ophthalmic veins, superficial middle cerebral veins, inferior cerebral veins, and the sphenoparietal venous sinuses. The venous blood then leaves the sinuses via the superior and inferior petrosal sinuses. These connections are clinically important as they **allow blood from the face to reach the cavernous sinuses** via the ophthalmic vein (Figure 7.6). Though occurrences are rare, infective thrombosis of the cavernous sinuses are well-described in medical literature and are largely due to facial furuncles within the "danger triangle" (Figure 7.6).[12]

The cavernous sinus also contains the following structures:

Contents	
Cranial nerves	5 cranial nerves/nerve branches: • Oculomotor nerve • Trochlear nerve • Ophthalmic nerve • Maxillary nerve • Abducens nerve
Autonomic nerves	Sympathetic plexus and fibres; parasympathetic fibres accompanying the oculomotor nerve
Artery	Cavernous segment of the internal carotid artery

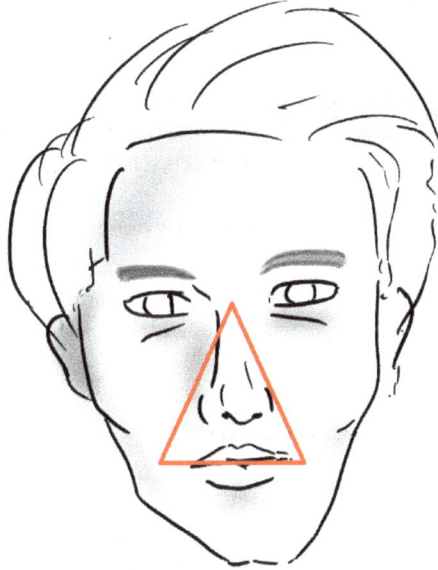

Figure 7.6. The "danger triangle". This area runs from the corners of the mouth to the nasal bridge. Venous drainage from this area communicates with cavernous sinus via the ophthalmic vein.

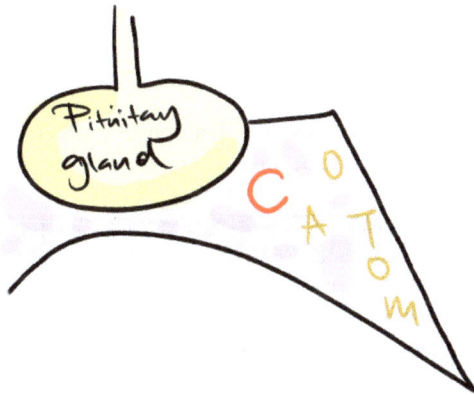

Figure 7.7. A simplified drawing of the cavernous sinus with its contents represented by the O TOM, CAT mnemonic.

Another way to remember the contents is with this mnemonic: OTOM, CAT. OTOM lists the contents along the lateral wall: the oculomotor and trochlear nerves superiorly, followed by the ophthalmic and mandibular nerves inferiorly. CAT lists the horizontal contents medio-laterally: the cavernous segment of the internal carotid artery, abducens, and trochlear nerve (Figure 7.7).

CSS represents a collection of signs and symptoms resulting from the partial or complete dysfunction of its contents. They may include:

Signs and Symptoms	Details
Binocular diplopia	Depending on the extent of involvement of the **oculomotor, trochlear,** and **abducens** nerve, the character of diplopia may vary. The presence of ptosis or impaired pupillary reactivity suggests dysfunction of the oculomotor nerve.
Ipsilateral facial numbness and hypoesthesia	Dysfunction of the **ophthalmic** and **maxillary** nerves result in numbness and hypoesthesia of the ipsilateral face.
Ipsilateral Horner's syndrome	Dysfunction of the third-order sympathetic fibers as they ascend with the internal carotid arteries results in ipsilateral Horner's syndrome. Practically speaking, it may be difficult to appreciate miosis and dilatory lag of the pupil when there is concomitant compromise of the parasympathetic fibres traveling with the oculomotor nerve.
Other Signs and Symptoms	
Look out for accompanying signs that hint at the nature of the underlying cause. Patients with underlying **carotid-cavernous fistula** may display chemosis (also seen in cavernous sinus thrombosis), pulsatile exophthalmos, proptosis, diplopia, and visual loss. Ocular bruit may be heard on auscultation over the eye. Tenderness over the paranasal sinuses or the presence of furuncles or wounds within the "danger triangle" may suggest an **infective cause of CSS**.	

There are many causes of cavernous sinus syndrome, of which tumours remain the commonest. The aetiologies may otherwise be broadly categorised into four big groups:

Aetiologies	Details

Tumours	The **commonest** group of aetiologies, they may be further subdivided into:
	• **Primary tumours**
	  ○ Tumours of the central nervous system (e.g., meningiomas, schwannomas of the cranial nerves)
	• **Secondary metastasis**
	  ○ Perineural spread from metastasis of distant malignancies (e.g., breast or lung cancers)
	• **Direct compression or invasion by tumours of neighbouring structures** (e.g., pituitary tumours, nasopharyngeal carcinoma)

Vascular pathologies	Vascular pathologies within the cavernous sinus include: • Carotid-cavernous aneurysm • Carotid-cavernous fistula • Cavernous sinus thrombosis

Aetiologies	Details
Infections	Infections of the cavernous sinus are often bacterial or fungal in nature. ***Staphylococcus aureus*** is a common bacterial cause of cavernous sinus infections. These microorganisms gain entry via spread from adjacent structures: skin infections over the "danger triangle", dental infections, or paranasal sinusitis. **Tuberculous** and **fungal** infections of the cavernous sinuses have also been described in the medical literature.[13]
Non-infectious inflammatory causes	Non-infective, granulomatous inflammatory processes are known to cause cavernous sinus syndrome. They include sarcoidosis, granulomatosis with polyangiitis (previously known as Wegener's granulomatosis), IgG4-related disorders, and Tolosa-Hunt syndrome (THS). THS is a poorly understood granulomatous inflammatory process that causes painful ophthalmoparesis and responds well to steroids. The diagnosis of THS may only be made after exclusion of a myriad of similar conditions. There are calls within the medical fraternity to re-look at this syndrome, as deeper understanding of other diseases (e.g., IgG4-related diseases) and advances in medical knowledge may warrant revisiting its pathologic characteristics as a clinical entity.[14]

Case Example for the Examination Candidate

A 50-year-old man presented with insidiously progressive right facial numbness and binocular diplopia. He denied having febrile or constitutional symptoms. Examination revealed the following:

- Incomplete right blepharoptosis
- Right eye displayed weakness of elevation, depression, adduction, and abduction
- Right facial hypoesthesia (CN V1 and V2 territories)

The deficits localise to the right cavernous sinus. The insidious progression is worrisome for space-occupying lesions, rendering acute causes such as cavernous sinus thrombosis and inflammation/infections less likely. At this point of time, you should look for signs that are supportive of your suspicion:

- Clinical features of endocrinopathies (e.g., acromegalic or cushingoid habitus) suggestive of a pituitary tumour
- Neurosurgical scars suggestive of prior intracranial structure abnormalities or malignancies
- Prior surgical scars (abdominal, thoracic, or breasts) suggestive of prior history of malignancy
- Examination of the neck and axilla for lymphadenopathy
- Chest examination for features of lung malignancies
- Breast examination for breast lumps
- Abdominal examination for features of gastrointestinal malignancies

Investigations you should consider include:

- MRI of the brain with gadolinium contrast
- Targeted imaging studies (e.g., CT scan of the thorax if lung malignancies are suspected)
- Appropriate endoscopic studies, for example:
  - Colonoscopy to evaluate for colorectal cancers
  - Nasopharyngoscopic evaluation of the posterior nasal space if nasopharyngeal cancers are suspected

E. Superior Orbital Fissure (SOF) and Orbital Apex (OCA) Syndromes

The SOF and OA syndromes will be discussed together. The OA is the posterior confluence of the four orbital walls. The SOF lies just anterior to the optic canal and is bordered by the greater and lesser sphenoid wings (Figures 7.8 and 7.9). The SOF is structurally important as it allows the

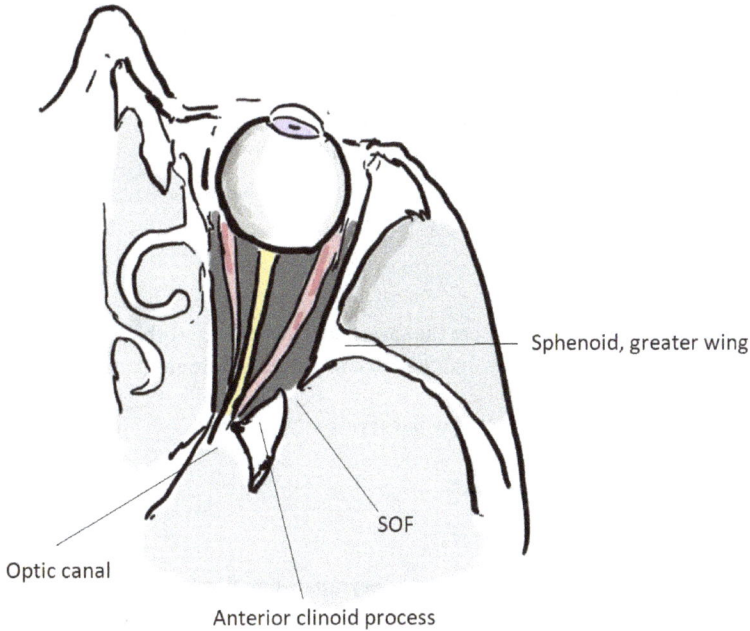

Figure 7.8.   The orbital apex (axial) showing the relative positions of the superior orbital fissure with the optic canal.

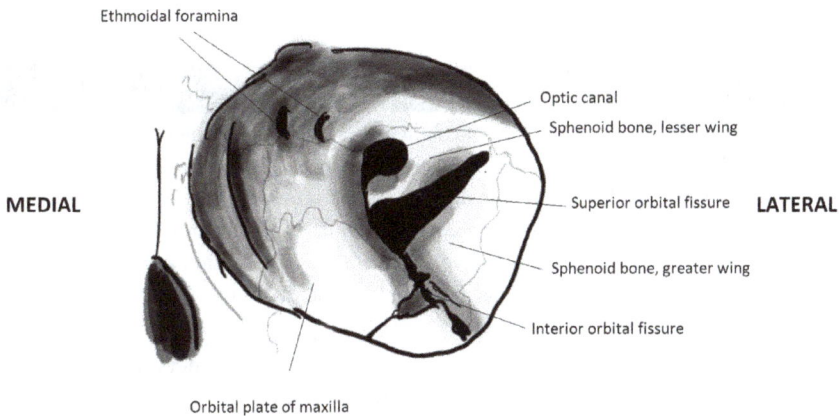

Figure 7.9.   The bony structure of the left orbital apex showing the positions of the SOF and optic canal in relation to other important structures.

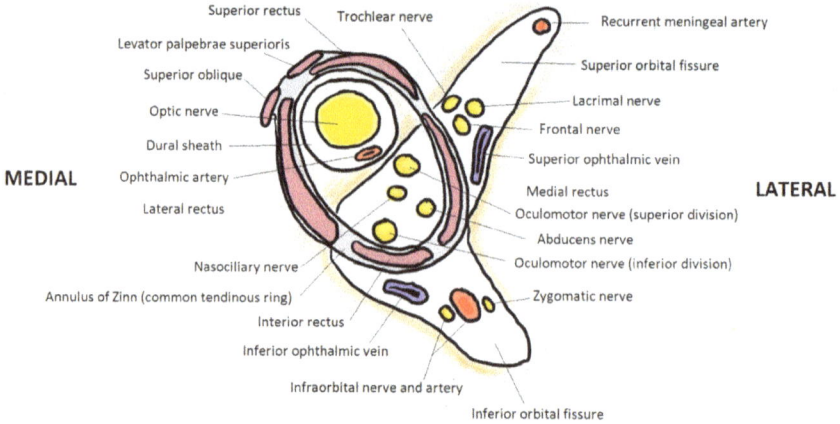

Figure 7.10.   Left OA showing the optic canal and superior and inferior orbital fissures in relation to their neurovascular contents.

passage of neurovascular structures from the cavernous sinus into the orbital cavity. These include **four major cranial nerves/branches** and their **accompanying autonomic fibres** (Figure 7.10):

1. **Oculomotor** nerve with accompanying **parasympathetic fibres**
2. **Trochlear** nerve
3. **Ophthalmic** nerve (trigeminal nerve)
   - Lacrimal nerve
   - Frontal nerve
   - Nasociliary nerve and accompanying **oculosympathetic fibres**
4. **Abducens** nerve

   SOF and OA syndromes describe the distinct collection of characteristic ipsilateral ocular and extraocular abnormalities due to dysfunction of their contents. OA syndrome differs from SOF syndrome by its additional involvement of the optic nerve (Figure 7.11).

Signs and Symptoms	Details
Ocular signs include: • Blepharoptosis • Ophthalmoparesis • Pupillary abnormalities • Loss of corneal reflex • Lacrimal hyposecretion	Pupillary abnormalities may be present due to involvement of the **parasympathetic** and/or **sympathetic** fibres. Compromise of the **oculomotor, abducens**, and **trochlear** nerves, whether individually or in combination, results in ophthalmoparesis and binocular diplopia. Lacrimal hyposecretion and loss of corneal reflex may be observed due to involvement of the **lacrimal nerve** (a branch of the ophthalmic nerve).
Extraocular signs include numbness over the CN V1 territory	Involvement of the **frontal and lacrimal nerves** resulting in hypoesthesia or anaesthesia over the ipsilateral half of the forehead.
In **orbital apex syndrome**, involvement of the optic canal and the optic nerve within results in **monocular impairment of vision** (Figure 7.11).	

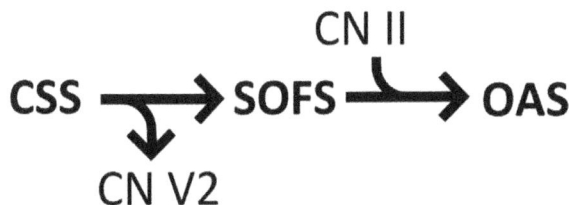

Figure 7.11.   Cavernous sinus, orbital apex, and superior orbital fissure syndromes may overlap due their mutual proximity. A helpful way to distinguish one from the other is to assess for involvement of maxillary and optic nerves. Abbreviations: CSS, cavernous sinus syndrome; SOFS, superior orbital fissure syndrome; OAS, orbital apex syndrome.

Due to their proximity, cavernous sinus, SOF, and OA syndromes are vulnerable to similar pathologies and insults. As such, do refer to the segment on cavernous sinus syndrome for a list of causes. It is important to note that a **traumatic fracture of the SOF is the commonest cause of SOF syndrome.**[13,14]

Case Example for the Examination Candidate
A 25-year-old man suffered facial injuries after falling down a flight of stairs. He had right periorbital ecchymosis and facial tenderness, and complained of diplopia. Examination of the patient revealed the following: • Right eye ophthalmoparesis • Right blepharoptosis • Hypoesthesia over the right half of the forehead • Preserved visual fields The patient's signs are consistent with a right SOF syndrome, with traumatic injury being the likely cause. This patient should be evaluated and treated in accordance with the principles described in the Advance Trauma Life Support protocol.

References

1. James G, *et al.* (1993) Cerebellopontine angle masses: radiologic-pathologic correlation. *Radiographics* **13**: 1131–1147.
2. Lalwani AK. (1992) Meningiomas, epidermoids, and other nonacoustic tumors of the cerebellopontine angle. *Otolaryngol Clin North Am* **25**: 707–708.
3. Heather E Moss. (2019) Eyelid and Facial Nerve Disorders. Liu, Volpe, and Galetta's *Neuro-Opthalmology (Third Edition)*.
4. Biswas SN, Ray S, Ball S, Chakraborty PP. (2018) Bruns nystagmus: an important clinical clue for cerebellopontine angle tumours. *BMJ Case Rep* 2018:bcr2017223378
5. Rao AB, Koeller KK, Adair CF. (1999) From the archives of the AFIP. Paragangliomas of the head and neck: radiologic-pathologic correlation. *Radiographics* **19**(6): 1605–1632.
6. Neo S, Lee KE. (2017) Collet-Sicard syndrome: a rare but important presentation of internal jugular vein thrombosis. *Practical Neurology* **17**: 63–65.
7. Hayward D, Morgan C, Emami B, Biller J, Prabhu VC. (2012) Jugular foramen syndrome as initial presentation of metastatic lung cancer. *J Neurol Surg Rep* **73**(1): 14–18.

8.   Amano M, Ishikawa E, Kujiraoka Y, Watanabe S, *et al.* (2010) Vernet's syndrome caused by large mycotic aneurysm of the extracranial internal carotid artery after acute otitis media — case report. *Neurol Med Chir (Tokyo).* **50**(1): 45–48.

9.   Ono N, Sakabe A, Nakajima M. (2010) [Herpes zoster oticus-associated jugular foramen syndrome]. *Brain Nerve* **62**(1): 81–84.

10. Jo YR, Chung CW, Lee JS, Park HJ. (2013) Vernet syndrome by varicella-zoster virus. *Ann Rehabil Med* **37**(3): 449–452.

11. Cherin P, De Gennes C, Bletry O, Lamas A, Launay M, Dubs A, Godeau P. (1992) Ischemic Vernet's syndrome in giant cell arteritis: first two cases. *Am J Med* **93**(3): 349–352.

12. Varshney S, Malhotra M, Gupta P, Gairola P, Kaur N. (2015) Cavernous sinus thrombosis of nasal origin in children. *Indian J Otolaryngol Head Neck Surg* **67**(1): 100–105. doi:10.1007/s12070-014-0805-4.

13. Peng Xia, *et al.* (2014) Septic cavernous sinus thrombosis caused by tuberculosis infection. *BMJ Case Rep* Nov 25; 2014:bcr2014206209.

14. Chen C-T, Chen Y-R. (2010) Traumatic superior orbital fissure syndrome: current management. *Craniomaxillofacial Trauma and Reconstruction* **3**(01): 9–16.

8

Approach to Diplopia

A. Introduction

Diplopia describes the perception two separate images when viewing a single object. The false image may be displaced **horizontally**, **vertically**, **oblique/angulated** or mixed, relative to the true image. The causes of diplopia may be broadly classified into **ophthalmological** or **neurological** aetiologies. This chapter will focus mainly on the latter. The extraocular muscles will thereafter be referred to by their abbreviations:

- Superior rectus: SR
- Medial rectus: MR
- Inferior rectus: IR
- Lateral rectus: LR
- Superior oblique: SO
- Inferior oblique: IO

B. Clinical History

Questions	Comments
Qn. 1: **Is the diplopia binocular or monocular?**	This is the **first step** of the neurolocalisation process. Instruct the patient to cover each one, one at a time, to achieve monocular vision. The diplopia is described as either **monocular** if it persists on covering of the other eye, or **binocular** if it is absent on covering of either eye (i.e., present only with binocular vision).
	In **monocular diplopia**, an ophthalmological cause is likelier, and may be due to refractive errors, corneal disorders, cataracts, injuries to the iris, and diseases within the humour, retinal detachments and macular disorders. An ophthalmological consultation will be helpful.
	Misalignments of the visual axes result in **binocular diplopia**, and are often indicative of an underlying neurologic disorder. Neurologic pathologies span widely across the neuro-axis (Figure 8.1): • **Muscles** (e.g. chronic progressive external ophthalmoplegia, and restrictive causes such as thyroid eye disease or muscular entrapment) • **Neuromuscular junction** (NMJ) (e.g. myasthenia gravis)

(Continued)

(*Continued*)

Questions	Comments
	• **Cranial nerves** (e.g., idiopathic cranial neuropathies, Miller Fisher syndrome) • **Brainstem: cranial nuclei and gaze centres** (e.g., internuclear ophthalmoplegia, one-and-a-half syndrome) 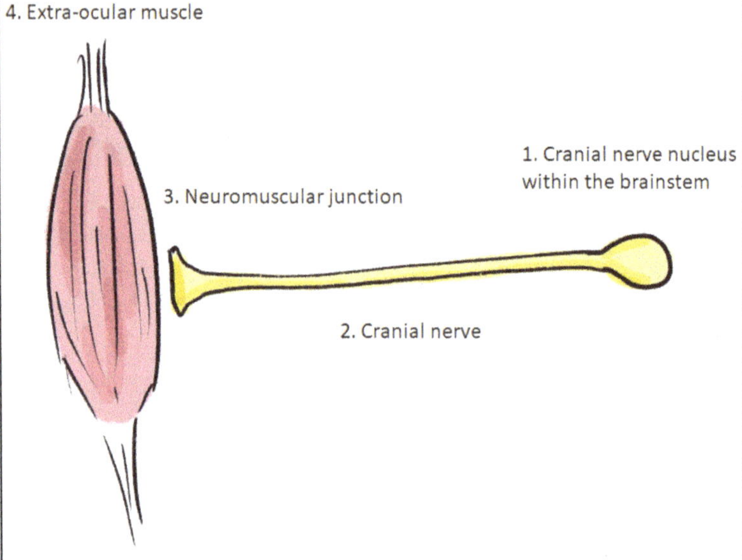 4. Extra-ocular muscle Figure 8.1. Schematic drawing of the "neural axis" mediating eye movement. Pathologies of binocular diplopia are often found along the axis. A distinction should be made between **bilateral monocular diplopia** and **binocular diplopia**, as they are not the same: in binocular diplopia, the diplopia resolves on occlusion of either eye, whereas in bilateral monocular diplopia, double vision persists regardless of whichever eye the patient occludes. **Bilateral monocular diplopia** may be due to bilateral ophthalmological abnormalities, or the rarer disorders of the visual cortices (e.g., palinopsia, cerebral polyopia).
Qn. 2: **How are the images mis-aligned, and in which direction of gaze is the separation of the images at its greatest?**	The separation of images is maximum in the **direction of the pure action of the pair of yoke muscles,** amongst which consist of the weak extraocular muscle (Figure 8.2). As such, how the images are separated (horizontal, vertical, oblique or mixed), and at which direction of gaze is the separation worst, provide important clues in identifying the culprit muscle.

Figure 8.1 labels: 1. Cranial nerve nucleus within the brainstem; 2. Cranial nerve; 3. Neuromuscular junction

(Continued)

Questions	Comments

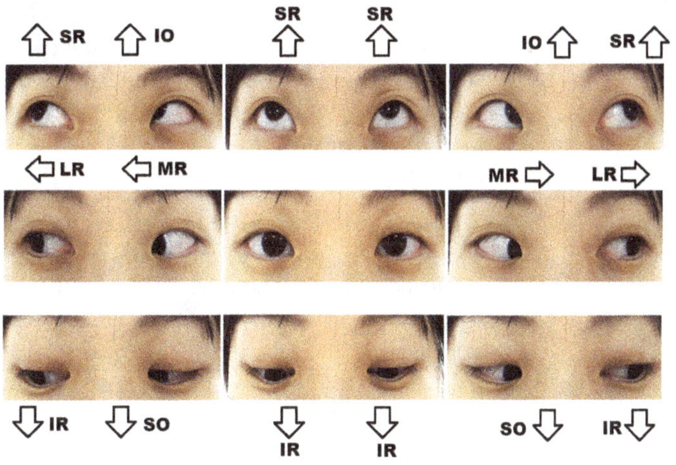

Figure 8.2. The main eye positions, showing the dominant muscles involved at that direction of gaze.

Horizontal diplopia

The presence of **binocular horizontal diplopia** suggests dysfunction of either the MR or LR muscles. The direction of gaze which worsens the diplopia helps differentiate the two. In the case of a patient with binocular horizontal diplopia when looking left, the symptomatic muscle is either the left LR or the right MR muscles.

The **aggravation** of diplopia with **near or far vision** provides additional clues in identifying the culprit extra-ocular muscle:

- **If the diplopia worsens when looking near**, this is suggestive of MR weakness due to its involvement in vergence. This, however, does not apply to patients with adduction weakness from internuclear ophthalmoplegia, as convergence is often spared.
- **If the diplopia worsens when looking far**, this is suggestive of LR weakness.

Vertical diplopia

The presence of **binocular vertical diplopia** suggests an imbalance of the supraductor and infraductor muscles, resulting in misalignment along the vertical axis. The four muscles of interest are:

- Supraductors: SR and IO
- Infraductors: IR and SO

Thankfully, these muscles have unique properties which can help us find the culprit:

- **SR** is the dominant supraductor when the eye is **abducted**, with **IO** being the dominant supraductor when the eye is **adducted**.

(Continued)

(Continued)

Questions	Comments
	• **IR** maximally infraducts the eye when in the **abducted** position, while **SO** maximally infraducts the eye when **adducted**.
	• **SO** and **IO** have additional roles in effecting ocular cyclotorsive movements:
	○ **SO**: incyclotorsion
	○ **IO**: excyclotorsion
	As such, in a patient with **left SO weakness** for example, his vertical diplopia will likely worsen when he looks towards his right, as the weakness of SO is maximally demonstrated with adduction of the left eye. The presence of an **angulated/oblique false image** hints at torsional misalignment, and is supportive of **SO** weakness.
Qn. 3: **Are there aggravating or relieving factors?**	Associated aggravating or relieving factors help trim the list of differential diagnoses. In myasthenia gravis, for example, the diplopia is often described as fatigable, worsening in severity with sustained eccentric gaze. A short period of rest may result in improvement of the diplopia.
Qn. 4: **Are there other pertinent associated or accompanying symptoms?**	Associated signs and symptoms will help with the localization process: • Involvement of other cranial nerves • Involvement of the long-tracts Please refer to **Chapters 6 and 7** for more details on brainstem localization and cranial nerve syndromes, respectively.

C. Physical Examination

Relying on the clues from the clinical history and symptoms, and with a list of differential diagnoses in mind, you may then proceed to examine the patient.

Examination Steps	Description
Inspection	This step has significant neurolocalisation value. Commit adequate time to thoroughly inspect the patient: • Make eye contact with the patient as you introduce yourself. ○ Is there misalignment of the eyes? ○ Is there accompanying blepharoptosis? ○ Is there facial weakness? ○ Does his speech sound normal? ○ Is there a feeding tube to suggest swallowing difficulties? ○ Is he moving one half of his body more than the other? • Observe how the patient looks at his surroundings — is the ocular misalignment more obvious when he looks at a certain direction? • Is there abnormal posturing of the head and neck?

Diplopia

Monocular
Ophthalmologic causes are likelier

Binocular
Neurologic causes are likelier

Unilateral monocular

Bilateral monocular

Muscle & surrounding soft tissue

- Restrictive eye disease:
  - Proptosis
  - Thyroid eye disease
  - Acromegaly
  - Traumatic entrapment
- Mitochondrial diseases (e.g. Chronic Progressive External Ophthalmoplegia)
- Muscular dystrophies

Neuromuscular Junction

- Myasthenia gravis

Cranial Nerve(s)

- Cranial nerve syndromes:
  - Isolated cranial neuropathy
    - Oculomotor nerve
    - Abducens nerve
    - Trochlear nerve
  - Gradenigo
  - Cavernous sinus
  - Super orbital fissure
  - Orbital apex
- Demyelinating polyneuropathies:
  - Miller Fisher syndrome

Brain and brainstem (Cranial nerve nuclei/fascicle)

- Thalamic esotropia
- Dysfunction of the PPRF-MLF:
  - Internuclear-ophthalmoplegia
  - One-and-a-half syndrome
- Brainstem stroke syndromes:
  - Weber's syndrome
  - Millard-Gubler syndrome

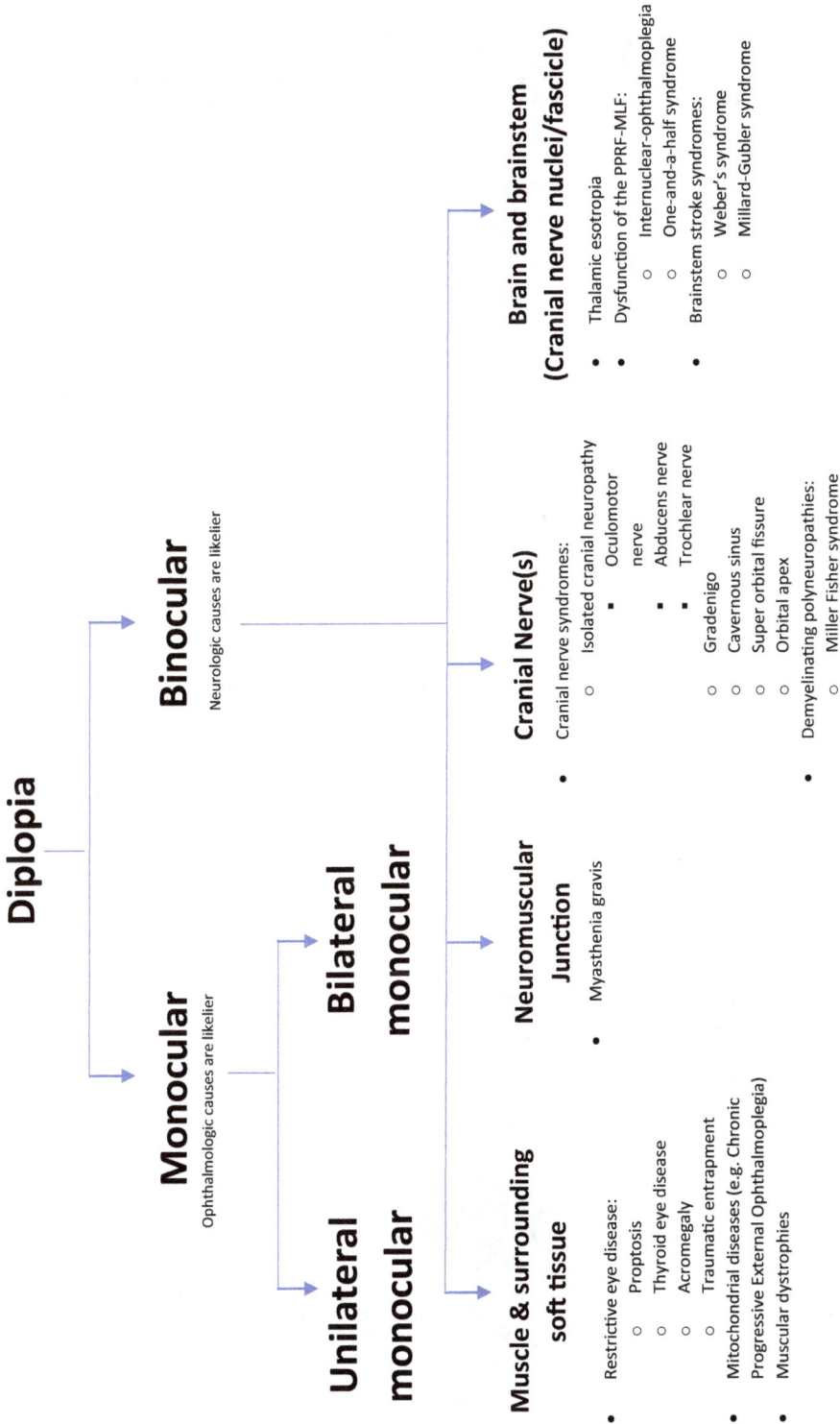

Flowchart 1. Approach to diplopia.

(Continued)

Examination Steps	Description
Hirschberg test	This is a simple bedside test to screen for ocular misalignment: • Shine a light at the patient's eyes • Observe how the light reflects off the patient's corneas • The reflection should lie within 0.5mm nasally from the midline of pupil • An asymmetry may suggest ocular misalignment (Figure 8.3) Although Hirschberg test is often used when examining a patient with binocular diplopia, its utility is impaired by its poor sensitivity: ocular deviation of about 7° is required to cause a 1mm shift of the light's reflection.[1] 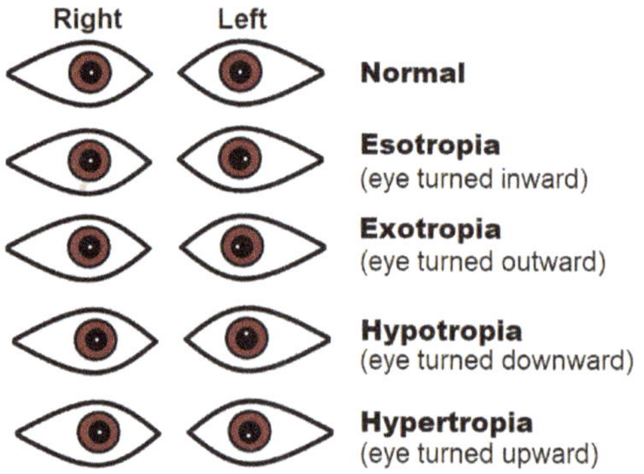 Figure 8.3. Hirschberg test, showing misalignment of the left eye.
Cover-uncover test	Another useful bedside test is the cover-uncover test.[2] An eye is covered for a few seconds, and observe the uncovered eye for shifts in fixation. Remove the occluder and note the presence of refixation movements when binocular viewing is re-established. Repeat the above steps on the other eye. The movement of the uncovered eye reveals the nature of the misalignment: • Moves nasally: exotropia • Moves temporally: esotropia • Moves up: hypotropia • Moves down: hypertropia (Figure 8.4) 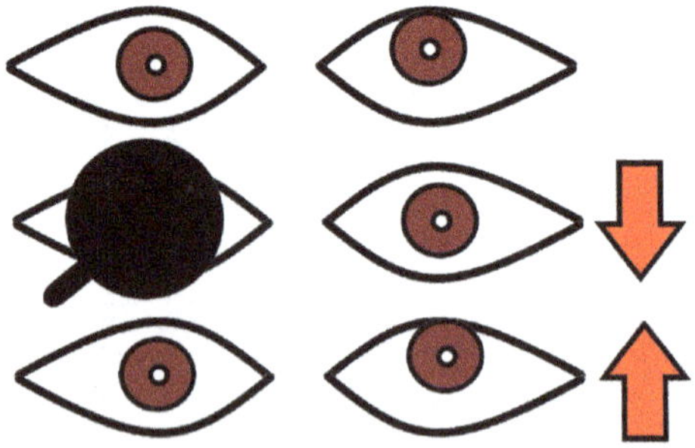 Figure 8.4. The cover-uncover test. Using the example of a patient with a hypertropic left eye. The vertical misalignment is demonstrated using the cover-uncover test.

(Continued)

Examination Steps	Description
Examination of ocular movement	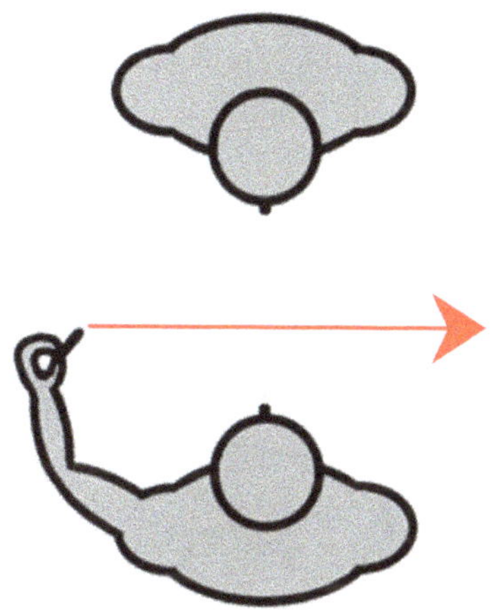 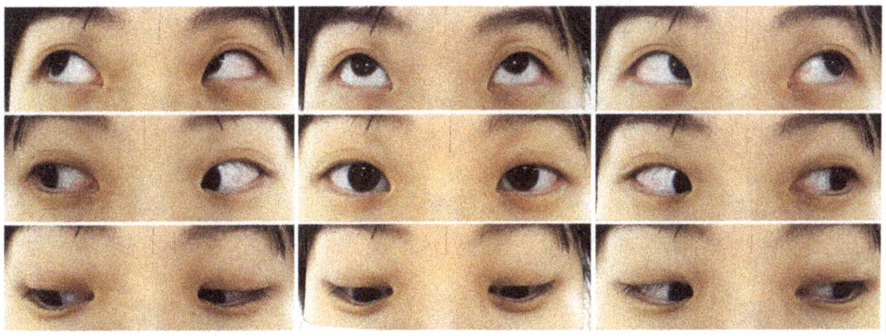 Slow pursuit and voluntary saccades should be assessed in the vertical and horizontal planes. The separation of images is maximum in the direction of the pure action of the pair of yoke muscles, amongst which consist of the weak extraocular muscle. As such, how the images are separated (horizontal, vertical, oblique or mixed), and at which direction of gaze is the separation maximal, provide important clues to the identity of the culprit muscle.

Smooth Pursuit

Smooth pursuit allows the patient to visually track a slowly moving object. Testing begins with the eyes at their primary positions. With patient fixating on an object, have him visually track the object as it is **slowly** moved along the horizontal and vertical planes.

"Look at the red hat pin. Track it with your eyes without moving your head"

Figure 8.5.   Examination of slow pursuit.

Figure 8.6.   Examination of slow pursuit involves bringing the eye to these nine positions.

(Continued)

(Continued)

Examination Steps	Description
	When the ocular misalignment is subtle and unobvious, you should **occlude the patient's eyes, one at a time**. Instruct the patient to inform you when the "outermost image" disappears on occluding that eye. Using the example of a patient with right LR weakness, ocular misalignment may not be easily evident in situations when the weakness is mild. With the patient looking to his right, proceed to occlude one eye at a time. Occlusion of the symptomatic right eye will result in the disappearance of the outer image. Pathologies that mechanically restrict the extraocular muscles can also cause binocular diplopia. In such cases, abrupt slowing/impairment of ocular movement occurs abruptly at the point of restriction. Such abruptness is not usually observed in neurologic causes of diplopia. **Voluntary Saccades** **Voluntary saccades** allow for quick shifts of gaze from a point to another (Figures 8.7 and 8.8). The assessment of visual saccades is an integral component of the neurologic examination, and should be performed in both the vertical and horizontal planes. Observe for the following: • **Initiation** of saccades • **Speed** of saccades • **Range** of movement • Saccadic **accuracy** 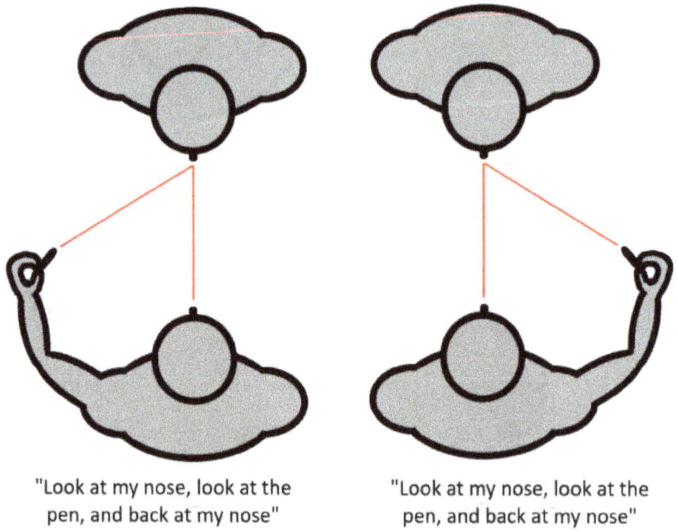 "Look at my nose, look at the pen, and back at my nose" "Look at my nose, look at the pen, and back at my nose" Figure 8.7. Examination of horizontal saccades.

(Continued)

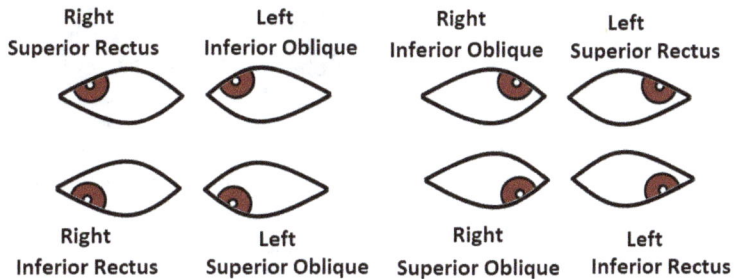

Examination Steps	Description
	  "Look at me." "Look up at the red hat pin." "Look back at me." "Look down at the red hat pin." "Look back at me." Figure 8.8. Examination of vertical saccades.

Park-Bielschowsky test (optional)[3]	When weakness of the SO is suspected in a patient with vertical diplopia, the **Park-Bielschowsky test** can be useful. In patients with vertical diplopia due to ocular misalignment, the fault lies in one of these four muscles — 2 supraductors and 2 infraductors (Figure 8.9):
	• Supraductors (elevate the eye)
	  o SR
	  o IO
	• Infraductors (depress the eye)
	  o IR
	  o SO
	
	Figure 8.9. Diagrammatic representation of the dominant supraductors/infraductors at that direction of gaze.

(Continued)

(Continued)

Examination Steps	Description

	At an **adducted position**, the oblique muscles play a larger role in elevating or infraducting the eyes. This is the result of their unique structures and insertions.
	• Main supraductor: IO
	• Main infraductor: SO
	
	At an **abducted position**, the recti muscles play a larger role in supra-ducting or infraducting the eyes:
	• Main supraductor: SR
	• Main infraductor: IR
	
	In addition, the oblique muscles also mediate torsional movements of the eyes, while the recti muscles do not:
	• Incyclotorsion: SO
	• Excyclotorsion: IO
	
	Figure 8.10. Excyclotorsion and incyclotorsion brought about by head roll.
	
	With this in mind, let's apply the Park-Bielschowsky test on a hypothetical patient who presents with binocular vertical diplopia.
	
	Step 1: Observe the eyes' positions at primary gaze
	
	The right eye appears higher than the left, and is thus described as "hyper-tropic". This can be demonstrated using the cover-uncover test. The vertical misalignment may be the result of weakness of the right eye's infraductors, or the left eye's supraductors. This leads us to **4 potential culprits**:
	• Right eye's infraductors:
	  ○ IR
	  ○ SO

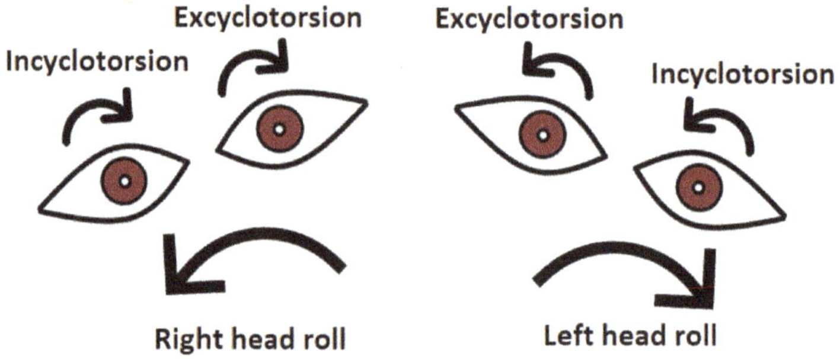

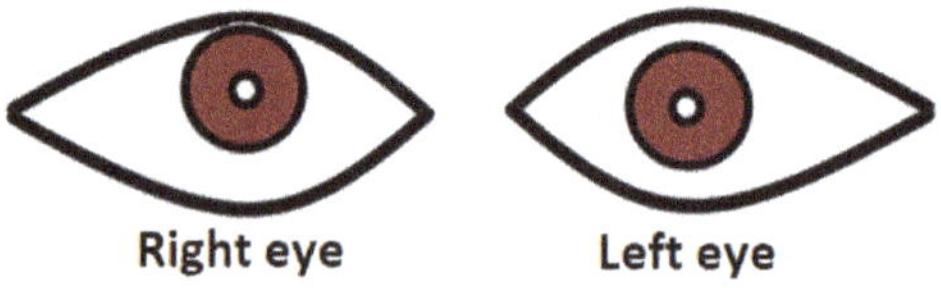

(Continued)

Examination Steps	Description
	• Left eye's supraductors: ○ SR ○ IO **Step 2:** Have the patient look left and right. At which direction of gaze did the misalignment or diplopia worsen? **Looking right** **Looking left** The misalignment worsened with the patient looking to his left. Knowing how the direction of gaze affects the relative contributions of the oblique and recti muscles in supraduction and infraduction, we can now narrow down to **2 culprits**: • Right eye's infraductors: ○ SO • Left eye's supraductors: ○ SR **Step 3:** Instruct the patient to roll his head left and right. At which side did the misalignment or diplopia worsen? **Right head roll** **Left head roll** In our patient, the ocular misalignment worsened when he rolled his head to his right. Knowing that oblique muscles are involved in cyclotorsive movements, we can conclude that the patient has weakness of his right **SO** muscle, and not the left SR. Normally, the SO mediates incyclotorsion of the eye. Impaired incyclotorsion results in misalignment of the eyes when the head is rolled towards the symptomatic side.

In summary, when approaching a patient with diplopia, our first task is to characterise the nature of the deficits using clues from the clinical history and symptoms. Clinical examination using adjunctive manoeuvres (Hirschberg's test, cover-uncover test) and the assessment of ocular movement will ultimately support the differential diagnoses you already have in mind. Be mindful of accompanying features (e.g., fatigability, long-tract deficits) which may be immensely helpful in the neurolocalisation process.

Tips for the Examination Candidate

Patients with diplopia commonly appear in the examinations. As such, a firm understanding of the approaches will serve to spare you unwanted surprises during these tests. Ask yourself these questions:

When we approach a patient with diplopia, we begin by answering a few questions:
1. Is the diplopia binocular or monocular?
2. How are the images aligned, and in which direction of gaze was the separation of the images at its greatest?
3. Are there aggravating or relieving factors?
4. Are there other pertinent associated or accompanying symptoms?

With these questions answered, you will be able to make better sense of the patient's signs!

References

1. Choi RY, Kushner BJ. (1998) The accuracy of experienced strabismologists using the Hirschberg and Krimsky tests. *Ophthalmology* **105**(7): 1301–1306.
2. Fung THM, Amoaku WMK. (2020) Strabismus and Orbit. In: Fung T., Amoaku W. (eds) Viva and OSCE Exams in Ophthalmology. Springer, Cham.
3. Bielschowsky A. (1935) A: Lecture on motor anomalies of the eyes: II. Paralysis of individual eye muscles. *Arch Ophthalmol* (Chicago) **13**(1): 33–59.

9

Oculomotor Nerve Palsy

A. Introduction

The oculomotor nerve is predominantly a **motor** nerve that conveys motor information from the oculomotor nuclear complex in the midbrain at the level of the superior colliculus to the extraocular muscles (superior rectus, inferior rectus, inferior oblique, and lateral rectus muscles) and the eyelids (levator palpabrae superioris). It also carries **parasympathetic** fibres along its course to the ciliary muscles and the pupils.

In the subsequent segments, the following structures will henceforth be referred by their abbreviations:

- Oculomotor nerve: CN III
- Abducens nerve: CN VI
- Edinger-Westphal: EWN
- Midbrain: MB
- Levator palpabrae superioris: LPS
- Superior rectus: SR
- Inferior rectus: IR
- Medial rectus: MR
- Inferior oblique: IO

B. Neurolocalisation in CN III Palsy

Palsy of the oculomotor nerve results in **blepharoptosis** and **ophthalmoparesis** of the ipsilateral eye with weakness of **adduction**, **supraduction**, and **infraduction**. When the weakness is severe enough, the eye may adopt a "down-and-out" position (Figure 9.1). Consequently, the patient will likely experience a mixed horizontal-vertical diplopia with or without a torsional component to the false-image. However, isolated adduction weakness of the affected eye should prompt you to consider the alternative diagnosis of **internuclear ophthalmoplegia** instead.

Oculomotor palsies may occur at the level of the **nucleus, fascicle,** or the **"peripheral" segment of the oculomotor nerve** (Figures 9.2 and 9.3). Diseases at different levels cause distinct clinical signs. As such, familiarity with these nuances is important for localisation of the lesion.

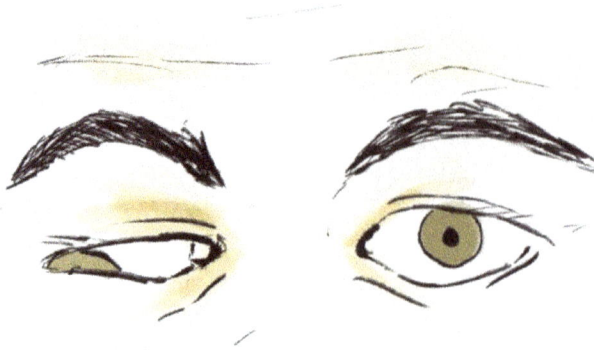

Figure 9.1.   Right-sided oculomotor nerve palsy with the right eye adopting a down-and-out position. There is accompanying blepharoptosis due to weakness of the LPS muscle.

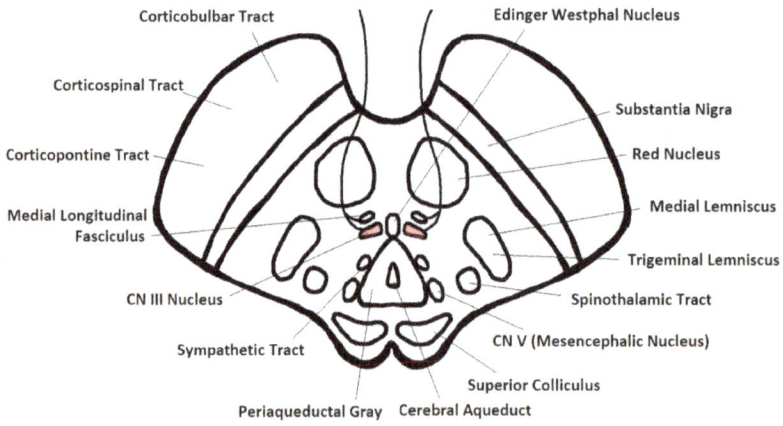

Figure 9.2.   Midbrain (axial) at the level of the superior colliculus. The oculomotor nuclei are highlighted in red.

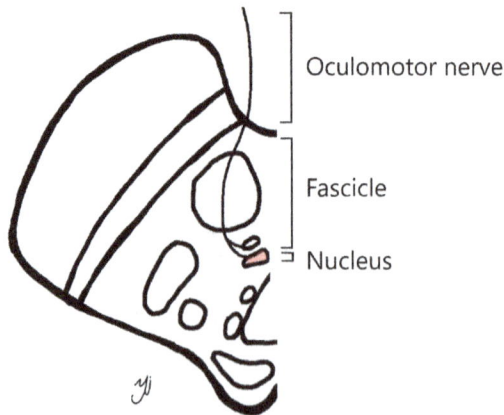

Figure 9.3.   Schematic drawing of the oculomotor nucleus, fascicular segment, and oculomotor nerve.

Level	Site	Description
Oculomotor nucleus complex	Midbrain	The oculomotor motor complex consists of multiple motor subnuclei, each serving an individual extraocular muscle, and a parasympathetic nucleus: • The MR, IR, and IO subnuclei serve their **ipsilateral** muscular counterpart. • The SR subnuclei sends fibres across the midline to the **contralateral** SR muscle. • A single subnuclei innervates **both** LPS. • A single nucleus (EWN) provides parasympathetic innervation to both pupils. Lesions at the oculomotor nucleus (also known as "nuclear palsies") usually result in: • **Adduction, infraduction, and extorsion** weakness of the **ipsilateral** eye due to weakness of the MR, IR and IO, respectively. • **Contralateral or bilateral supraduction weakness** due to weakness of the contralateral or both SRs. Because the fibres destined for the contralateral SR decussate early upon leaving the SR subnuclei, structural lesions in the vicinity often affect both the departing and the contralateral decussating SR fibres, causing bilateral supraduction failure. • **Bilateral blepharoptosis** due to weakness of both LPS. • **Bilateral dilated and poorly reactive pupils** due to loss of parasympathetic innervation if the EWN is involved.
Oculomotor fascicle	MB tegmentum	The fascicle passes near important **descending** and **ascending long tracts** as it travels anteriorly and exits at the interpeduncular fossa. Lesions within the midbrain tegmentum cause typical and well-described midbrain syndromes, which are dependent on the extent of the involvement of neighbouring long tracts.

Syndrome	Structures Involved	Clinical Signs
Weber's syndrome	CN III fascicle Cerebral peduncle	Ipsilateral CN III palsy Contralateral hemiparesis
Benedikt's syndrome[1]	CN III fascicle Red nucleus	Ipsilateral CN III palsy Contralateral tremor or ataxia[1,2]
Claude's syndrome[1]	CN III fascicle Red nucleus Superior cerebellar peduncle	Ipsilateral CN III palsy Contralateral tremors and ataxia[1,2]
Nothnagel's syndrome[2]	CN III fascicle Superior cerebellar peduncle	Ipsilateral CN III palsy Ipsilateral ataxia

(Continued)

(Continued)

Level	Site	Description
		The emphasis here, however, is not to learn these syndromes by heart, but to appreciate how the presence of long tract signs help localize lesion at the brainstem.
Oculomotor nerve		CN III exits between the **superior cerebellar** and **posterior cerebral arteries,** enters the subarachnoid space, moves parallel to the **posterior communicating artery,** and travels through the **cavernous sinus** before entering the eye via the **superior orbital fissure.** It then divides into the **superior** and **inferior** divisions. • The **superior division** innervates the LPS and SR muscles. • The **inferior division** innervates the IR, IO, and MR muscles. Palsy may occur from lesions occurring anywhere along its peripheral path:

Site	Comments
Arachnoid space	This is where compression by the arterial aneurysms occur.
Meninges	Metastatic meningeal disease can result in CN III palsies, especially when there are concomitant palsies of other cranial nerves, constitutional symptoms or a history of active malignancies.
Cavernous sinus	Additional findings of: • Deficits of CN IV, V1, V2, and VI • Horner's syndrome See Chapter 7 for details.
Superior orbital fissure and orbital apex	Additional findings of: • Deficits of CN IV, V1, and VI • Horner's syndrome • CN II in orbital apex syndrome See Chapter 7 for details.
Isolated	See below for details.

Isolated CN III palsies are often further subdivided into "**surgical third**" or "**medical third**".[3]

"**Surgical third**" implies palsies due to extrinsic **compression** by a structural abnormality, classically an aneurysm of the posterior communicating artery.[3] The parasympathetic fibres are situated superficially on the superio-medial aspect of the oculomotor nerve (Figure 9.4), and are thus vulnerable to lesions compressing from a superio-medial to infero-lateral direction, such as a aneurysm of the posterior communicating artery.

(Continued)

Level	Site	Description
		"Medical third" implies **non-compressive** mechanisms such as ischemia.[3] The core of the nerve is most vulnerable to ischemia, sparing the superficially located parasympathetic fibres. Pupillary reactivity is traditionally described to be normal in these patients.

C. Isolated CN III Palsy — Clinical Challenges

Challenges	Details
How do we differentiate between "medical third" and "surgical third" palsies?	There is no clinical diagnostic method that can perfectly classify CN III palsies into "medical third" or "surgical third". However, there are clinical features and clues that may be helpful. Features in favour of an ischemic CN III palsy ("medical third") include:[3] <table><tr><td>**Patient factors**</td><td>Age >40 years old Presence of ischemic risk factors</td></tr><tr><td>**Disease characteristics**</td><td>Isolated oculomotor nerve palsy Complete palsy Complete sparing of the pupil Pupil remain spared beyond 10 days No further deterioration beyond 3 weeks</td></tr><tr><td>**Recovery**</td><td>Recovery within 3-6 months No features of aberrant regeneration</td></tr></table>
Can compression of the CN III spare the pupils?	Yes. About 10% of patients with CN III palsy due to compressive aetiologies have reactive pupils.[4] The parasympathetic fibres lie supero-medially and are prone to compression by aneurysms of the posterior communicating artery. However, if the lesion compresses from another direction, the parasympathetic fibres may be spared. Figure 9.4. Schematic drawing of the right oculomotor nerve showing the relative positions of the motor and parasympathetic fibres.

(Continued)

(Continued)

Challenges	Details
How do we differentiate CN III palsy from ocular myasthenia?	Accompanying features are often helpful in differentiating between ocular myasthenia and CN III palsy:

Ocular Myasthenia	CN III Palsy
Commonly bilateral	Commonly unilateral
Weak eye closure due to weakness of the orbicularis oculi	Eye closure is spared due to preserved orbicularis oculi
Compensatory lid retraction	No compensatory lid retraction
Fatigable	Not fatigable

Challenges	Details
What are the worrisome peripheral causes of CN III palsy?	These causes of peripheral CN III palsy (i.e. distal to the nucleus and fascicle) should be considered depending on the clinical context: 1. Cerebral aneurysms 2. Uncal herniation • Compression of the oculomotor nerve along its subarachnoid segment as the uncus herniates downwards below the tentorium cerebelli. 3. Giant cell arteritis 4. Pituitary apoplexy 5. Cavernous sinus infections It is noteworthy that although the incidence of cranial nerve palsy in nasopharyngeal carcinoma may be as high as 20%, isolated oculomotor nerve involvement as in initial manifestation is exceedingly rare.[8]

D. Investigations

Patients with third nerve palsies will likely require **magnetic resonance imaging** of the brain. Of course, an urgent computed tomography scan will be more appropriate in patients suspected of having an uncal herniation. Additional consideration for **vascular imaging** or **dedicated scans** of the cavernous sinuses, orbital apices, or posterior nasal space are appropriate if localisation at the cavernous sinus or orbital apex is suspected.

    Assessment of control of **cardiovascular risk factors** are helpful and appropriate **infective** or **autoimmune** assays may be required depending on the prevailing clinical suspicion.

Tips for Examination Candidates
When you encounter a patient with CN III palsy in your examination: • Look for involvement of other cranial nerve deficits   o Does it fit into one of the cranial nerve syndromes (e.g., cavernous sinus syndrome, superior orbital fissure syndrome etc.)?

(Continued)

Tips for Examination Candidates
• Examine the limbs for 'long-tract signs'   o Presence of sensorimotor or cerebellar deficits may be suggestive of a fascicular CN III palsy Once the diagnosis of isolated CN III palsy is made, the subsequent line of questioning will often focus on distinguishing "medical third" from "surgical third" palsies. It is advisable to not be stubbornly committed to one over the other as efferent pupillary defect may be seen in up to 20–25% of vasculopathic ("medical third") CN III palsies, while normal pupils are not uncommon in cases of "surgical third" palsies.[4–7]

References

1. Liu GT, Crenner CW, Logigian EL, *et al*. (1992) Midbrain syndromes of Benedikt, Claude, and Nothnagel: Setting the record straight. *Neurology* **42**: 1820–1822.
2. Glaser JS, Bachynski B. (1990) Infranuclear disorders of eye movement. In: Glaser JS, ed. Neuro-ophthalmology. 2nd ed. Philadelphia: JB Lippincott, p. 374.
3. Modi P, Arsiwalla T. (2019) Cranial Nerve III Palsy. In: StatPearls [Internet]. Treasure Island (FL): StatPearls Publishing; 2020 Jan–
4. Jacobson DM. (2001) Relative pupil-sparing third nerve palsy: etiology and clinical variables predictive of a mass. *Neurology* **56**(6): 797–798.
5. Jacobson DM. (1998) Pupil involvement in patients with diabetes-associated oculomotor nerve palsy. *Arch Ophthalmol* **116**: 723–727.
6. Dhume KU, Paul EK. (2013) Incidence of pupillary involvement, course of anisocoria and ophthalmoplegiain diabetic oculomotor nerve palsy. *Indian J Ophthalmol.* **61**(1): 13–17.
7. O'Connor PS, Tredici TJ, Green RP. (1983) Pupil-sparing third nerve palsies caused by aneurysm. *Am J Ophthalmo* **95**(3): 395–397.
8. Lee AW, Foo W, Law SC, *et al*. (1997) Nasopharyngeal carcinoma: presenting symptoms and duration before diagnosis. *Hong Kong Med J* **3**: 355–361.

10

Abducens Nerve Palsy

A. Introduction and Anatomy

The abducens nucleus is at the dorsomedial aspect of the pons just anterior to the fourth ventricle. Its motor fibres travel anteriorly in close proximity to important ascending and descending tracts before exiting at the ventral surface of the **pontomedullary junction**. As it enters the subarachnoid space, it adopts an "S" shaped course, first bending to ascend alongside the bony clivus before making a second turn to pierce the dura mater and enter the **Dorello's canal** under the **petroclinoid ligament** (Gruber's ligament). The abducens nerve (CN VI) has the **longest subarachnoid course** of the cranial nerves.[1]

Over the tip of the petrous apex, it exits the Dorello's canal to enter the **cavernous sinus**. Here, it travels towards the eye with the oculomotor, ophthalmic, and trochlear nerves, leaving the cavernous sinus through the **superior orbital fissure** before finally coming in contact with the lateral rectus muscle (Figure 10.1).

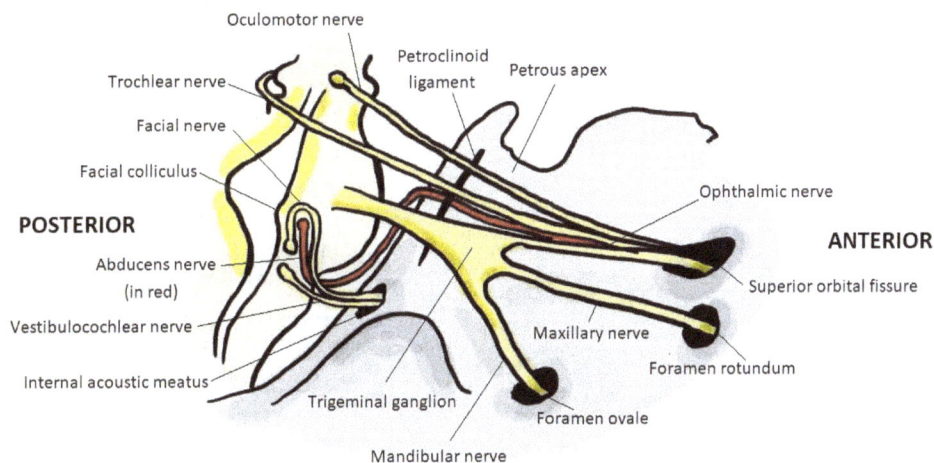

Figure 10.1.   Simplified diagram of the site of the abducens nucleus and the course of the abducens nerve (in red), showing its anatomical relationship to neighbouring structures.

In addition to transmitting motor information to the lateral rectus, the abducens nucleus also communicates with the contralateral oculomotor nucleus (medial rectus sub-nucleus) via the medial longitudinal fasciculus, a pathway that is integral to mediating the horizontal conjugate gaze.

In the subsequent segments, the following structures will henceforth be referred by their abbreviations:

- Abducens nerve: CN VI
- Lateral rectus: LR

B. The Clinical Signs of CN VI Palsy

Palsy of the abducens nerve weakens the ipsilateral LR, impairing the eye's ability to abduct. At its primary position, the patient may display an **esotropic** gaze. When looking horizontally towards the affected side, the patient may experience worsening of the binocular horizontal diplopia (Figure 10.2). The diplopia may be more troubling when he looks far and less so when he looks at something near (e.g., reading a book).

There may be times when the esotropia is not easily evident despite the patient experiencing binocular horizontal diplopia. It is then useful to have the patient look towards the symptomatic side and appreciate the presence of two images — the **"inner/true image"** and the **"outer/false image"**. The "outer/false image" will disappear on occluding the affected eye. Figure 10.3 explains how the false outer image is generated.

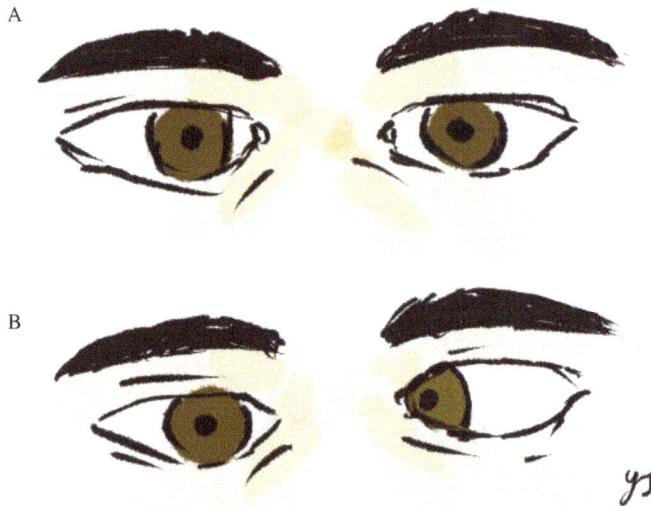

Figure 10.2.   Right CN VI palsy. A: The right eye is mildly esotropic when the patient looks forward. B: Abduction weakness of the right eye is obvious when the patient attempts to look to his right.

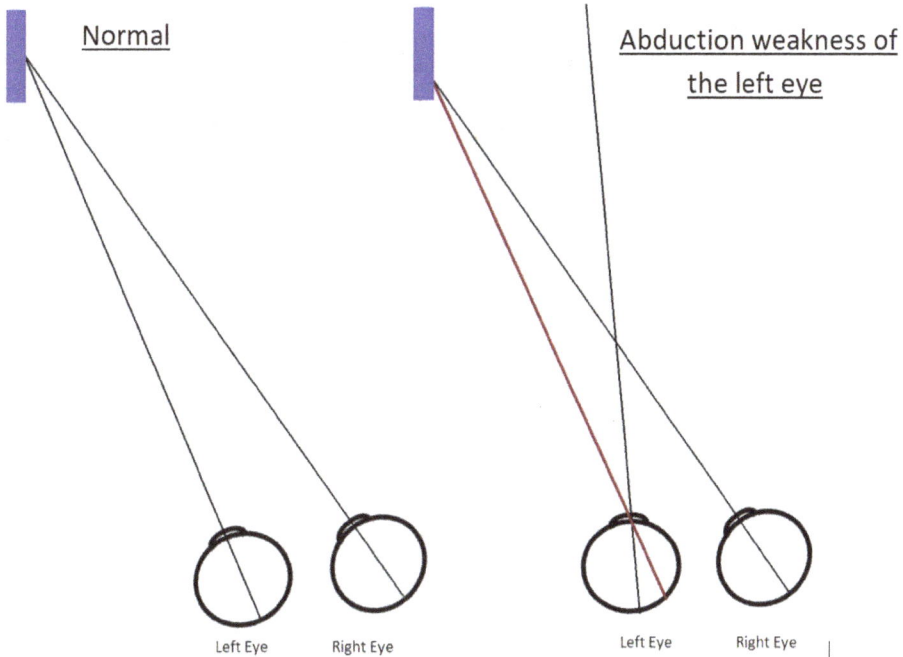

Figure 10.3. This drawing shows how the false outer image is generated in a patient with abduction weakness of the left eye. Under normal circumstances, the object's image falls onto the foveas of both eyes and the patient is able to perceive a single image. When the left eye's abduction is impaired, the image of the object hits the retina medial to the fovea. This causes the visual processing centres to perceive the image as being lateral to the actual object, resulting in the generation of a false outer image.

C. The Six Syndromes of the Sixth Cranial Nerve[1]

CN VI palsies may be broadly grouped into six syndromes, dependent on the location of the insult along the course of the nerve:[1]

1. Brainstem
2. Subarachnoid
3. Petrous apex
4. Cavernous sinus
5. Orbital apex and superior orbital fissure
6. Idiopathic

Location	Description
Brainstem	The abducens nucleus is located in the dorsomedial aspects of the pons with a long fascicular segment as it travels forward in close proximity to other important brainstem structures and tracts. As such, a small insult within the pons can result in different constellations of signs and symptoms.

(Continued)

(Continued)

Location	Description		

Pontine Syndrome	Structures Involved	Clinical Signs
Millard-Gubler syndrome[2]	Abducens nerve Facial nerve Corticospinal tract	Weak abduction of ipsilateral eye Ipsilateral hemifacial weakness Contralateral hemiparesis
Raymond syndrome[2,3]	Abducens nerve Corticospinal tract	Weak abduction of ipsilateral eye Contralateral hemiparesis
Foville syndrome[2,4]	Abducens nerve Facial nerve Corticospinal tract Medial lemniscus Paramedian pontine reticular formation	Weak abduction of ipsilateral eye Ipsilateral hemifacial weakness Contralateral hemiparesis and sensory deficits (dorsal column domains) Congjugate gaze palsy

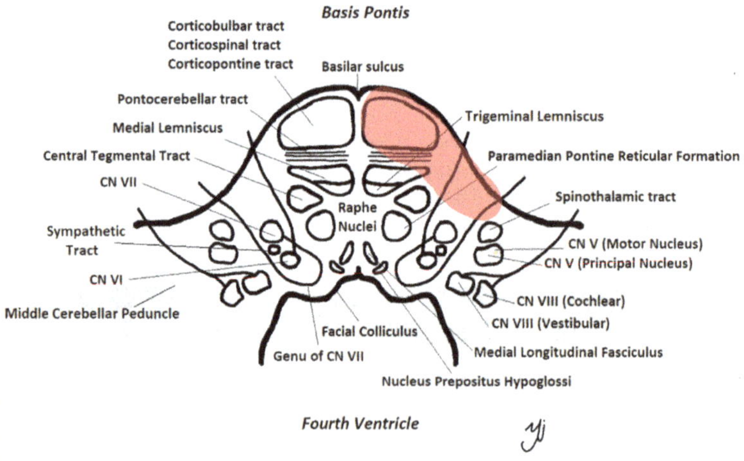

Figure 10.4.   Pons (axial view). Millard-Gubler syndrome: the likely location of the causative lesion is coloured in red.

Subarachnoid	CN VI has a **long subarachnoid cause** and is therefore vulnerable to increases in **intracranial pressure** and **disorders of the meninges** such as meningeal metastatic disease.[1]

(Continued)

Location	Description
Petrous apex	As the nerve traverses within the **Dorello's canal**, it is vulnerable to disorders of the petrous apex. A condition that comes to mind is the **Gradenigo syndrome**, classically described as a triad of otitis media, facial pain, and CN VI palsy. Inflammation of the petrous part of the temporal bone results in impairment of the abducens and trigeminal nerves. Other clinical symptoms include photophobia, pain, and fever.
Cavernous sinus	Disorders of the cavernous sinus may cause ipsilateral CN VI palsy with accompanying palsies of the oculomotor, trochlear, ophthalmic, and maxillary nerves. Ipsilateral Horner's syndrome may also be present, as the oculosympathetic fibres travels within the cavernous sinus alongside the internal carotid artery. Causes of cavernous sinus syndrome include: • **Vascular abnormalities**: arteriovenous malformations, fistulas, and sinus thrombosis. • **Inflammation**: infections, granulomatous inflammatory disorders. • **Invasive disease**: pituitary tumours, nasopharyngeal carcinoma, tumours of the base of skull). Cavernous sinus syndrome is discussed in Chapter 7.
Orbital apex and superior orbital fissure	Orbital apex syndrome describes a constellation of nerve palsies involving the optic, oculomotor, abducens, and nasociliary nerves. Due to their mutual proximity, causes of orbital apex and superior orbital fissure syndromes are similar to cavernous sinus syndromes. Due to their mutual proximity, **the causes of orbital apex and superior orbital fissure syndromes are similar to cavernous sinus syndromes**. Both syndromes are discussed in Chapter 7.
Isolated CN VI palsy	Isolated CN VI palsy should be considered, when found in the absence of additional long tract signs and palsies of the other cranial nerves. Common causes of isolated sixth nerve palsy may be broadly grouped into: 1. **Ischemic:** • Ischemic neuropathy is amongst the common aetiologies of isolated CN VI palsy in adults, and may be due to established vascular risk factors, arteriosclerosis.[1] 2. **Traumatic**[5] 3. **Idiopathic**

D. Investigations

Most patients with sixth nerve palsies will require **magnetic resonance imaging** of the brain. Additional consideration for **vascular imaging** or **dedicated scans** of the cavernous sinuses, orbital apices, or posterior nasal space are appropriate if localisation at the cavernous sinus or orbital apex is suspected.

Assessment of control of **cardiovascular risk factors** are helpful and appropriate infective or autoimmune assays may be required depending on the prevailing clinical suspicion. Do not forget to consult our otorhinolaryngologist colleagues, especially when the patient is at risk of having nasopharyngeal carcinoma.

Tips for Examination Candidates

Patients with abducens nerve palsies do appear in our professional examinations. Though it is clinically easy to demonstrate, diligence must be exercised in searching for other cranial neuropathies or concomitant long tract deficits to help you localise the lesion along its extensive path. It is important to note that idiopathic sixth nerve palsies are diagnoses of exclusion and should not be your topmost diagnosis when in discussion with the examiners.

Reference

1.   Azarmina M, Azarmina H. (2013) The six syndromes of the sixth cranial nerve. *J Ophthalmic Vis Res* **8**(2): 160–171.
2.   Hubloue I, Laureys S, Michotte A. (1996) A rare case of diplopia: medial inferior pontine syndrome or Foville's syndrome. *Eur J Emerg Med* **3**: 194–198.
3.   Zaorsky NG, Luo JJ. (2012) A case of classic raymond syndrome. *Case Rep Neurol Med* **2012**: 583123.
4.   Foville A. (1858) Note sur une paralysie peu connue de certains muscles de l'oeil, et sa liaison avec quelques points de l'anatomie et la physiologie de la protibérance annulaire. *Bull Soc Anat Paris* **33**: 393–414.
5.   Holmes JM, Droste PJ, Beck RW. (1998) The natural history of acute traumatic sixth nerve palsy or paresis. *J AAAPOS* **2**(5): 265–268.

11

Approach to Blepharoptosis

A. Introduction

Blepharoptosis (ptosis of the eyelids) describes the clinical finding of droopy eyelids. They may represent a part of a larger constellation of clinical signs, and a good understanding of the mechanisms behind the elevation of our eyelids is vital to our search for the underlying pathology. Herein, the terms "blepharoptosis" and "ptosis" will be used interchangeably.

The elevation of the eyelids involves three muscles:

Muscle	Description
Levator palpabrae superioris muscle (LPS)	• **Arises** from the lesser wing of the sphenoid bone. • **Inserts** into the eyelid and tarsal plate. • **Innervated** by the superior division of the oculomotor nerve (CN III). • **Voluntary elevation** of the eyelids.
Superior tarsal muscle	• **Arises** from the underside of the levator palpebrae superioris muscle. • **Inserts** into the superior tarsal plate. • **Innervated** by third-order oculosympathetic fibres. • **Involuntary** elevation of the eyelids under conditions of high sympathetic activity (e.g., fear). Works in tandem with the inferior tarsal muscle, which depresses the lower eyelid during periods of high sympathetic activity.
Frontalis muscle (frontal belly of the occipitofrontalis muscle)	• **Innervated** by the facial nerve (CN VII). • **Indirectly assists** in elevating the eyelids by pulling on the neighbouring soft tissue.

B. Clinical Description of Blepharoptosis

We need to characterise the blepharoptosis as best as we can. Description of the patient's blepharoptosis should include the following details:

	Questions	Description
1.	Unilateral or bilateral?	**Unilateral** ptosis may hint at a focal pathology, while bilateral involvement makes a diffuse/systemic process more likely. In **bilateral** ptosis, do take note of any **asymmetric** involvement. Asymmetric bilateral ptosis can occur in myasthenia gravis, and may be misinterpreted as unilateral blepharoptosis.
2.	Partial or complete?	Complete ptosis occurs when the eye is fully closed, and can occur from paralysis of the LPS muscle due to CN III palsy.
3.	Fatigable? Does it fluctuate?	If the blepharoptosis is fatigable, or improves with rest, neuromuscular junction disorders such as myasthenia gravis should be suspected.
4.	What about the pupils?	The presence of a miotic pupil or a mydriatic and poorly-reactive pupil can indicate ipsilateral Horner's syndrome or CN III palsy, respectively.
5.	What about the extraocular motility?	Dependent on the pattern of involvement, extraocular dysmotility with ptosis can be in multiple conditions such as CN III palsy, myasthenia gravis, complex progressive external ophthalmoplegia (CPEO) or even thyroid eye diseases.

C. Causes of Blepharoptosis

The causes of blepharoptosis are grouped into three main categories.

Causes	Description
Congenital	There are many congenital causes of ptosis, from simple congenital ptosis to the wildly-complex blepharophimosis syndrome, and not forgetting the absolutely bizarre Marcus-Gun Jaw Winking syndrome. Thankfully, they are rarely encountered in our professional examinations, and will not be discussed in this chapter.
Acquired	Acquired causes of ptosis may be broadly divided into the following five groups (Figure 11.1). **Diseases in bold** are discussed in greater detail as they are commonly encountered in the wards and in our professional examinations.

(Continued)

Causes	Description

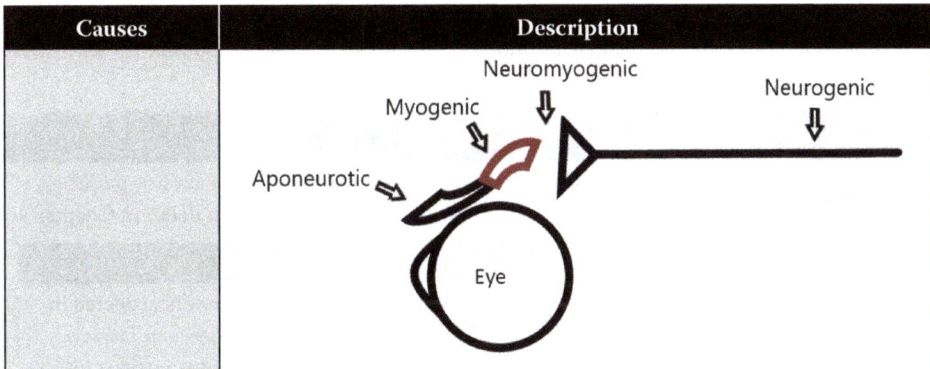

Figure 11.1. Schematic drawing representing four of the five groups of causes of acquired blepharoptosis.

Groups	Diseases
Neurogenic	• **Third nerve palsy** • **Horner's syndrome** • Cerebral ptosis
Neuromyogenic Neuromuscular junction disorders	• **Myasthenia gravis** • Botulism
Myogenic	• **Myopathies** (e.g., myotonic dystrophy, ocular myopathies, oculo-pharyngeal dystrophy)
Aponeurotic Defect in the levator aponeurosis in the presence of normal muscle	• Senile ptosis: Ageing-related levator dehiscence with stretching and thinning of the aponeurosis • Post-operative ptosis • Blepharochalasis: Relapsing-remitting recurrent eyelid inflammation, resulting in stretching, damage, and atrophy of the soft tissue • Post-traumatic dehiscence of the aponeurosis
Others	• Periorbital soft tissue swelling • Periorbital tumours • Periorbital scarring (cicatricial ptosis)

Causes	Description
Pseudoptosis	The term pseudoptosis describes the "appearance of ptosis" in the absence of neurologic, muscular, neuromuscular, and Aponeurotic abnormalities. Causes include **micro-ophthalmos, anophthalmos, enophthalmos**, etc.

Let's now focus on the selected neurogenic, neuromyogenic, and myogenic causes of blepharoptosis. As mentioned earlier, because these conditions appear frequently in the neurology wards as well as in our professional examinations, a greater degree of familiarity with these conditions is paramount.

Localisation	Aetiology	Description	
Neurogenic	Oculomotor nerve (CN III) palsy • Nucleus • Fascicle • Nerve	CN III palsy results in weakness of the levator palpebrae superioris. CN III palsy is discussed in detail in Chapter 9.	
		Questions	
		Unilateral or bilateral? Symmetry	Unilateral involvement is expected in CN III palsy of the nerve or fascicle. Palsy of the oculomotor nucleus (i.e., nuclear third) results in bilaterally symmetric ptosis.
		Complete or partial?	Variable, dependent on the underlying cause.
		Fatigable?	No
		Pupils?	Dependent on the involvement of the parasympathetic pathway to the ipsilateral eye, loss of pupillary reactivity of may be present.
		Extraocular motility?	CN III palsy is usually accompanied by ophthalmoparesis of the same eye due to weakness of the medial rectus, superior rectus, and inferior oblique muscles.
		Other features:	In nuclear and fascicular CN III palsy, accompanying long tract signs may be present.
	Horner's syndrome	Oculosympathetic denervation results in weakness of both the superior and inferior tarsal muscles while sparing the levator palpebrae superioris. This results in a mild/partial ptosis of the upper eyelid with elevation of the lower eyelid, commonly described as **upside-down ptosis** or **inverse ptosis**. Horner's syndrome is discussed in Chapter 12.	
		Questions	
		Unilateral or bilateral?	Usually unilateral
		Complete or partial?	Partial, mild, inverse
		Fatigable?	No
		Pupils?	Ipsilateral miosis
		Extraocular motility	Normal in isolated Horner's syndrome.

(Continued)

Localisation	Aetiology	Description	
		Questions	
		Others features:	Concomitant cranial nerve palsies and long tract signs may be seen in diseases involving the first-order neuron. Lower cervical radiculopathy or brachial plexopathy can occur pathologies involving the second-order neuron.
Neuromyogenic	Myasthenia gravis	Myasthenia gravis is an immune-mediated disorder with impairment of neuromuscular transmission. Fatigability is the signature feature, and weakness of eye closure due to involvement of the orbicularis oculi muscle often co-exists.	
		Questions	
		Unilateral or bilateral? Symmetric or asymmetric?	Usually bilateral. Asymmetric involvement of the eyelids may cause the ptosis to falsely appear unilateral.
		Complete or partial?	Variable
		Fatigable?	Yes
		Pupils?	The pupils should remain uninvolved.
		Extraocular motility?	Ophthalmoparesis may be present, and can mimic isolated cranial neuropathies, gaze palsies and internuclear ophthalmoplegia.
		Others:	Look out for: • Eye closure weakness • Facial weakness • Dysarthria and dysphagia • Neck and truncal weakness • Respiratory difficulties • Limb weakness and fatigability
Myogenic	Myopathies	Myopathies can cause blepharoptosis if the facial and levator muscles are also affected, usually in accompaniment with other features of facial weakness (e.g., expressionless appearance, tented mouth in myopathic facies).	

(Continued)

(Continued)

Localisation	Aetiology	Description	
		Questions	
		Unilateral or bilateral? Symmetric or asymmetric?	Bilateral, and usually symmetric
		Complete or partial?	Varied
		Fatigable?	No
		Pupils?	The pupils should remain uninvolved.
		Extraocular motility?	In mitochondrial diseases such as CPEO, ophthalmoparesis will be present.
		Others:	Look out for: • Facial weakness • Dysarthria and dysphagia • Neck and truncal weakness • Respiratory difficulties • Weakness and wasting of the limbs
		Interestingly, facial weakness is exceedingly rare in dermatomyositis and polymyositis. As such, ptosis is rare in these patients.	

Tips for Examination Candidates
In the course of your preparations, you will likely encounter patients with blepharoptosis. There are many causes of ptosis, but thankfully, the top four causes you will likely encounter in your examinations are: 1. Oculomotor nuclear/nerve palsy 2. Horner's syndrome 3. Myasthenia gravis 4. Myopathies They each boast unique distinguishing features which can help you tell them apart. Do take some time to familiarise yourself with these conditions before your examinations, and you will be more than ready to face them. Regardless of the underlying cause of ptosis, the quintessential first step is to be able to adequately describe the ptosis: • Unilateral vs. bilateral? If bilateral, is it symmetric? • Partial or complete ptosis? • Fatigable? Fluctuating? • Are the pupils involved? • Is there ocular dysmotility?

12

Horner's Syndrome

A. The Sympathetic Pathways of the Head and Neck

Failure of the sympathetic innervation to the head and neck regions results in the constellation of clinical signs known as Horner's syndrome. It constitutes an assemblage of physical signs, including the triad of blepharoptosis, miosis, and anhidrosis.

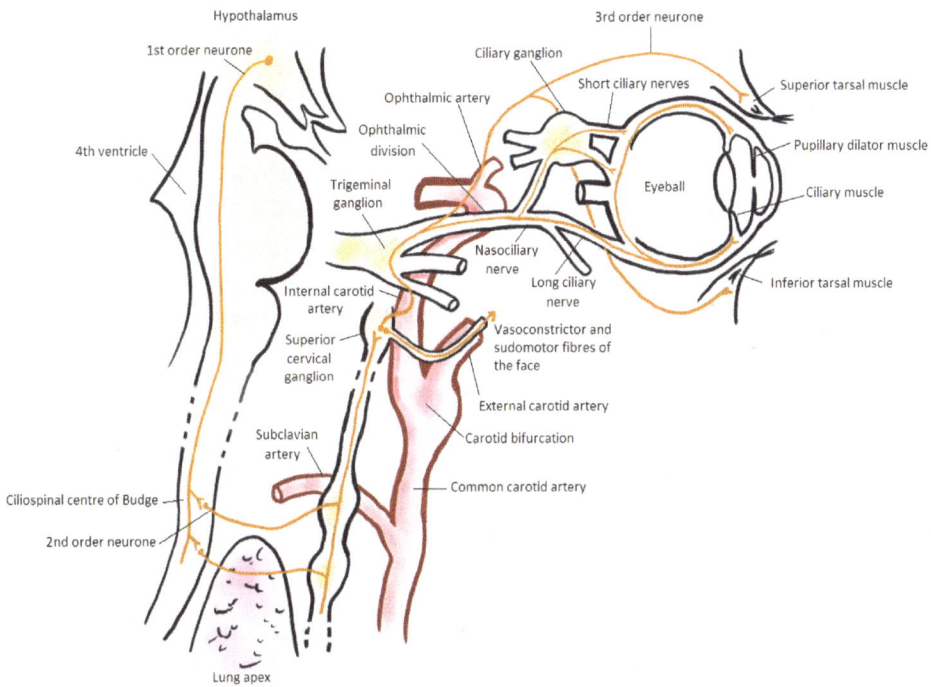

Figure 12.1. Detailed schematic drawing of the sympathetic pathway to the head and neck.

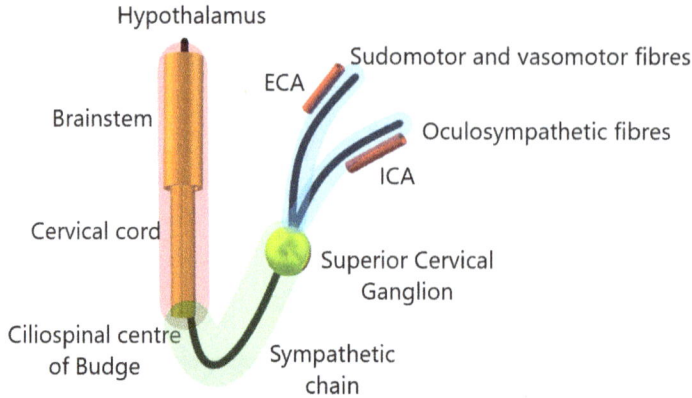

Figure 12.2.   Simplified drawing of the sympathetic pathway to the head and neck. Pink = first-order (central) neuron, green = second-order (pre-ganglionic) neuron, blue = third-order (post-ganglionic) neuron.

The sympathetic pathway is arranged into three orders:

Pathway	Description
First-order (central)	Begins at the hypothalamus • Travels caudally through the brainstem and the cervical cord • Synapses at the intermediolateral cell columns within the **C8-T1 level** of the cervical cord (**ciliospinal centre of Budge**).
Second-order (preganglionic)	Preganglionic neurons leave the cord to ascend within the **sympathetic chain**, traveling near the pulmonary apex before synapsing at the **superior cervical ganglion**. The superior cervical ganglion is situated at the bifurcation of the common carotid artery.

Third-order (post-ganglionic)	Begins at the **superior cervical ganglion**:
	• **Vasomotor** and **sudomotor** fibres of the face:
	  o Ascend the **external carotid artery** (ECA).
	• **Oculosympathetic** fibres:
	  o Ascend the **internal carotid artery** (ICA).
	  o Travel within the cavernous sinus with the ICA.
	  o Join the ophthalmic nerve (CN V1) as it enters the orbit to supply the **pupillary dilators**, and the **superior** and **inferior tarsal muscles**.

It is noteworthy that **"Müller's muscle"** refers not only to the superior tarsal muscle, as the orbitalis muscle and circular fibres of the ciliary muscle are similarly named. It is thus better to avoid using this term at all, so as to minimize ambiguity and confusion.

B. Clinical Signs of Horner's Syndrome

The clinical signs of Horner's syndrome are easy to comprehend. The failure of the sympathetic pathways to the head and neck leads to the classic triad of:

1. Blepharoptosis (inverse ptosis)
2. Miosis
3. Anhidrosis

The eyes, being the terminal "target" of oculosympathetic innervation, are often affected regardless of the level of insult. As such, our initial goal is to demonstrate the features of oculosympathetic failure.

Physical Signs	Description and Comments
Inverse ptosis (Figure 12.3)	Due to impaired sympathetic output to the superior and inferior tarsal muscles, the palpebral fissure appears smaller from a **ptotic upper eyelid** and an **elevated lower eyelid**.[1] Concomitant elevation of the lower eyelid is uncommon in other causes of blepharoptosis, and its presence is suggestive of Horner's syndrome. Normal Inverse ptosis with miosis Figure 12.3. The image on the left depicts a normal eye; the image on the right illustrates the appearance of an inversely ptotic eye with accompanying miosis.
Miosis, anisocoria, and dilatory lag	Decreased sympathetic stimulation of the pupillary dilators results in **miosis** and **anisocoria** (unequal pupillary sizes). Vary the ambient lighting and observe for changes in pupillary sizes: • **Anisocoria worsens in darkness** → sympathetic failure ○ The normal pupil dilates in darkness. ○ Weakness of the pupillary dilator on the symptomatic side prevents appropriate pupillary dilatation, exacerbating the anisocoria. Dilatory weakness of the affected pupil may be further exhibited by demonstrating the presence of **dilatory lag**: • With the penumbra of your torch, illuminate the patient's eyes just enough to visualise the pupillary sizes. • Instruct your assistant to darken the room. • Observe for **dilatory lag.** ○ A normal pupil should dilate within 5 seconds.[2] ○ A delay in dilatation is indicative of oculosympathetic failure.

(Continued)

(Continued)

Physical Signs	Description and Comments
Additional localising findings	The sympathetic tract divided into three different orders (Figures 12.1 and 12.2): 1. First-order neuron 2. Second-order neuron 3. Third-order neuron **Localisation along the first-order neuron** should be suspected if there are additional features of brainstem disease or cervical myelopathy. Lateral medullary syndrome is one such example of sympathetic failure at the level of the first-order neuron, showing both long tract signs and cranial nerve deficits Additionally, anhidrosis of the ipsilateral face and body may be present. **Localisation along the second-order neuron** should be suspected if there are concomitant involvement of the C8-T1 roots or the brachial plexus. It is not unheard of for a mass lesion to physically compress the second-order neuron along its course. A Pancoast tumour is one such example. Proceed to examine the following areas: • **Supraclavicular fossa**: Fullness in this area suggests an apical mass. • **Cervical lymph nodes**: Cervical lymphadenopathy suggests an underlying head, neck, or lung malignancy. • **Upper limbs** for sensorimotor deficits. Ipsilateral hemifacial anhidrosis may be also present, providing additional localising clues. **Disease along the third-order neuron** may occur together with other cranial neuropathies. Using the example of cavernous sinus syndrome, Horner's syndrome may be observed together with palsies of the ipsilateral oculomotor, trochlear, abducens, ophthalmic and maxillary nerves.
What about enophthalmos?	Enophthalmos describes the posterior displacement of the eyeball as a result of weakness of the sympathetically innervated orbitalis muscle. This explanation is, however, not widely accepted. Recent literature describes the "enophthalmos" as being an illusory consequence of the narrowed palpebral fissure, rather than the actual posterior displacement of the eyeball.[3,4]

C. Aetiologies

The causes of Horner's syndrome may be broadly classified into three categories based on the location of the sympathetic pathway:

Locations	Example of Causes
First-order neuron (central)	1. Hypothalamic disorders: • Stroke • Tumours 2. Brainstem disorders: • Brainstem stroke syndromes (e.g., lateral medullary syndrome) • Demyelinating diseases • Brainstem tumours 3. Cervical cord disorders: • Trauma • Syringomyelia • Spinal cord tumours (intramedullary) • Myelitis • Vascular malformations
Second-order neuron (pre-ganglionic)	1. Brachial plexus diseases • Trauma • Inflammation • Malignant infiltration[5] • Radiation 2. Structural abnormalities around the pulmonary apex • Pancoast tumour • Mediastinal tumours • Cervical rib 3. Vascular abnormalities • Carotid disease — dissection, aneurysm[6,7] o Carotid artery dissection should be strongly considered if there is concomitant headache or preceding trauma to the head • Subclavian artery aneurysm[8]
Third-order neuron (post-ganglionic)	1. Superior cervical ganglion disorders • Trauma • Iatrogenic injury (surgical neck dissection) 2. Diseases of the ICA • Aneurysm • Dissection • Arteritis (e.g., giant cell arteritis)[9,10] 3. Diseases of the cavernous sinus, superior orbital fissure, or orbital apex • Pituitary tumours • Nasopharyngeal carcinoma • Cavernous sinus thrombosis or inflammation

D. Diagnostic Tests

The intents of the diagnostic tests are to:

1. **Confirm** the diagnosis
2. **Localise** the lesion
3. Look for the **underlying cause**

Intention of Tests	Description
Confirmation of oculosympathetic failure	This involves the administration of **4% cocaine** (Figure 12.4) or **0.5%/1% apraclonidine** (Figure 12.5) eye drops. Cocaine **inhibits reuptake of norepinephrine** at the synaptic cleft. Administering cocaine eye drops will have the following effects: • **The normal eye**, being able to secrete norepinephrine at the synaptic cleft, will experience accentuation of the sympathetic tone at the pupillary dilator muscles, enhancing the dilation of the pupils. The maximum response is seen around 45 to 60 minutes. • **The abnormal eye**, unable to secrete norepinephrine at the synaptic cleft, will be minimally affected by the 4% cocaine. As there is either no or minimal norepinephrine at the synaptic cleft to begin with, the effect of a reuptake inhibitor will be insignificant. • The final result is the **worsening of the anisocoria**. Figure 12.4. The abnormal eye is marked with a red asterisk. Before administration of cocaine eye drops, the abnormal eye is miotic. After administering cocaine eye drops, the abnormal pupil remains unchanged while the normal pupil dilates further, exacerbating the anisocoria. **Apraclonidine** is a **weak $\alpha 1$ receptor agonist**. Administration of apraclonidine eye drops will have the following effects: • The **normal eye** will appear unchanged. • Sympathetic denervation of the **abnormal eye** causes up-regulation of α_1 receptors on the pupillary dilator muscles, rendering them supersensitive to apraclonidine, causing marked dilatation of the pupils, and resulting in **reversal of the anisocoria**.

(Continued)

Intention of Tests	Description
	Before apraclonidine / After apraclonidine Figure 12.5. Effect of apraclonidine eye drops. The abnormal eye is marked with a red asterisk. On administration of apraclonidine eye drops to both eyes, the normal pupil remains unchanged while the abnormal pupil dilates larger than the normal pupil, resulting in the reversal of anisocoria.

Localisation of dysfunction
  a. Post-ganglionic
  b. Central or pre-ganglionic
	Administration of **1% hydroxyamphetamine** will help to localise the dysfunction along the sympathetic pathway. **1% hydroxyamphetamine**, a sympathomimetic agent, **potentiates the release of norepinephrine** by the third-order neurons into the synaptic cleft, causing pupillary dilatation. If the post-ganglionic neuron is intact — that is, the lesion is lying along the first- or second-order neurons — pupillary dilatation will be observed in that eye. If the post-ganglionic neurone is dysfunctional, pupillary dilatation will not be seen, thus localising the lesion along the third-order neuron (Figure 12.6 and 12.7).
	
	 Before hydroxyamphetamine / After hydroxyamphetamine
	
	Figure 12.6. Effect of hydroxyamphetamine eye drops on a patient with disease along the third-order neuron. The abnormal eye is marked with a red asterisk.

(Continued)

(*Continued*)

Intention of Tests	Description
	Before hydroxyamphetamine ... After hydroxyamphetamine Figure 12.7. Effect of hydroxyamphetamine eye drops on a patient with disease along the first- or second-order neuron. The abnormal eye is marked with a red asterisk.
Search for the underlying cause	Upon localisation of the lesion, imaging studies will be dependent on the level of disease:

Level of Dysfunction	Suggested Tests
First-order neuron	• MRI of the brain • MRI of the cervical cord
Second-order neuron	• MRI of the cervical cord, and/or neck • MRI of the brachial plexus • CT of the thorax • Chest X-ray
Third-order neuron	• MRI of the brain • MRI of the posterior nasal space • Invasive or non-invasive angiography of the arteries of the head and neck • Ultrasound of the carotid arteries

---

Tips for the Examination Candidate

Oculosympathetic failure seldom occurs in isolation. Look for further clues in your physical examination to help you characterise the underlying clinical syndrome and localise the offending lesion. Plan your examination well so that you have adequate time to examine the cranial nerves, upper limbs, neck, and chest when appropriate.

When Horner's syndrome is suspected:
• Demonstrate the **clinical features of oculosympathetic failure**:
  o Presence of upside-down ptosis
  o Miosis of the abnormal pupil with dilatory lag in darkness
  o Anisocoria that worsens in darkness
• Look for **additional clinical findings** that may hint at the "level" of the lesion and the likely cause of the dysfunction.

The clinical features of Horner's syndrome are summarized below:

Site of Lesion	Accompanying Neurological Signs	Pattern of Anhidrosis
First-order (central)	Features of brainstem dysfunction: • Altered consciousness • Cranial neuropathies • Long-tract signs Features of cervical myelopathy	Ipsilateral hemiface, and body
Second-order (pre-ganglionic)	Features of C8/T1 radiculopathy: • Hand weakness and numbness • Atrophy of the hand muscles Features of brachial plexopathy: • Varying patterns of monolimbic sensorimotor deficits, dependent on the extent of dysfunction Supraclavicular fossa fullness and cervical lymphadenopathy	Ipsilateral hemiface
Third-order (post-ganglionic)	Cranial neuropathies, depending on the clinical syndrome.	Perspiration unaffected

After going through the steps listed above, proceed with the following:
- Use the eye drops to:
  - **Demonstrate** the presence of oculosympathetic failure of the eye
  - **Localise** the lesion: third-order vs. first- and second-order neurons
- With the help of imaging studies, evaluate for **underlying causes**

References

1. Nielsen PJ. (1983) Upside down ptosis in patients with Horner's syndrome. *Acta Ophthalmo (Copenh)* **61**(5): 952–957.
2. Pilley SF, *et al.* (1975) Pupillary 'dilatation lag' in Horner's Syndrome. *Brit J Ophthal* **59**: 731.
3. Loewenfeld IE. (1999) The Pupil: Anatomy, physiology, and clinical applications, Volume 1. Boston: Butterworth-Heinemann; 2v.
4. Daroff R. (2005) Enophthalmos is not present in Horner syndrome. *PLoS Med* **2**(4): e120.
5. Rai W, Olcese V, Elsheikh B, Stino AM. (2019) Horner's syndrome as initial manifestation of possible brachial plexopathy neurolymphomatosis. *Front Neurol* **10**: 4.
6. Creavin ST, Rice CM, Pollentine A, Cowburn P. (2012) Carotid artery dissection presenting with isolated headache and Horner syndrome after minor head injury. *Am J Emerg Med* **30**(9): 2103.E5–2103.E7.
7. McCorry D, Bamford J. (2004) Painful Horner's syndrome caused by carotid dissection. *Postgrad Med J* **80**: 164.
8. Levent E, *et al.* (2001) A rare cause of Horner's syndrome: Subclavian artery aneurysm. *Respiration* **68**(6): 620.
9. Shah A, Paul-Oddoye A, Madill S, *et al.* (2007) Horner's syndrome associated with giant cell arteritis. *Eye* **21**: 130–131.
10. Bromfield EB, Slakter JS. (1988) Horner's syndrome in temporal arteritis. *Arch Neurol* **45**: 604.

13

Internuclear Ophthalmoplegia and the One-and-a-Half Syndrome

A. Introduction

Internuclear ophthalmoplegia (INO) is a disorder of conjugate gaze due to a defect along the medial longitudinal fasciculus (MLF), resulting in impaired adduction of the affected eye. As its name suggests, INO describes the clinical syndrome of **ophthalmoplegia/ophthalmoparesis** secondary to a defect in the **internuclear** communication (the MLF) between the **abducens nucleus** and the **medial rectus subnucleus** of the contralateral oculomotor nucleus. INO should be considered a differential diagnosis in patients with isolated adduction weakness of the eye.

B. Paramedian Pontine Reticular Formation (PPRF) and the Medial Longitudinal Fasciculus (MLF) (Figures 13.1, 13.2 and 13.3)

The MLF is a pair of well-defined white matter tracts traveling through the dorsomedial brainstem, just **ventral to the cerebral aqueduct** (at the midbrain) and the **fourth ventricle** (at the pons). It provides internuclear relay between the abducens nucleus and the contralateral medial rectus subnucleus of the oculomotor nucleus.

The MLF is a major component in the control of horizontal conjugate gaze. It is part of the final common pathway of three conjugate eye movements (saccades, pursuit, and vestibulo-ocular reflex), but is not involved in ocular vergence, a fact that has localising implications.

Upon receiving signals to initiate horizontal saccades or pursuit from higher cortical centres the **paramedian pontine reticular formation (PPRF)** activates the ipsilateral abducens nucleus. The signal is transmitted to the ipsilateral lateral rectus muscle via the ipsilateral abducens motor neuron and concurrently to the contralateral medial rectus subnucleus via the MLF. The entire process is more extensive, involving other pontomedullary structures and gaze-holding centres, and will not be discussed in this book.

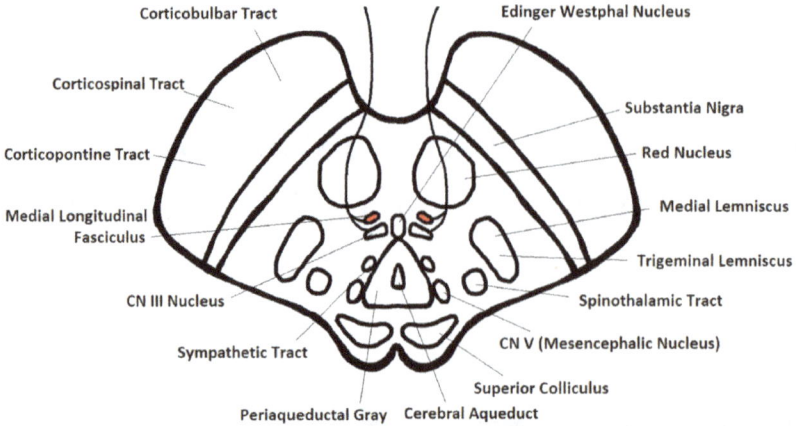

Figure 13.1.   Midbrain (axial). The MLF is coloured red, showing its relative position to the neighbouring midbrain structures.

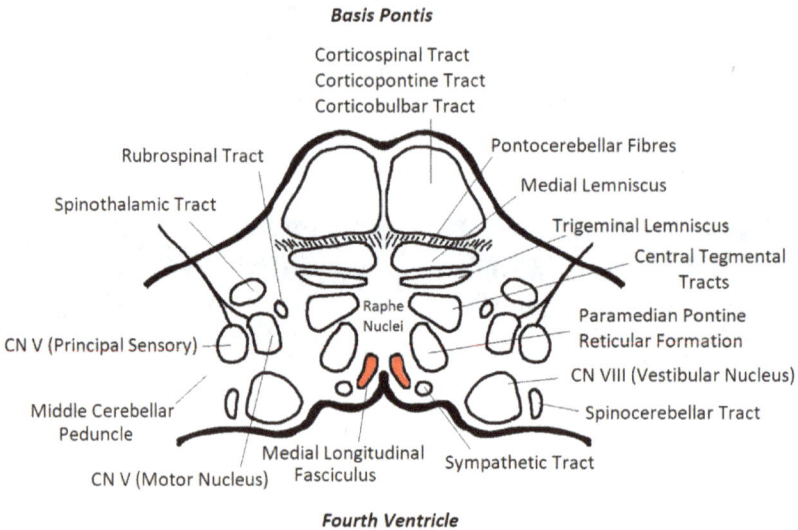

Figure 13.2.   Pons (axial). The MLF is coloured red, showing its relative position to the other pontine structures.

C. Internuclear Ophthalmoplegia (INO) — the Clinical Signs

During attempts at horizontal gaze, the following are observed (Figure 13.4):

1. **Slowing or impaired adduction** of the eye on the side of the lesion (cardinal sign)
2. **Dissociated gaze-evoked horizontal nystagmus** of the contralateral abducting eye
   - The manifestation of Herring's law of equal innervation
   - Increased stimulus to the poorly adducting medial rectus muscle results in concomitantly increased stimulus to its yoke muscle (contralateral lateral rectus)[1]
   - This results in horizontal nystagmus of the contralateral/abducting eye

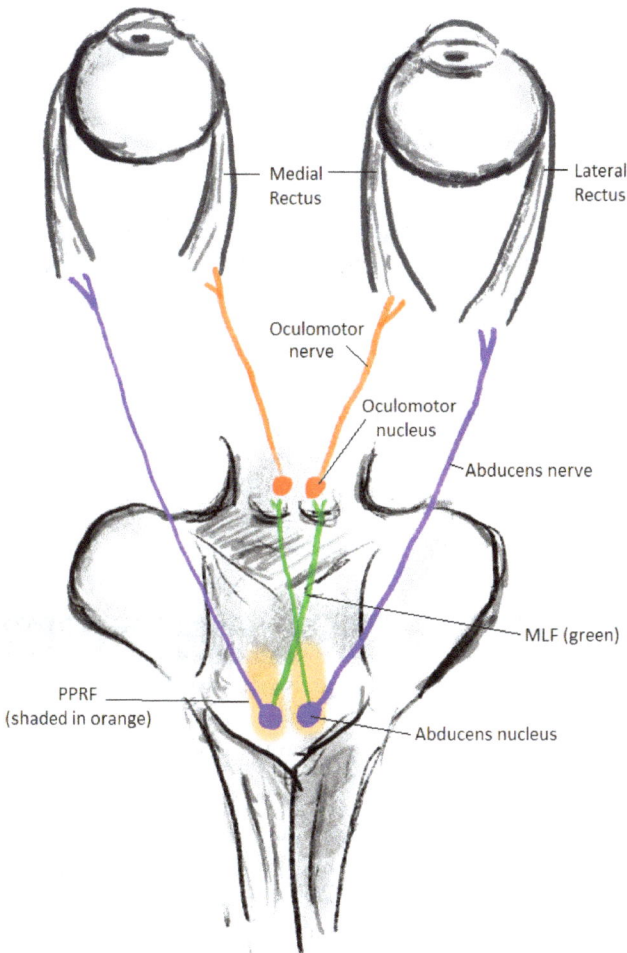

Figure 13.3.   Brainstem (coronal). This schematic drawing illustrates the PPRF-MLF system, showing its individual components and their connections in mediating horizontal conjugate eye movements.

The signs of INO are best demonstrated by the testing of saccades.[2] If the patient shows signs of isolated monocular adduction weakness during slow pursuit, the next logical step will be to assess the patient's horizontal saccades, so that you may better demonstrate the signs of INO. Once the clinical signs of INO are clearly demonstrated, the following two tasks are imperative in the neurolocalisation process:

1. Assess ocular **convergence**.
2. Look for accompanying features of **brainstem involvement**.

Right Eye   Left Eye

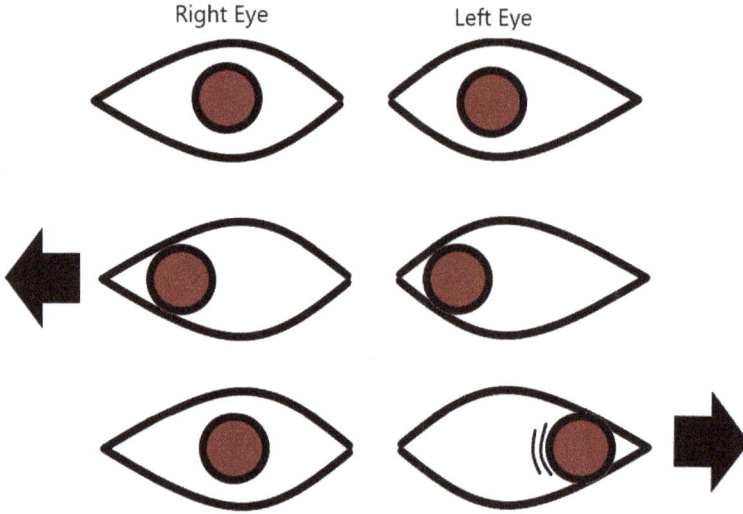

Figure 13.4.   Eye movements in a patient with right INO, due to a lesion along the right MLF.

Examination Steps	Comments	
Assessment of ocular convergence	The assessment of ocular convergence helps to: 1. Localise the lesion along the MLF 2. Distinguish INO from myasthenia gravis and partial oculomotor nerve palsy	
	Localise the lesion	The pathways mediating ocular vergence are unique from those involved in horizontal saccades, pursuit, and vestibulo-ocular reflex: • Ocular vergence **does not involve the MLF**. • The pathway mediating ocular vergence is less extensive than the others, with its "control centre" sitting within the **midbrain's pretectal area** in close proximity to the oculomotor nuclei and MLF. In most INOs, convergence of the eyes is often spared. However, if convergence is also impaired, it may imply a lesion along the MLF high in the midbrain at the level of the superior colliculus, where the vergence centre resides.[3]

(Continued)

Examination Steps	Comments	
	Distinguish INO from myasthenia gravis and partial oculomotor nerve palsy	Conditions such as myasthenia gravis, and incomplete oculomotor nerve palsy can cause "pseudo-INO" through their impairment of ocular movement.[4] However, the relative preservation of convergence rules out oculomotor nerve palsy and myasthenia gravis. Because myasthenia gravis and oculomotor nerve palsies are "peripheral" causes of ocular weakness (neuromuscular junction and cranial nerve, respectively), the impaired adduction should be equally prominent during both horizontal gaze and convergence.
Looking for concomitant long-tract signs and cranial neuropathies	INO can occur either in isolation or as part of a constellation of signs. The MLF courses extensively through the brainstem and is thus vulnerable to insults. The presence of other concomitant cranial neuropathies or long-tract signs can further pinpoint the location of the lesion within the brainstem. Neurolocalisation within the brainstem is discussed in **Chapter 6.**	

D. Causes of INO

Categories	Description
Ischemia/ infarction	• About 1/3 of INO are caused by infarctions. • These are more common in the older patients. • These are commonly unilateral, although cases of bilateral INO have been described.[5]
Demyelinating diseases of the CNS	• About 1/3 of INO are caused by demyelinating diseases like multiple sclerosis. • These are more common in younger patients and are more likely bilateral (WEBINO: wall-eyed bilateral internuclear ophthalmoplegia).[5]
Less common causes	• Infections (e.g., herpes zoster, syphilis, borreliosis etc.)[6,7] • Head trauma • Brainstem structural abnormalities (e.g., Chiari malformations, brainstem tumours)[5] • Systemic vasculitis • Metabolic disorders (e.g., Wernicke's encephalopathy)[5,8] • Neurogenerative disorders (e.g., progressive supranuclear palsy)

The more common causes of INO are multiple sclerosis and infarction of the brainstem. Despite the inconvenient symptoms, the prognosis is generally good.[9,10] However, this is also dependent on the underlying aetiology, with some (e.g., infarctions) faring better than others (e.g., tumours).

E. One-and-a-Half Syndrome

Less common than INO, the one-and-a-half syndrome is the result of the dysfunction of both the PPRF and the MLF. As explained above, the PPRF plays an important role in horizontal conjugate gaze — the left PPRF mediates horizontal conjugate gaze of both eyes towards the left. Diseases of the PPRF result in impaired horizontal conjugate gaze (pursuit and saccades) towards the ipsilateral side.[11]

In one-and-a-half syndrome, when both the right PPRF and MLF are diseased for example, the right eye will have difficulties abducting and adducting when looking right and left, respectively, while the left eye will only have difficulty adducting when looking towards the right, thus the name "one-and-a-half".

Location of Disease	Clinical Signs (Figure 13.5)
Right PPRF	The patient is unable to initiate conjugate gaze to his right
Right MLF	The patient is unable to adduct his right eye to the left on leftwards gaze

The presence of one-and-a-half syndrome localises the lesion at the **paramedian regions of the pontine tegmentum**,[11] where the PPRF is situated. The aetiologies are similar to that of INOs (Section D).

Right Eye   Left Eye

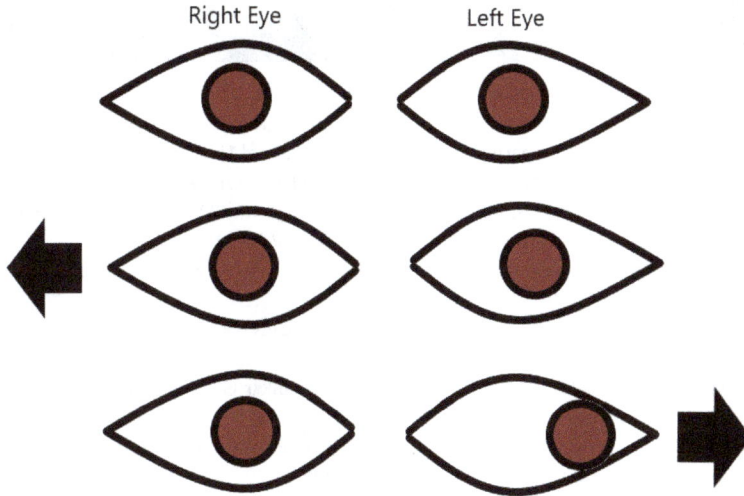

Figure 13.5.   Eye movements in a patient with right one-and-a-half syndrome.

Diseases of the PPRF and MLF can occur concurrently with other cranial neuropathies, resulting in syndromes with rather unimaginative names (facial follicular, 8 and a half syndrome,[12] 13 and a half, 15 and a half, 16 and a half syndromes, so on and so forth). These will not be discussed in this chapter, but for our advanced readers who are passionate in the clinical art of neurology, do feel free to read up on these syndromes!

Tips for Examination Candidates

INO is not uncommon in the professional examinations. You should feel a sense of optimism when encountering a patient with INO for the following reasons:

1. You **already know what to do**!
   - Demonstrate INO while testing for saccades,
   - Assess ocular convergence, and
   - Evaluate for concomitant cranial neuropathies or long tract signs.
2. You've **clinically localised the lesion with some degree of precision**, without an MRI scan.
3. The underlying cause is most likely either a stroke, or demyelinating diseases of the CNS such as multiple sclerosis.
   - Brainstem infarction is more likely if the patient is elderly or has significant cardiovascular risk factors.
   - Demyelinating diseases (e.g., multiple sclerosis) should be strongly considered, especially when the patient is young.
   - Do not forget to consider the rarer causes as well, depending on the patient's clinical history.

That's it! You've nothing to fear!

References

1. Feroze KB, Wang J. (2020) *Internuclear Ophthalmoplegia*. StatPearls Publishing, Treasure Island.
2. Niestroy A, Rucker JC, Leigh RJ. (2007) Neuro-ophthalmologic aspects of multiple sclerosis: Using eye movements as a clinical and experimental tool. *Clin Ophthalmol* **1**(3): 267–272.
3. Cogan D. (1970) Internuclear ophtlamoplegia, atypical and atypical. *Arch Ophthalmol* **84**: 583–589.
4. Khanna S, Liao K, Kaminski HJ, Tomsak RL, Joshi A, Leigh RJ. (2007) Ocular myasthenia revisited: insights from pseudo-internuclear ophthalmoplegia. *J Neurol* **254**: 1569–1574.
5. Kean JR. (2005) Internucluear ophthalmoplegia: unusual causes in 114 of 410 patients. *Arch Neurol* **62**(5): 714–715.
6. Keane JR. (2005) Internuclear ophthalmoplegia: unusual causes in 114 of 410 patients. *Arch Neurol* **62**(5): 714–717
7. Paramanadam V, Perumal S, Jeyaraj M, Velayutham S, Shankar G. (2016) Herpes Zoster internuclear ophthalmoplegia. *Neuroimmunol Neuroinflammation* **3**: 102–103.
8. De La Paz MA, Chung SM, McCrary JA. (1992) Bilateral internuclear ophthalmoplegia in a patient with Wernicke's encephalopathy. *J Clin Neuroophthal* **12**(2): 116–120.
9. Wu YT, Cafiero-Chin M, Marques C. (2015) Wall-eyed bilateral internuclear ophthalmoplegia: a review of pathogenesis, diagnosis, prognosis and management. *Clin Exp Optom* **98**(1): 25–30.
10. Eggenberger E, *et al.* (2002) Prognosis of ischemic internuclear ophthalmoplegia. *Ophthalmology* **109**(9): 1676–1678.
11. Martyn CN, Kean D. (1988) The one-and-a-half syndrome: Clinical correlation with a pontine lesion demonstrated by nuclear magnetic resonance imaging in a case of multiple sclerosis. *Br J Ophthal* **72**: 515–517.
12. Eggenberger E. (1998) Eight-and-a half syndrome: one-and-a half syndrome plus cranial nerve VII palsy. *J Neuroophthalmo* **18**: 114–116.

14

Approach to Unilateral Facial Weakness

A. Introduction

Facial nerve palsies present with characteristic patterns of facial weakness which are important to recognise. Supranuclear facial palsies, also known as upper motor neuron (UMN) facial palsies, result in weakness of the contralateral lower quadrant of the face. Facial nerve or nuclear palsies, also known as lower motor neuron (LMN) facial palsies, cause weakness over the ipsilateral half of the face. The commonest cause of acute unilateral facial nerve palsy is Bell's palsy.[1]

B. Anatomy of the Facial Nerve

The facial nucleus is functionally divided into **dorsal** and **ventral** components. The **dorsal component** receives input from **bilateral motor cortices** and provides motor output to the ipsilateral upper quadrant of the face. The **ventral component** receives input from the **contralateral motor cortex**, and provides motor output to the ipsilateral lower quadrant of the face. This unique manner of innervation results in the distinctive patterns of UMN and LMN facial palsies (Figure 14.1).

From the facial nucleus, the nerve fascicle forms a loop around the abducens nucleus through a bulge at the facial colliculus (Figure 14.2), before exiting the pons at the anterolateral aspect of the pontomedullary junction together with the vestibulocochlear nerve. From here, it is joined by **parasympathetic** fibres from the pontine **superior salivatory nucleus** via the **intermediate nerve**, as well as fibres carrying **special sensory** information from the anterior 2/3 of the tongue to the **solitary nucleus**.

The nerve then enters the **facial canal** via the **internal acoustic meatus,** adopts a serpentine course through which it gives off motor, sensory and parasympathetic branches, before exiting at the **stylomastoid foramen** to give off its 5 major branches — the **temporal, zygomatic, buccal, marginal mandibular** and **cervical branches.**

Its course within the facial canal may be anatomically divided into 3 parts (Figure 14.3) — the **labyrinthine, tympanic** and **mastoid segments.**

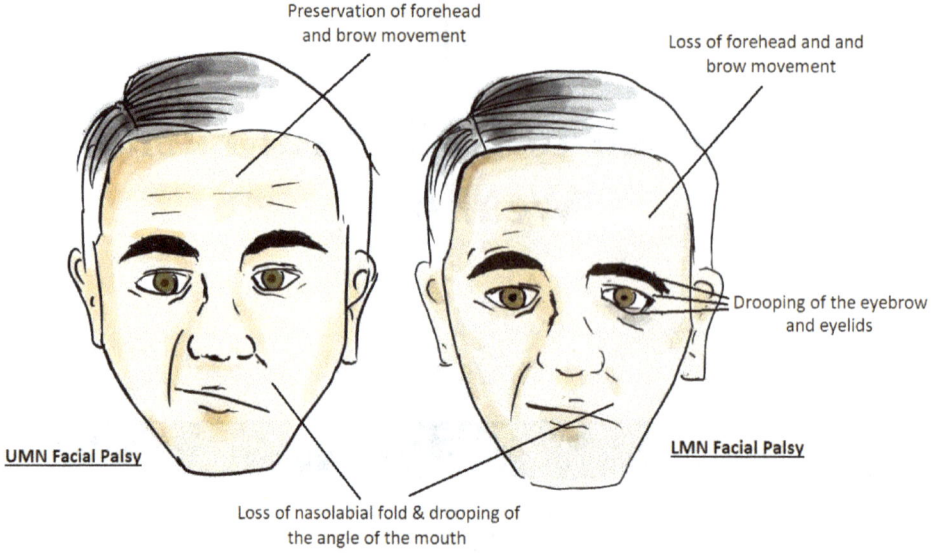

Preservation of forehead
and brow movement

Loss of forehead and and
brow movement

Drooping of the eyebrow
and eyelids

UMN Facial Palsy

LMN Facial Palsy

Loss of nasolabial fold & drooping of
the angle of the mouth

Figure 14.1.   The patterns of facial weakness in UMN and LMN facial palsies.

ANTERIOR

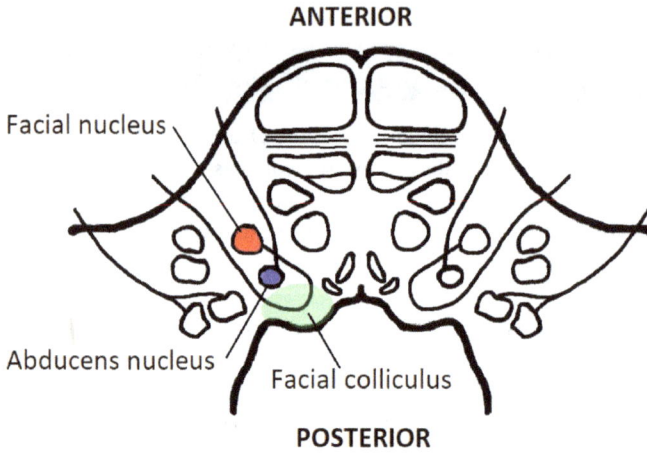

Facial nucleus

Abducens nucleus   Facial colliculus

POSTERIOR

Figure 14.2.   Schematic drawing of the pons along its axial plane. The facial colliculus is shaded green.

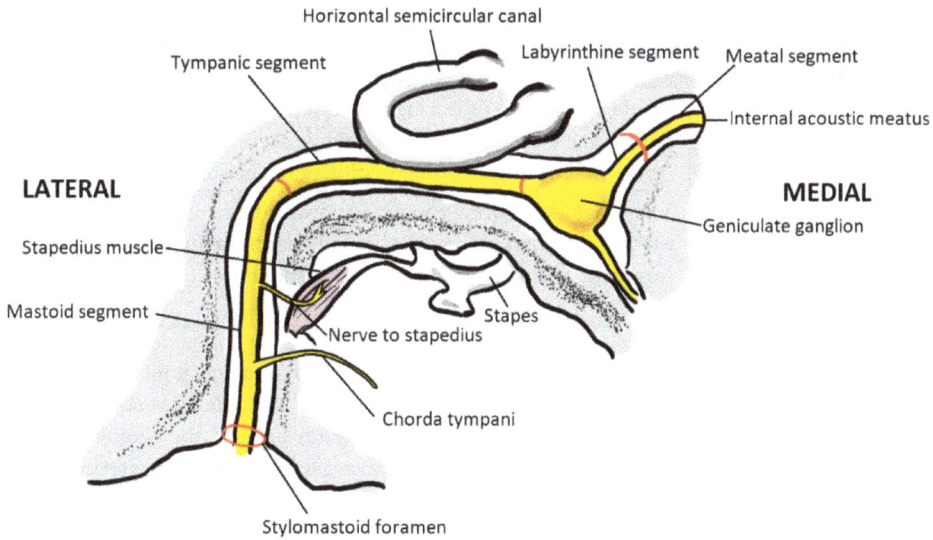

Figure 14.3.   Schematic drawing of the facial nerve within the facial canal.

Facial Canal Segment	Description (Figure 14.4)
Labyrinthine	The shortest of the 3 segments, the facial nerve forms a bend, forming the **facial geniculum**, with "genu" being the Latin word for "knee". It is here where the **geniculate ganglion** resides. The geniculate ganglion plays a major role in the conveying parasympathetic fibres from the **superior salivatory nucleus** to the secretory glands of the head:

Subsequent Path After Leaving the Geniculate Ganglion	Target Gland
Greater petrosal nerve ↓ Pterygopalatine ganglion ↓ Zygomatic nerve (CN V2) ↓ CN V1 branch to lacrimal gland	Lacrimal gland
Greater petrosal nerve ↓ Pterygopalatine ganglion ↓ CN V2 nasal branches	Glands of the nasal mucosa
Chorda tympani ↓ Submandibular ganglion ↓ Lingual nerve (CN V3)	Submandibular and sublingual glands

(Continued)

(Continued)

Facial Canal Segment	Description (Figure 14.4)
Tympanic	The facial nerve runs through the tympanic cavity, a space containing the three ossicles of the middle ear. It is here that the facial nerve is vulnerable to inflammation of the middle ear (otitis media).
Mastoid	The facial nerve forms another bend within the mastoid segment, as it travels inferiorly to exit the skull via the **stylomastoid foramen**. The nerve to stapedius and the chorda tympani branches off from the facial nerve within this segment.

As the facial nerve leaves the facial canal via the stylomastoid foramen, it gives off the **posterior auricular nerve**, which provides motor innervation to the **auricularis posterior** muscle via the auricular branch and the **occipitalis** muscle (occipital belly of the occipitofrontalis muscle) via the occipital branch. Another motor branch emerges to supply the **posterior digastric** muscles.[2]

Moving anteriorly within the parotid gland leads to the parotid plexus, dividing into 5 motor branches to supply the muscles of facial expression:

Branch	Muscle	Function
Temporal	Frontalis (or the frontal belly of the occipitofrontalis muscle[2])	Elevation of eyebrows Wrinkling of the forehead
	Orbicularis oculi muscle	Eye closure
	Procerus muscle	Draws the skin between the eyebrows downwards, resulting in an expression of anger
	Corrugator supercilia muscle	Draws the eyebrows medially and downward, resulting in a frown
Zygomatic	Orbicularis oculi muscle	Eye closure
Buccal "The smile nerve"	Buccinator muscle	Flattening of the cheeks to assist in mastication
	Risorius muscle	Smirking
	Levator labii superioris and levator labii superioris alaeque nasi muscles	Elevation of upper lip Smiling
	Orbicularis oris muscle	Pursing the lips Blowing a kiss
Marginal mandibular	Depressor labii inferioris muscle	Depresses the corners of the lower lip
	Mentalis muscle	Elevates and protrudes the lower lip
Cervical	Platysma muscle	Depresses and widens the corners of the mouth when tensed, forming a grimace

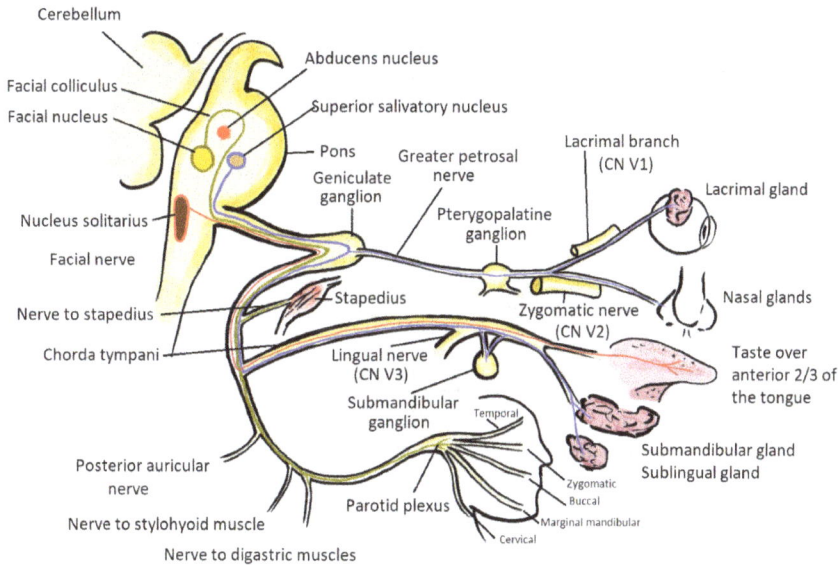

Figure 14.4.   Schematic drawing of the facial nucleus and nerve.

There are many mnemonics that can be used to help you remember these 5 motor branches, with **"To Zanzibar by My Car"** being my favourite. Zanzibar is a region within Tanzania, which is steeped in history, blessed with abundant wildlife, and remains on my bucket list of travel destinations.

Last but not least, the facial nerve also receives **general somatic afferents** from the concha and a small area behind the ear.

C. Clinical Assessment of a Patient with Unilateral LMN Facial Palsy

Examination of a patient with unilateral facial weakness involves the following steps:

Examination Steps	Steps in Detail	Description in Detail
Inspection	Inspect the patient's face as you greet him	As you interact with the patient, observe for facial asymmetry. This may range from subtle asymmetry of the nasolabial fold, diminished eye blink, and presence of Bell's phenomenon to frank paralysis of the facial muscles and paralytic ectropion.
Instruct the patient to:	Elevate the eyebrows or wrinkle the forehead	This tests the **frontalis** and **corrugator muscles.** Unilateral weakness may result in asymmetrical elevation of the eyebrows and wrinkling of the forehead.

(Continued)

(Continued)

Examination Steps	Steps in Detail	Description in Detail
	Close eyes tightly	This tests the **orbicularis oculi** muscle. Unilateral weakness of this muscle causes lagophthalmos (incomplete eye closure), and Bell's phenomenon may be observed. In severe cases, paralytic ectropion can be evident. Interestingly, the asymmetrical nasolabial fold may be accentuated on attempting eye closure. Be sure not to miss this clue.
	Puff up cheeks	This tests the **buccinator** muscles.
	Pucker lips	This tests the **orbicularis oris** muscle.
	Smile or grimace	There are four main muscles that maintain the nasolabial fold: • **Zygomaticus major** • **Zygomaticus minor** • **Levator labii superioris** • **Levator labii superioris alaeque nasi** These 4 muscles are tested when the patient smiles, grimaces, or attempts to show his or her teeth. Of note, grimacing depresses the corners of the mouth and concomitantly activates the **platysma**. The platysma is innervated by the cervical branch of the facial nerve. The presence of asymmetrical platysmal contraction is thus evident in patients with ipsilateral facial weakness (Platysma sign).[3] Interestingly, the platysma is also innervated by the high cervical cord, and platysma weakness has also been reported in patients with high cervical cord pathologies.[4]
Examination of other cranial nerves		The examination of the other cranial nerves is discussed in **Chapter 5.** It is important to assess the patient for sensorineural hearing loss, as 40% of patients with Ramsay-Hunt syndrome (zoster oticus) have concomitant involvement of the vestibulocochlear nerve.[5]
Examination of the neighbouring regions (Figure 14.5)	Occipital region	Inspect for surgical scars. If present, they may represent prior surgeries involving the structures of the posterior cranial fossa.
	Mastoid region	Examine for redness or tenderness over the mastoid area, which serve as clinical signs of mastoiditis.

(Continued)

Examination Steps	Steps in Detail	Description in Detail
	External ear and external acoustic meatus	Inspect the external ear (especially the concha) and external acoustic meatus for vesicles.
	Tympanic membrane	Using an otoscope, visually inspect the tympanic membrane for features of otitis media.
	Region around the angle of the jaw	Observe for surgical scars or skin changes from prior radiotherapy.
	Parotid gland and overlying skin	Examine the parotid gland for signs of an underlying parotid tumour. Presence of swelling, redness and tenderness are features of parotitis or parotid abscesses, which are rare causes of facial nerve palsy.[6]
	Oral cavity	Examine the walls of the oropharynx and the tongue for vesicular rash or ulcerations.
	Eyes	Facial weakness may be complicated by exposure keratopathy of the eye, especially when eye closure is impaired. Observe for conjunctival injection or chemosis.
	Skin of the head and neck	In rare cases, regional skin cancers (especially **squamous cell carcinoma**[5,7]) may metastasize to the parotid gland, causing facial palsies.
	Cervical lymph nodes	Regional cervical lymph nodes should be examined. An enlarged lymph may suggest underlying lymphomatous, malignant or inflammatory processes.
Further examination	Upper and lower limbs for long-tract deficits: • Sensory • Motor • Cerebellar	
Other findings	Other neurologic findings that may be present include: • Absent or diminished ipsilateral blink response to corneal reflex testing, • Ipsilateral hyperacusis due to weakness of the stapedius muscle. • Loss or altered sense of taste over the anterior 2/3 of the ipsilateral half of the tongue.	

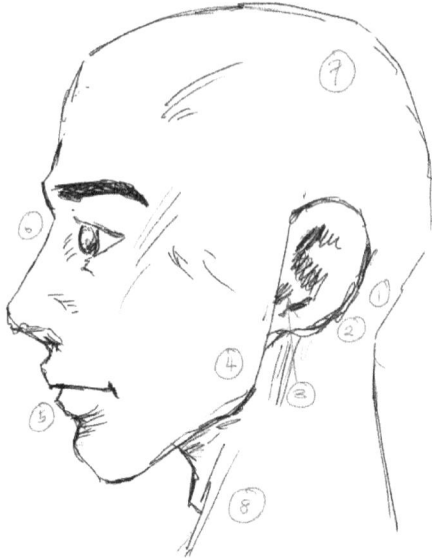

Figure 14.5.   Schematic drawing of the side of the face, showing the regions of interest when examining patients with ipsilateral LMN facial palsy. The numerals are ordered in sequence, demonstrating the suggested flow of examination steps: (1) occiput, (2) mastoid area, (3) examination of the external ear, external acoustic meatus and the tympanic membrane, (4) angle of the jaw and parotid gland, (5) oral cavity, tongue and palate, (6) eyes — sclera and blink reflex, (7) skin over the head and neck, and (8) cervical lymph nodes.

Traditionally, localisation along the facial nerve's path follows the **topognostic principle** — if a lesion lies distal to the origin of a particular branch of the facial nerve, that branch in question will be spared. For example, if the facial palsy occurs at the region of the parotid glands, sense of taste should be preserved and hyperacusis should be absent. This is because the chorda tympani and the nerve to the stapedius muscle branch off within the facial canal prior to the parotid gland. However, recent medical literature has revealed that topognostic tests are fraught with discrepancies, limiting their neurolocalisation value.[1] As described by Tan's team, these limitations could be the result of inherent differences in vulnerability of selected branches to injury, or from a multifocal disease process.[1]

D. Causes of LMN Facial Palsy

Bell's palsy is the commonest diagnosis given to patients with isolated LMN facial weakness. It remains a diagnosis of exclusion, and up to 40% of patients with LMN facial palsy can be attributed to other causes:[5]

• Trauma, inclusive of temporal bone fractures and iatrogenic surgical injuries
• Ramsay-Hunt syndrome (zoster oticus)
• Neoplasms — cerebellopontine angle tumours, primary parotid tumours, squamous cell carcinoma
• Infections — otitis media, otomastoiditis, parotid abscesses, Lyme disease
• Others: Sjögren's syndrome,[8,9] neurosarcoidosis[10]

Because facial palsies from other causes tend to have poorer clinical outcomes when untreated, clinical assessment of patients should be geared towards the identification of "red flags" — clinical symptoms or signs suggestive of another aetiology other than Bell's palsy. The 6 **red flags**[1,5] are:

1. Paediatric patients
2. Head or facial trauma
3. Long-tract signs (sensory, motor, or cerebellar deficits)
4. Involvement of other cranial nerves
5. Facial pain
6. Features suggesting an underlying cancerous lesion: gradual onset, persistent facial weakness more than 6 months, ipsilateral hearing loss, suspicious head or neck lesions, or history of known regional cancers

Appropriate referrals and imaging studies should be performed upon detection of these red flags.

E. Bell's Palsy

The commonest cause of LMN facial palsy, the peak incidence of Bell's palsy occurs between the ages of 15 to 50 years, with similar reported incidences between both genders.[1,5] Susceptible groups at risk of Bell's palsy include the **elderly, diabetics**, patients with **hypothyroidism**, and **pregnant women** in their third trimester.[7] Currently, the accepted pathogenic mechanism behind Bell's palsy is the reactivation of latent **herpes simplex virus 1 (HSV-1) within the geniculate ganglion**. The consequent inflammation results in the compression of the facial nerve within the proximal labyrinthine segment of the facial canal, leading to the clinical features of ipsilateral hemifacial weakness.[7]

The typical presentation of Bell's palsy involves the sudden appearance of hemifacial weakness, with rapid deterioration within a few hours and often reaching the maximum facial weakness within 2 days.[8] It is not uncommon for patients to experience discomfort over the ipsilateral ear, concomitant hyperacusis, reduced lacrimation and altered taste.[7,11]

There are many grading systems to assess the severity of facial weakness, but the House-Brackmann grading system is accepted by the American Academy of Otolaryngology-Head and Neck Surgery as a standardised and reliable way to describe facial function.[7,12]

Laboratory tests and neuroimaging studies are not routinely required, except when the red-flag features are present or when the recovery is protracted beyond 3 weeks despite appropriate treatment.[7]

Management of Bell's palsy involves the early administration of **corticosteroids** and **prevention of corneal complications** due to lagophthalmos. Aimed at reducing the inflammation of the facial nerve early in the disease, the efficacy of prednisolone was satisfactorily demonstrated in a Cochrane review of over 1,500 patients by Salinas *et al*. Beyond improvement of facial motor functions, corticosteroids have also displayed utility in reducing motor synkinesis from aberrant facial nerve regeneration.[14] The role of antivirals remains controversial in the treatment of Bell's palsy, with trials showing no to modest benefit of antivirals alone or when used concurrently with corticosteroids.[7,15,16]

Bell's palsy is usually **self-limiting**, with most patients recovering fully within 3 weeks, although cases of protracted weakness of up to 9 months have been reported.[17] Recovery may not be perfect, and facial synkinesis is a common complication.

House-Brackmann Grading Scale[7,13]

Grade	Severity	Description
I	None	Normal facial function in all areas.
II	Mild	Slight weakness noticeable on close inspection. Normal symmetry and tone at rest. Complete eye closure with minimal effort.
III	Moderate	Obvious weakness but not disfiguring. Normal symmetry and tone at rest. Complete eye closure with effort. Mouth is slightly weak with maximal effort.
IV	Moderately severe	**Obvious weakness with disfiguring asymmetry.** Normal symmetry and tone at rest. **Incomplete closure of the eye.** Mouth asymmetry with maximal effort.
V	Severe	Barely perceptible movement of the facial muscles. Asymmetry is obvious at rest. Incomplete eye closure. Slight movement of the mouth with maximal effort.
VI	Total paralysis	No facial movement.

Tips for Examination Candidates

Patients with hemifacial weakness commonly appear in our professional examinations. Although Bell's palsy remains the commonest cause of isolated hemifacial weakness, you are more likely to encounter patients with hemifacial weakness from other causes. Patients are often selected weeks or months prior to the examination. Given the self-limiting nature of Bell's palsy, it is difficult to ensure that the deficits are still present on the day of your examination.

Your are also unlikely to encounter patients with active Ramsay Hunt Syndrome (Zoster oticus) with fresh vesicles in an examination due to the inherently contagious nature of this disease.

References

1. Tan AK, Hanom Annuar F. (2011) A systemic approach to facial nerve paralysis. *Opthalmology* **2**(4): WMC001856.
2. "m. occipitofrontalis". Terminologia Anatomica: TA98. 1998.
3. Leon-Sarmiento FE, Prada LJ, Torres-Hillera M. (2002) The first sign of Babinski. *Neurology* **59**(7): 1067.
4. Ogawa Y, Sakakibara R. (2005) Platysma sign in high cervical lesion. *J Neurol Neurosurg Psychiatry* **76**: 735.
5. Masterson L, Vallis M, Quinlivan R, Prinsley P. (2015) Assessment and management of facial nerve palsy. *BMJ* **351**: h3725.
6. Andrews JC, Abemayor E, Alessi DM, Canalis RF. (1989) Parotitis and facial nerve dysfunction. *Arch Otolaryngol Head Neck Surg* **115**(2): 240–242.
7. Zandian A, Osiro S, Hudson R, Ali IM, Matusz P, Tubbs SR, Loukas M. (2014) The neurologist's dilemma: a comprehensive clinical review of Bell's palsy, with emphasis on current management trends. *Med Sci Monit* **20**: 83–90.
8. Zhang W, Shi J, Guo J. (2019) Bilateral facial paralysis as a rare neurological manifestation of primary Sjögren's syndrome: Case-based review. *Rheumatol Int* **39**(9): 1651–1654.
9. Ashraf VV, Bhasi R, Kumar RP, Girija AS. (2019) Primary Sjögren's syndrome: case-based review. *Rheumatol Int* **39**(9): 1651–1654.
10. Hoyle JC, Jablonski C, Newton HB. (2014) Neurosarcoidosis: clinical review of a disorder with challenging inpatient presentations and diagnostic considerations. *Neurohospitalist* **4**(2): 94–101.
11. De Seta D, Mancini P, Minni A, Prosperini L, De Seta E, Attanasio G, Covelli E, De Carlo A, Filipo R. (2014) Bell's palsy: symptoms preceding and accompanying the facial paresis. *Sci World J* **2014**: 801971.
12. Reitzen SD, Babb JS, Lalwani AK. (2009) Significance and reliability of the House-Brackmann grading system for regional facial nerve function. *Otolaryngol Head Neck Surg* **140**(2): 154–158.
13. House KW, Brackmann DE. (1985) Facial nerve grading system. *Otolaryngol Head Neck Surg* **93**(2): 146–147.
14. Salinas RA, Alvarez G, Daly F, Ferreira J. (2010) Corticosteroids for Bell's palsy (idiopathic facial paralysis). *Cochrane Database Syst Rev* **17**(3): CD001942.
15. Numthavaj P, Thakkinstian A, Dejthevaporn C, Attia J. (2011) Corticosteroid and antiviral therapy for Bell's palsy: a network meta-analysis. *BMC Neurol* **11**: 1.
16. Quant EC, Jeste SS, Muni RH, Cape AV, Bhussar MK, Peleg AY. (2009) The benefits of steroids versus steroids plus antivirals for treatment of Bell's palsy: a meta-analysis. *BMJ* **339**: b3354.
17. Wolfson AB. (2009) *Narwood-Nuss' Clinical Practice of Emergency Medicine*, 5th ed. Lippincott Williams & Williams, Philadelphia.

15

The Median Nerve

A. Introduction (Figure 15.1)

As the median nerve is a major nerve of the upper limb, a degree of familiarity is necessary (Figure 15.1). Here, we will look at its anatomy, discuss the appropriate sensorimotor assessments, and explore the clinical correlations using a few examples.

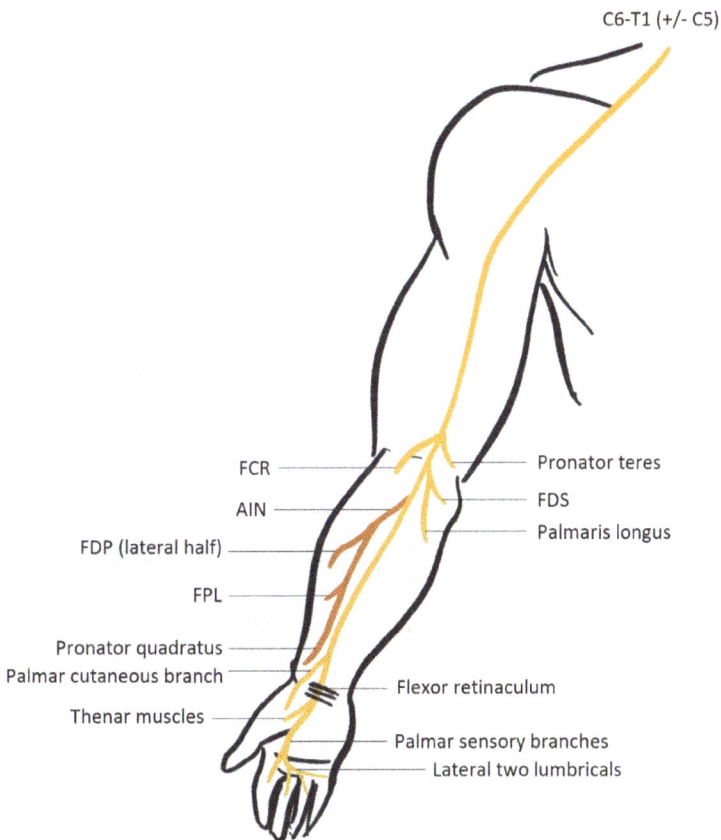

Figure 15.1.   The median nerve and its branches. Abbreviations: FCR, flexor carpi radialis; FDS, flexor digitorum superficialis; AIN, anterior interosseous nerve (in orange); FDP, flexor digitorum profundus; FPL, flexor pollicis longus.

B. Anatomy

The median nerve contains fibres from the **C6–T1 roots** (some variants receive contribution from the C5 root). It has no sensorimotor contributions at the arm. As it travels distally, it enters the anterior compartment of the forearm via the cubital fossa, giving its first branch to supply the **pronator teres** muscle. Just a short distance away, nerve fibres supplying the **palmaris longus**, the **flexor digitorum superficialis** (FDS), and the **flexor carpi radialis** (FCR) leave the median nerve for their respective muscles.

Further down, the median nerve gives off the **anterior interosseous nerve** (AIN) to supply the lateral half of the **flexor digitorum profundus** (FDP), the **flexor pollicis longus** (FPL), and the **pronator quadratus**. Finally, it gives off the **palmar cutaneous branch** to supply the skin over the lateral palm, before entering the hand beneath the flexor retinaculum via the carpal tunnel. Here, it gives off the **recurrent branch** and the **palmar digital branch**. The recurrent branch supplies the thenar muscles, while the palmar digital branch innervates the lateral two lumbricals, and the skin over the palmar surface and fingertips of the lateral three and a half digits. The thenar muscles include the **abductor pollicis brevis** (APB), the **opponens pollicis** (OP) and the **flexor pollicis brevis** (FPB) muscles.

C. Motor Function

The median nerve provides vital motor innervation of the forearm and hand. The table below provides a summary of the important muscles supplied by the median nerve and their corresponding actions.

Site	Muscle	Main Action
Anterior forearm	Pronator teres	Forearm pronation.
	Flexor carpi radialis	Flexion of the wrist.
	Palmaris longus	Minor flexor of the wrist.
	Flexor digitorum brevis	Flexion of the PIPJs of all fingers
	Flexor digitorum profundus (lateral half) — by AIN	Flexion of the index and middle fingers' DIPJs.
	Flexor pollicis longus — by AIN	Flexion at the thumb's IPJ.
	Pronator quadratus — by AIN	Minor pronator of the forearm.
Hand	Lateral two lumbricals	Flexion of the index and middle fingers' MCPJ, with concomitant extension of the IPJs.
	Opponens pollicis	Thumb opposition.
	Abductor pollicis brevis	Thumb abduction.
	Flexor pollicis brevis	Flexion at the thumb's MCPJ.

Abbreviations: AIN, anterior interosseous nerve; MCPJ, metacarpophalangeal joint; IPJ, interphalangeal joint; PIPJ, proximal interphalangeal joint; DIPJ, distal interphalangeal joint.
Note: Although the flexor pollicis brevis muscle is predominantly innervated by the median nerve, its medial head is supplied by the ulnar nerve. Avoid confusing our learners, this is omitted here.

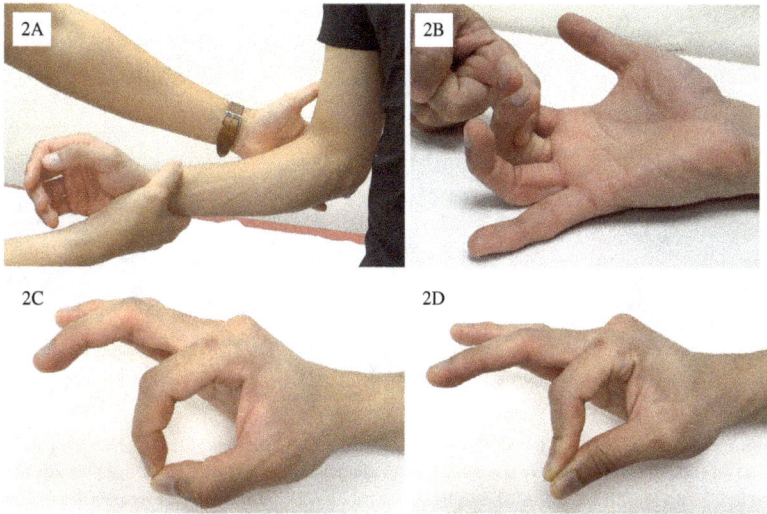

Figure 15.2.   Examination technique of the muscles innervated by the median nerve. The pronator teres is best tested with the elbow flexed at 90°, as the patient attempts to pronate the forearm against resistance (2A). The FDS is assessed by having the patient flex the fingers at the PIPJs against resistance (2B). The "OK" sign (2C) allows you to quickly assess the AIN by testing the integrity of the FPL, and the FDP to the index finger. Dysfunction of these two muscles impairs flexion of the index finger at the DIPJ and thumb at the IPJ, causing the volar surfaces of the distal phalanges to come into contact instead of the fingertips (2D).

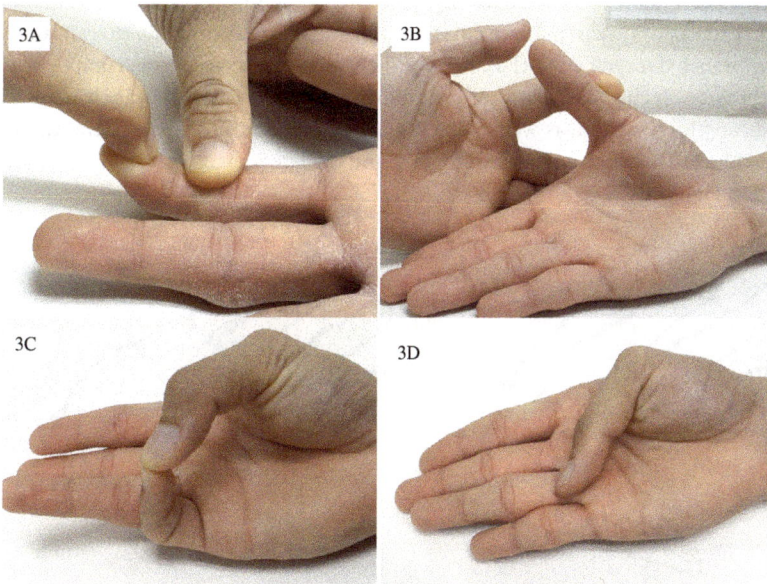

Figure 15.3.   Examination technique of the muscles innervated by the median nerve. The lateral half of the FDP is tested by instructing the patient to flex his index or middle finger at the DIPJ against resistance (3A). The APB is best assessed by having the patient abduct the thumb against resistance as shown (3B). Thumb opposition is shown in 3C. Thumb flexion at the MCPJ is mediated by the FPB and is demonstrated in 3D.

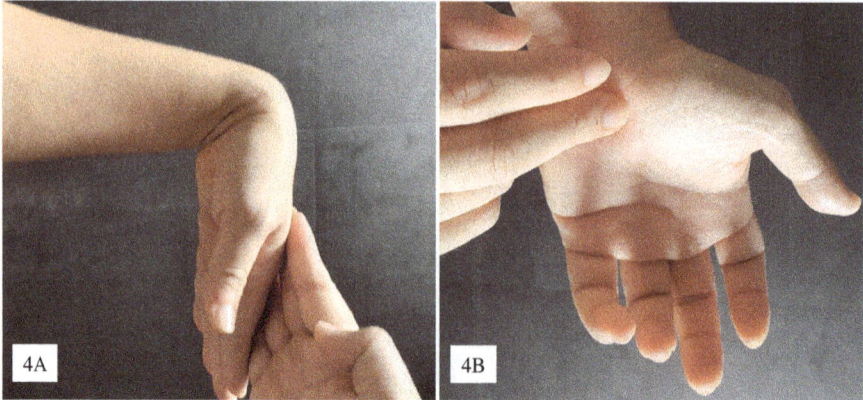

Figure 15.4. The Phalen's test (4A) is a provocative test for carpal tunnel syndrome, during which the patient flexes the wrist for 30–60 seconds. The test is positive if numbness or tingling sensation is elicited in the symptomatic hand. The test is reported to be 57–68% sensitive, and 58–73% specific for carpal tunnel syndrome.[1] The reverse Phalen's test (not shown) involves extending the patient's wrist for a minute and is an acceptable alternative to the traditional Phalen's test.[2] The Tinel's sign (4B) is also helpful when assessing a patient with carpal tunnel syndrome. Gently tap the patient's wrist over the flexor retinaculum as shown. The sign is present if paraesthesia is elicited in the symptomatic hand. The sensitivity and specificity of this test is at 36–50% and 77%, respectively.[1]

D. Sensory Function

The median nerve does not contribute significantly to the sensation to the arm and forearm, with its first sensory branch (**palmar cutaneous branch**) innervating the lateral palmar region. This nerve branch does not enter the carpal tunnel and is thus spared from compressive neuropathies at the wrist, such as carpal tunnel syndrome. The **palmar digital branch** arises within the hand, and supplies the palm, as well as the ventral surface and tips of the lateral three and half digits (the thumb, the index and middle fingers, and the lateral half of the ring finger). These are illustrated in Figure 15.5.

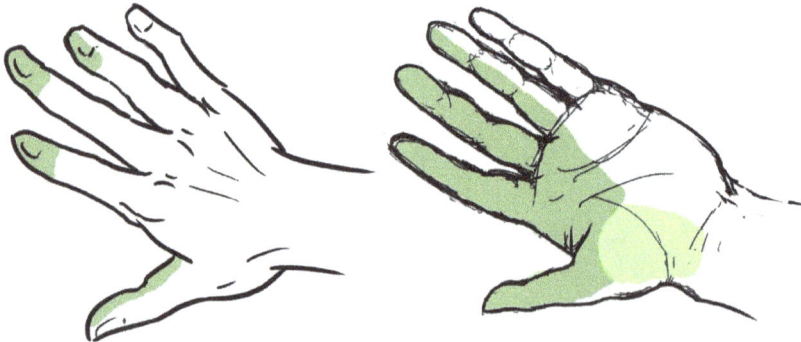

Figure 15.5.   The sensory territory of the median nerve. The areas supplied by the palmar cutaneous branch (light green) and the palmar digital branch (dark green) are shown here.

E. Clinical Examples

Focal lesions of the median nerve may occur anywhere along its path, and the pattern of deficits can allow us to localise the lesion. Here, we discuss the clinical symptoms and signs of median neuropathy at three different sites.

Site of Disease	Description of Signs and Symptoms	Diagnosis
At or above the elbow	**Motor:** • Weak forearm pronators • Wrist flexion weakness due to weakness of the FCR • Weak flexion of all PIPJs • Weak flexion of index and middle fingers' DIPJs **Sensory:** • Numbness over the lateral palm, inclusive of the thenar eminences • Numbness of the ventral surface and tips of the lateral three and half fingers (thumb, index and middle fingers, and the lateral half of the ring finger) **Others:** • Hand of Benediction when making a fist	The clinical symptoms suggest a proximal lesion along the median nerve, likely at or above the elbow. This is reflected by the weakened pronator teres muscle, which is the most proximal muscle supplied by the median nerve. A supracondylar humeral fracture is a good example of an injury that can damage the median nerve along its proximal segment. The **Hand of Benediction** may be seen in proximal median neuropathies when the patients attempt to make a fist. Although the FDS to all fingers are affected, the flexion of the index and middle fingers are further confounded by the involvement of the lateral FDP, resulting in a disparity of finger flexion between the medial two fingers and the index and middle fingers.
At the forearm	**Motor:** • The extent of weakness depends on the proximity of the lesion. Lesions distal to the elbow likely will spare the forearm pronators, while lesions that are further distal may spare the muscles innervated by the AIN. **Sensory:** • Variable, depending on the proximity of the lesion.	Traumatic lacerations over the forearm can result in such palsies. **AIN syndrome**, though rare, is worthy of mention. AIN is a pure motor branch, innervating the pronator quadratus, FPL, and the FDP's lateral half. Isolated palsy of the AIN results in weakness of the

(Continued)

(*Continued*)

Site of Disease	Description of Signs and Symptoms	Diagnosis
		above muscles, without concomitant sensory complaints. Patients may be unable to demonstrate the "OK" sign. Classical causes of AIN syndrome include inflammatory and compressive diseases.[3]
At the wrist	**Motor:** • Weakness of the thenar muscles (thumb flexion, abduction, and opposition) • Weakness of the lateral two lumbricals **Sensory:** • Numbness and tingling of lateral portions of the hand, sparing the thenar eminences **Others (Figure 15.4):** • Tinel's sign may be present • Phalen's manoeuvre may be positive	**Carpal tunnel syndrome** describes the compressive neuropathy of the median nerve within the carpal tunnel. Although often seen in otherwise healthy individuals, it may be a complication of conditions like pregnancy, diabetes mellitus and acromegaly. When severe and chronic enough, wasting of the thenar muscles may be observed. Sensory sparing of the thenar eminence reflects the departure of the palmar cutaneous branch, before the median nerve enters the carpal tunnel.

Quick Reference	
Spinal roots	C6-T1, +/− C5
Motor function	The median nerve innervates the flexor and pronator muscles within the forearm's anterior compartment, with the exception of the ulnar-innervated medial half of the FDP, and the flexor carpi ulnaris. At the hand, the nerve supplies the thenar muscles (APB, OP, and FPB) and the lateral two lumbricals.
Sensory function	The median nerve supplies the sensation over the palm as shown (Figure 15.5). It has no sensory contributions above the wrist.

References

1. Wipperman J, Goerl K. (2016) Carpal tunnel syndrome: diagnosis and management. *Am Fam Physician* **94**(12): 993–999.
2. Werner RA, Bir C, Armstrong TJ. (1994) Reverse Phalen's maneuver as an aid in diagnosing carpal tunnel syndrome. *Arch Phys Med Rehabil* **75**(7): 783–786.
3. Aljawder A, Faqi MK, Mohamed A, Alkhalifa F. (2016) Anterior interosseous nerve syndrome diagnosis and intraoperative findings: A case report. *Int J Surg Case Rep* **21**: 44–47.

16

The Ulnar Nerve

A. Introduction

The ulnar nerve plays a major role in the innervation of the forearm and hand. Here, we will look at its anatomy, discuss the appropriate sensorimotor assessments, and explore the clinical correlations using a few examples.

B. Anatomy (Figure 16.1)

The ulnar nerve contains fibres from the **C8 and T1 roots**. It has no sensorimotor contribution at the arm. It descends medially down the arm, passing posterior to the bony medial epicondyle (**retro-epicondylar groove**), rendering it vulnerable to extrinsic compression. It then enters the cubital tunnel into the forearm. The **cubital tunnel** is often erroneously associated with the retro-epicondylar groove, but these are entirely different structures. It is formed by a thick transverse band between the humeral and ulnar heads of the **flexor carpi ulnaris** (FCU), the olecranon, the elbow's joint capsule, and medial collateral ligament. Here, the ulnar nerve travels deep to the FCU, before breaking off into two muscular branches to supply the FCU and the **medial half of the flexor digitorum profundus** muscles.

The ulnar nerve does not provide sensory innervation to the forearm. As it nears the wrist, the **dorsal cutaneous branch** and the **palmar cutaneous branch** are given off at the forearm to supply the skin over the dorso-medial hand and over the hypothenar eminence (Figure 16.4), respectively. It then travels superficial to the flexor retinaculum to enter the hand through the Guyon's canal, where it gives off the **superficial and deep branches** to provide sensorimotor innervation to the hand. The deep branch supplies the **hypothenar group of muscles**, the **palmar and dorsal interossei** (PI and DI), the **adductor pollicis** (AP), and the **medial two lumbricals**. The hypothenar muscles include the **abductor digiti minimi** (ADM), **opponens digiti minimi** (ODM), and **flexor digiti minimi brevis** (FDMB).

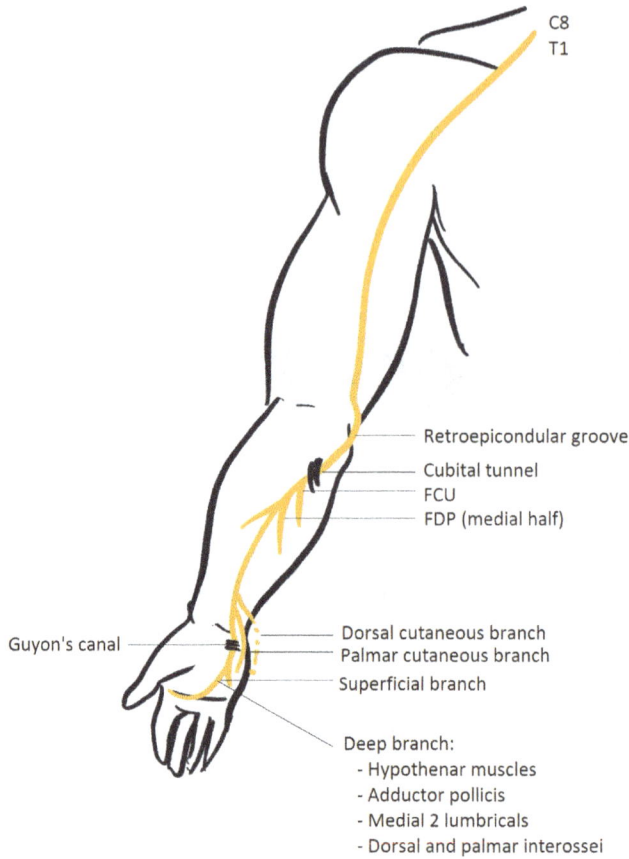

Figure 16.1. The ulnar nerve, its branches, and the pertinent anatomical landmarks. Abbreviations: FCU, flexor carpi ulnaris; FDP, flexor digitorum profundus.

C. Motor Function

Site	Muscle	Main Action
Forearm	Flexor carpi ulnaris (Figure. 16.2)	Flexion of the medial wrist.
	Flexor digitorum profundus, medial half	Flexion of the ring and little fingers' DIPJ.
Hand	Hypothenar muscles • ADM • ODM • FDMB	ADM: abduction of the little finger. ODM: opposition of the little finger. FDMB: flexion of the little finger's MCPJ.

(Continued)

Site	Muscle	Main Action
	Dorsal interossei	Abduction of the index and ring fingers.
	Palmar interossei	Adduction of the index, ring, and little fingers towards the middle finger.
	Adductor pollicis	Adduction of the thumb.
	Medial two lumbricals	Flexion of the ring and little fingers' MCPJ, with concomitant extension of the IPJs.

Abbreviations: ADM, abductor digiti minimi; ODM, opponens digiti minimi; FDMB, flexor digiti minimi brevis; MCPJ, metacarpophalangeal joint; PIPJ, proximal interphalangeal joint; DIPJ, distal interphalangeal joint.

Note: Although the flexor pollicis brevis muscle is predominantly innervated by the median nerve, its medial head is supplied by the ulnar nerve. To avoid confusing our learners, this is omitted here.

D. Sensory Function

The ulnar nerve does not contribute to the sensation to the arm and forearm. However, two important sensory branches are given off at the forearm — **dorsal cutaneous and the palmar cutaneous branches**. The dorsal cutaneous sensory branch provides sensory innervation over the dorsolateral aspect of the hand, while the palmar branch supplies the skin over the hypothenar eminence. Distal to the Guyon's canal, the **superficial branch** provides sensory innervation over the ventral surface and tips of the little finger and the medial half of the ring finger (Figure 16.4).

E. Clinical Examples

Focal lesions of the ulnar nerve may occur anywhere along its path, and the pattern of deficits allows us to localise the lesion. Here, we discuss the clinical symptoms and signs of ulnar neuropathy at two different sites.

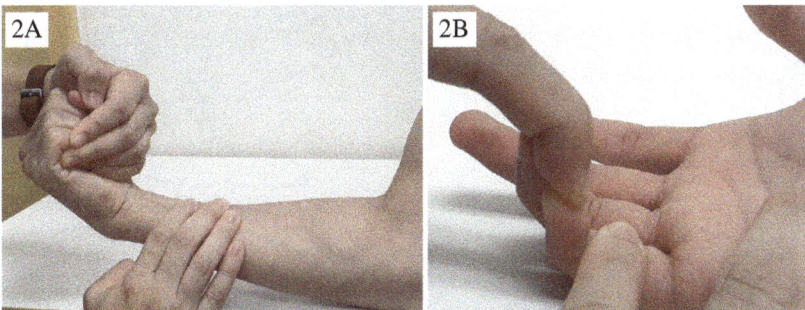

Figure 16.2. To test the FCU, flex the wrist against resistance in an ulnar direction (2A).[1] The medial half FDP is tested by instructing the patient to flex his or her ring or little finger at the DIPJ against resistance (2B).

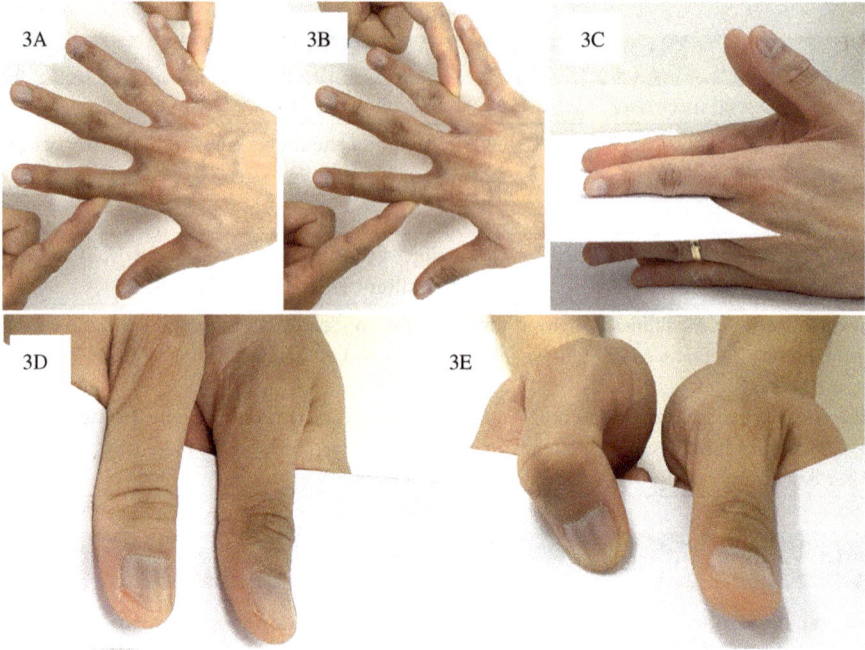

Figure 16.3.   Finger abduction (3A, 3B) is best tested against resistance at the PIPJs. Because the dorsal interossei muscles do not insert onto the little finger, abduction of the fifth digit is mediated by the ADM. As such, 3B tests only the dorsal interossei, while 3A tests the ADM as well. Testing of finger adduction is shown in 3C. The adductor pollicis muscle is tested by having the patient pinch a piece of paper strongly between the thumb and index fingers (3D). In ulnar neuropathies, the flexor pollicis longus substitutes the weakened adductor pollicis, causing the thumb to flex at the IPJ. This is known as the Froment's sign (3E).

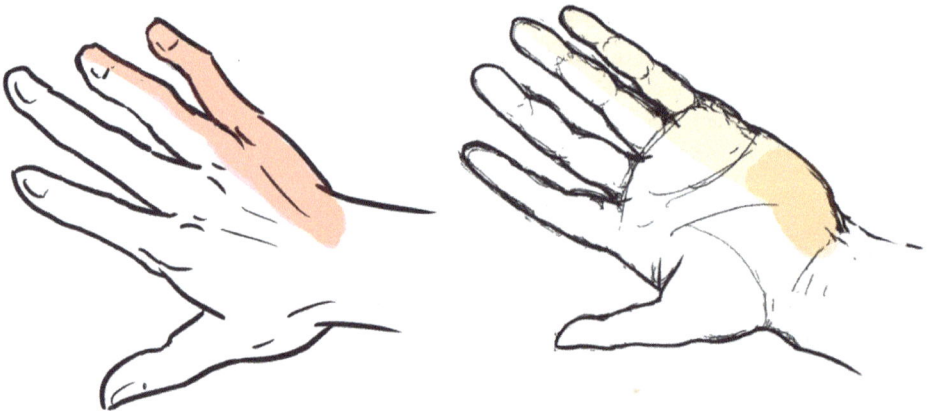

Figure 16.4.   The sensory territory of the ulnar nerve. The areas supplied by the dorsal cutaneous branch (red), palmar cutaneous branch (orange) and the superficial branch (pale orange) are shown here.

(Continued)

Site of Disease	Description of Signs and Symptoms	Diagnosis

At or above the elbow	**Motor:**
	• Weak flexion of the wrist due to weakness of the FCU, with accompanying abduction of the wrist as the median nerve innervated flexor carpi radialis is spared.
	• Weak flexion of the little and ring finger's DIPJs.
	• Weakness of the hypothenar muscles.
	  ○ Weak opposition of the little finger.
	  ○ Weak abduction of the little finger.
	• Weak abduction of the ring and index fingers.
	• Weak adduction of the fingers.
	
	Sensory:
	• Numbness over the ventro-medial and dorso-medial aspects of the hand, the little finger, and the medial half of the ring finger (Figure 16.4).
	
	Others:
	• Ulnar claw-hand (clawing of the little and ring fingers).
	• Wartenberg's sign.
	• Froment's sign (Figure 16.3).
		The signs suggest a proximal lesion along the ulnar nerve, likely at or above the elbow. This is reflected by the involvement of the FCU, which is the most proximal muscle supplied by the ulnar nerve. Fractures of the humerus (supracondylar or medial epicondylar) and compression within the retro-epicondylar groove or the cubital tunnel are possible causes.
		
		The **"ulnar claw"** describes the claw-like appearance of the symptomatic hand when the patient attempts to extend his or her fingers. The little and ring fingers are hyperextended at their MCPJs, while their DIPJs and PIPJs remain flexed due to the weakened lumbricals and interossei, which insert into the extensor hood and normally play a role in extending the interphalangeal joints.
		
		Wartenberg's sign describes the abduction of the little finger due to the unopposed action of finger extensors in the presence of weakened palmar interossei muscles.
		Froment's sign may be seen when a patient with ulnar neuropathy attempts to strongly pinch a piece of paper between his or her thumb and index fingers, during which the thumb of the symptomatic hand inadvertently flexes at the interphalangeal joint. During the test, the flexor pollicis longus (innervated by the median nerve) substitutes the weakened adductor pollicis, causing the thumb to flex.[2]

At the wrist	**Motor:** • Weakness of the hand's intrinsic muscles innervated by the ulnar nerve (see above). ○ Wrist flexion is strong as the FCU is spared.	The signs reflect the involvement of the ulnar nerve's distal branches, while sparing the more proximal branches. Sensory preservation over the hand's dorsum and the hypothenar eminence places the lesion at the wrist.

(Continued)

(Continued)

Site of Disease	Description of Signs and Symptoms	Diagnosis
	o Flexion of the little and ring fingers' DIPJs remain strong, as the medial half of the FDP is spared. **Sensory:** • Numbness over the ventral surface and tips of the little finger, as well as the medial half of the ring finger (Figure 16.4). **Others:** • Ulnar claw-hand. • Wartenberg's sign. • Froment's sign (Figure 16.3).	In patients with ulnar neuropathies, the **ulnar paradox** describes the observation that the clawing appears paradoxically milder in proximal lesions, and more severe in distal lesions. This is due to the paralysis of the medial half of the FCP from proximal lesions, resulting in weakened flexion of the ring and little fingers, causing the hand to appear less clawed.

Quick Reference	
Spinal roots	C8, T1
Motor function	Within the forearm, the ulnar nerve supplies the FCU and the medial half of the FDP. At the hand, the nerve supplies the hypothenar muscles (ADM, ODM, FDMB), the AP, the medial two lumbricals, and the interossei muscles.
Sensory function	The median nerve supplies the sensation over the palm as shown (Figure 16.4). It has no sensory contributions above the wrist.

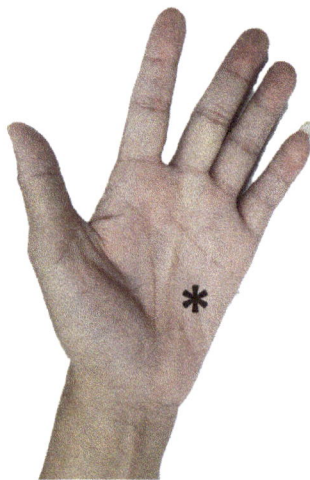

Figure 16.5.   The left hand of a patient with long-standing ulnar neuropathy at the left elbow, showing obvious atrophy of the hypothenar muscles (asterisk), while the thenar eminence (supplied by the median nerve) is relatively spared.

References

1. Andrews K, Rowland A, Pranjal A, Ebraheim N. (2018) Cubital tunnel syndrome: anatomy, clinical presentation, and management. *J Orthop* **15**(3): 832–836.
2. Konin JG, Wiksten D, Isear JA Jr, Brader H. (2006) *Special Tests for Orthopedic Examination*, 3rd ed. SLACK Incorporated, Thorofare.

17

The Radial Nerve

A. Introduction

The radial nerve plays a major part in the sensorimotor innervation of the arm. Here, we will look at its anatomy, discuss the appropriate sensorimotor assessments, and explore the clinical correlations using a few examples.

B. Anatomy (Figure 17.1)

The radial nerve contains fibres from the **C5 and T1 roots**. It has sensorimotor contributions at the arm, the forearm, and the hand. It arises from the posterior cord of the brachial plexus together with the axillary nerve. Just before the **spiral groove**, the nerve sends off motor branches to the long and lateral heads of the triceps brachii and a sensory branch to the posterior arm (**posterior cutaneous nerve to the arm**). Descending down the spiral groove, it gives off motor branches to supply the medial head of the **triceps brachii**, as well as sensory branches to the lateral arm (**lower lateral cutaneous nerve of the arm**) and the posterior forearm (**posterior cutaneous nerve of the forearm**). Upon exiting the spiral groove, it sends motor branches to the **brachialis** (also innervated by the musculocutaneous nerve), the **brachioradialis**, and the **extensor carpi radialis longus** (ECRL).

The radial nerve travels anterior to the lateral epicondyle to enter the forearm through the cubital fossa, giving rise to the **superficial** and **deep branches**. The superficial branch provides sensory innervation over the dorsolateral hand (Figure 17.6). The extensor carpi radialis brevis (ECRB) is supplied by the deep branch (see below) proximal to the supinator muscle, but there are other anatomical variations to its innervation. The deep branch then pierces and supplies the **supinator** muscle, continuing as the **posterior interosseous nerve** (PIN) thereafter. The PIN provides motor innervation to the extensors of the wrist and fingers. These include the **extensor digitorum communis** (EDC), **extensor carpi ulnaris** (ECU), **extensor digiti minimi** (EDM), **extensor indicis proprius** (EIP), and the **muscles surrounding the snuff box** (Figure 17.5) — **abductor pollicis longus** (APL), **extensor pollicis brevis** (EPB), and **extensor pollicis longus** (EPL).

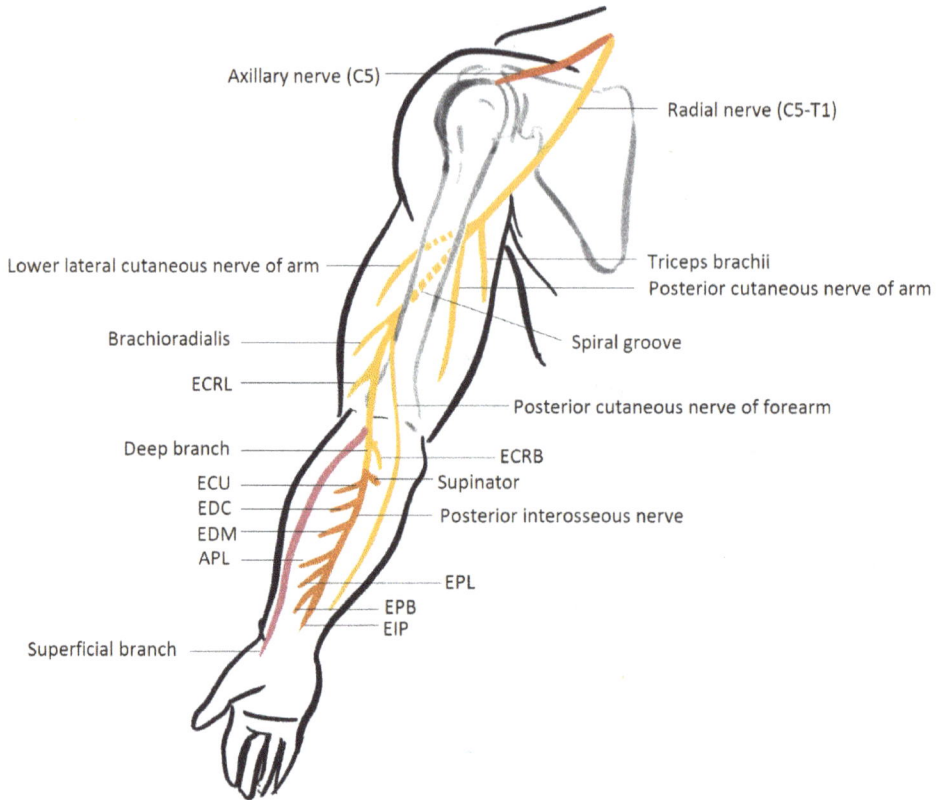

Figure 17.1.   The radial nerve, its branches, and the pertinent anatomical landmarks. Abbreviations: ECRL, extensor carpi radialis longus; ECRB, extensor carpi radialis brevis; ECU, extensor carpi ulnaris; EDC, extensor digitorum communis; EDM, extensor digiti minimi; APL, abductor pollicis longus; EPL, extensor pollicis longus; EPB, extensor pollicis brevis; EIP, extensor indicis proprius.

C. Motor Function

The radial nerve provides motor innervation to the muscles in the arm, forearm and hand. The table below provides a summary of the important muscles supplied by the radial nerve, as well as their corresponding actions.

Site	Major Muscles	Main Action
Arm	Triceps brachii	Extension of the elbow.
Elbow	Brachioradialis (Figure 17.2)	Flexion of the elbow, with the forearm in mid-pronation (neutral position).
Forearm	Extensor carpi radialis longus	Extension of the wrist.
	Extensor carpi radialis brevis*	
	Supinator	Supination of the forearm.

(Continued)

Site		Major Muscles	Main Action
	Innervated by PIN	Extensor carpi ulnaris	Extension of the wrist.
		Extensor digitorum communis	Extension of the index, middle, ring and little fingers' MCPJs. Extension at the DIPJ and PIPJ is also assisted by the lumbricals and the interossei muscles.
		Extensor digiti minimi	Extension of the little finger.
		Extensor indicis proprius	Extension of the index finger.
		Extensor pollicis brevis	Extension of the thumb at the MCPJ and CMCJ.
		Extensor pollicis longus	Extension of the thumb at the MCPJ, CMCJ and IPJ. Although the extensor pollicis brevis, attached to the extensor pollicis longus tendon, can extend the thumb's IPJ, only the extensor pollicis longus is capable to achieving full extension at that joint.
		Abductor pollicis longus	Abduction of thumb at the CMCJ.

Abbreviations: PIN, posterior interosseous nerve; MCPJ, metacarpophalangeal joint; PIPJ, proximal interphalangeal joint; DIPJ, distal interphalangeal joint; CMCJ, carpo-metacarpal joint; IPJ, interphalangeal joint.
*The ECRB has multiple anatomical variations to its innervating branch, which may originate from the radial nerve proper, the PIN, or the superficial branch itself.[1]

D. Sensory Function

The radial nerve supplies sensory innervation to the arm, forearm and hand. At the arm, the radial nerve sends off the lower lateral cutaneous nerve of the arm, posterior cutaneous nerve to the arm, and the posterior cutaneous nerve of the forearm. At the forearm, the nerve sends off the superficial branch, providing sensory innervation to the dorsolateral hand.

E. Clinical Examples

Focal lesions of the radial nerve may occur anywhere along its path, and the pattern of deficits can allow us to localise the lesion. Here, we discuss the clinical symptoms and signs of radial neuropathy at different sites.

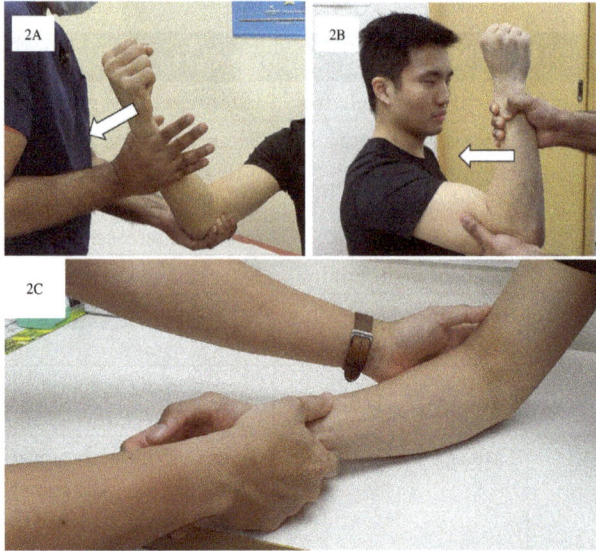

Figure 17.2.   The examination of the triceps brachii, brachioradialis, and supinator muscles are shown in 3A, 3B and 3C, respectively. When assessing the brachioradialis (2B), the patient is instructed to flex the elbow with his or her forearm in mid-pronation (neutral position). To test the supinator, place the elbow in extension with the forearm in mid-pronation and instruct the patient to supinate against resistance. Extension at the elbow is necessary when testing the supinator muscle, as the biceps brachii muscle is the primary supinator when the elbow is flexed.

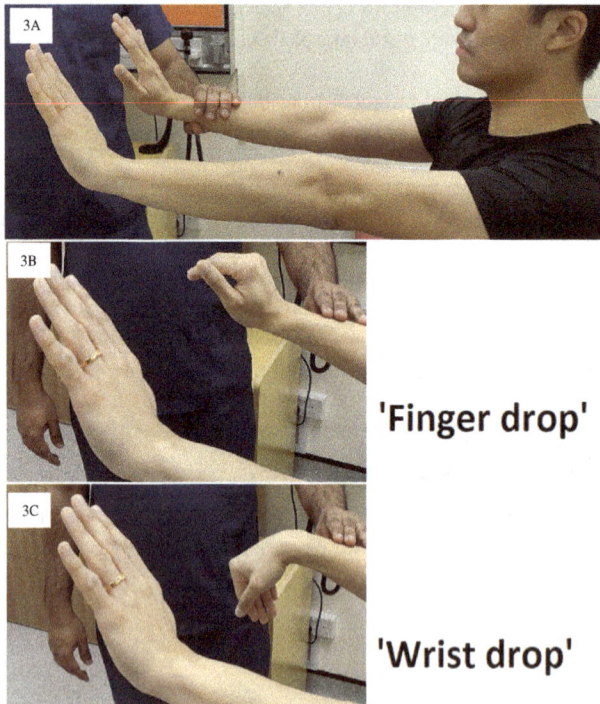

'Finger drop'

'Wrist drop'

Figure 17.3.   The radial nerve's integrity may be easily screened by having the patient extend the fingers and wrists as shown in 3A. Weakness of the finger or wrist extensors may result in "finger drop" or "wrist drop", respectively. However, these signs are not limited to radial neuropathy, and may be seen in other pathologies such as Guillain-Barré syndrome.[2]

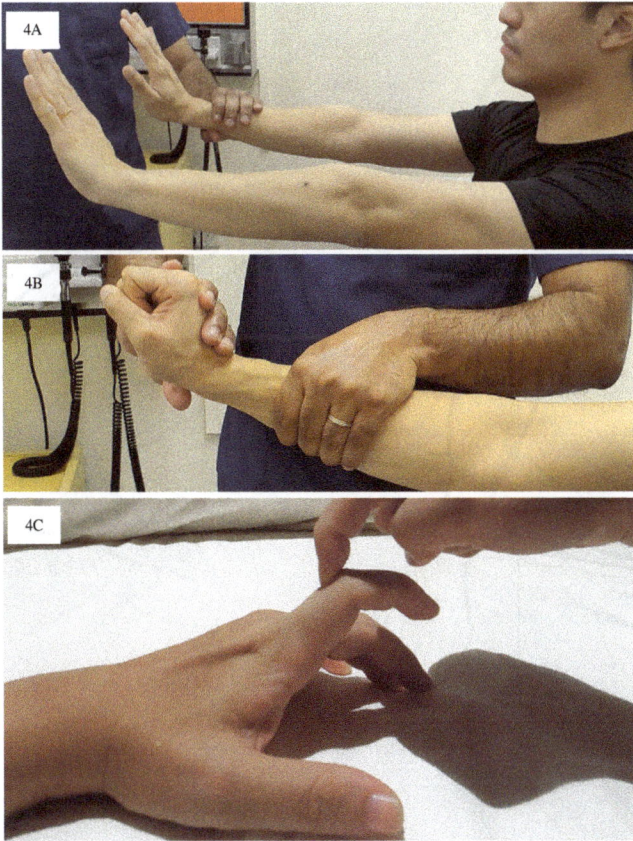

Figure 17.4. The assessment of the wrist extensors is shown in 4A and 4B, while the testing of finger extensors (in this case, the index finger) is shown in 4C.

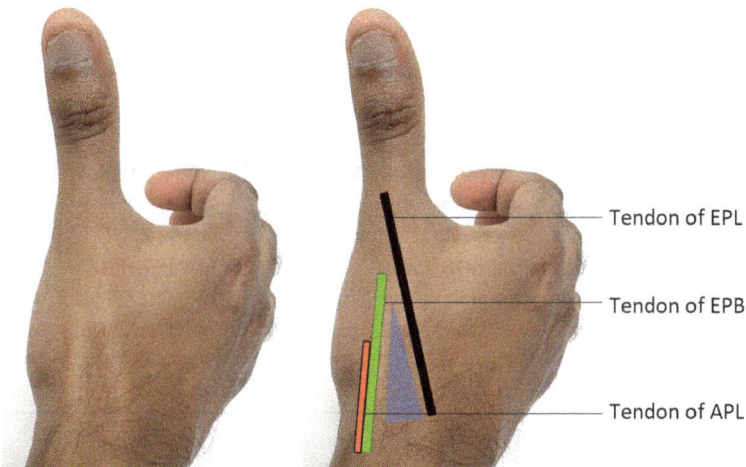

Tendon of EPL

Tendon of EPB

Tendon of APL

Figure 17.5. The anatomical snuff box (shaded blue) is bordered by the tendons of the extensor pollicis longus (EPL), extensor pollicis brevis (EPB), and abductor pollicis longus (APL) muscles. These muscles are innervated by the posterior interosseous nerve (PIN).

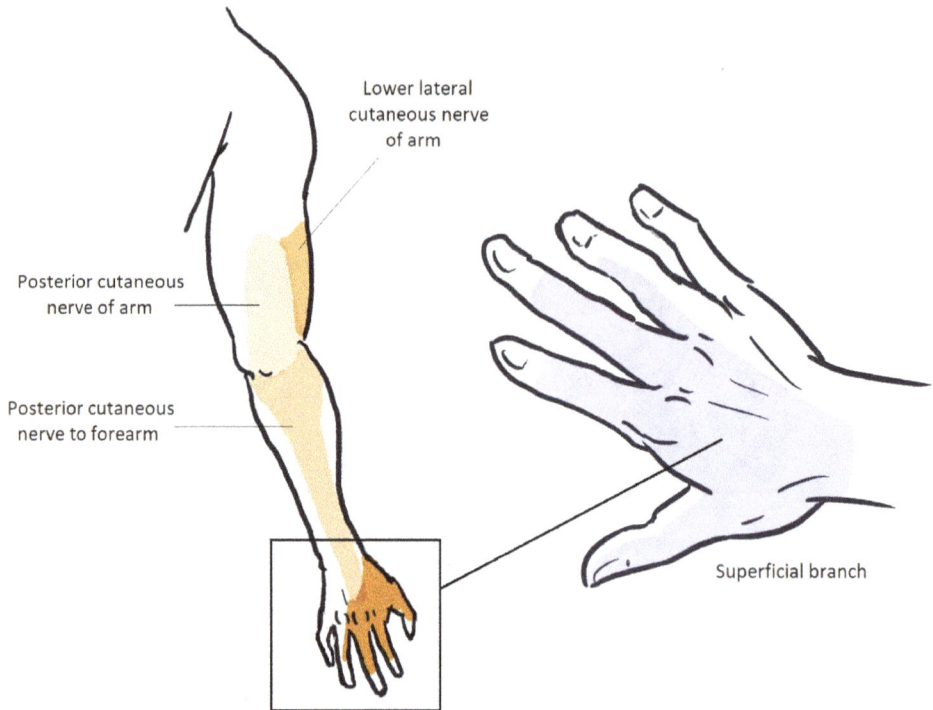

Figure 17.6.   The sensory territories of the radial nerve and its branches.

Site of Disease	Description of Signs and Symptoms	Diagnosis
Axilla	**Motor:** • Weak elbow extension due to weakness of the triceps brachii • Weak flexion of the elbow, when half-pronated, due to weakness of the brachioradialis • "Wrist drop" due to weakness of the wrist extensors (ECU, ECRL, ECRB) • Finger drop due to weakness of the finger extensors (EDC, EIP, EDM) • Thumb extension weakness, with impairment of thumb abduction, due to weakness of the thumb extensors (EPB, EPL) and the APL respectively	The clinical symptoms and signs point to a proximal lesion, at least above the spiral groove. This is reflected by the involvement of the proximal branches. It is pertinent to examine the deltoids as well. Concomitant weakness of shoulder abduction may be indicative of simultaneous axillary neuropathy, which when present is suggestive of a lesion at the posterior cord of the brachial plexus.

(Continued)

Site of Disease	Description of Signs and Symptoms	Diagnosis
	Sensory: • Numbness over the lower lateral arm, the posterior arm, the posterior forearm, and the dorsolateral hand (Figure 17.6). **Others:** • "Wrist drop" (see above) • "Finger drop" (see above)	
Arm	**Motor:** The pattern of weakness is nearly similar to that of a lesion at the axilla. Where they differ, however, is the extent of weakness in the triceps brachii muscles. Because the branches to the lateral and long heads depart before the spiral groove, lesions within the groove can thus result in milder elbow extension weakness when compared to lesions above the spiral groove. **Sensory:** The pattern of numbness may be similar to that of a lesion at the axilla. However, the posterior cutaneous nerve of the arm branches proximal to the spiral groove and may thus be spared in lesions within the groove. **Others:** • "Wrist drop" sign • "Finger drop" sign	The radial nerve is wound tightly around the humerus within the spinal groove and is thus vulnerable to damage from **fractures of the humeral shaft** and extrinsic compression against the bone. The term "Saturday night palsy" refers to a compressive radial neuropathy due to extrinsic pressure over the medial arm, pressing the radial nerve against the humerus. This historically involves an intoxicated person resting his arm against a hard surface.[3]
Forearm	There are two noteworthy clinical syndromes at the forearm: 1. PIN syndrome 2. Wartenberg's syndrome, or cheiralgia paresthetica **PIN syndrome** (supinator syndrome) describes the clinical symptoms and signs caused by palsy of the posterior interosseous nerve. Far rarer than carpal tunnel syndrome, PIN syndrome results in weakness in finger extension (at the MCPJ) and thumb extension due to involvement of the EDC, EIP, EDM, EPL and EPB. Thumb abduction and wrist extension may be less weak despite the involvement of the APL and ECU, due to sparing of the APB (innervated by the median nerve) and the ECR (branches to the ECRB and ECRL are proximal to the PIN). Therefore, the "wrist drop" sign is absent in PIN syndrome, although radial	

(Continued)

(Continued)

Site of Disease	Description of Signs and Symptoms	Diagnosis
	deviation of the wrist may be observed when wrist extension is attempted. The commonest site of compression is at the arcade of Frohse, formed by the proximal edge of the supinator muscle. **Wartenberg's syndrome** refers to the clinical symptoms and signs in a patient with disease of the superficial branch of the radial nerve. As this is a sensory nerve, the patient will experience sensory deficits over the dorsolateral aspect of the hand. Because of its superficial position, it is vulnerable to extrinsic compression at the wrist and forearm, and the patient may report a history of prior trauma to that area (e.g., tight handcuffs, watches, wrist bands, etc.).	

F. Something Extra: Differentiating Cortical Hand from Palsy of the Radial Nerve

Wrist extension weakness leading to a "wrist drop" may be due to peripheral (e.g., radial nerve palsy) and central causes (e.g., ischemic strokes). In the case of an ischemic stroke, infarction of the hand area on the motor cortex's homunculus can result in isolated hand weakness ("cortical hand") leading to a "wrist drop". To differentiate between central and peripheral causes, instruct the patient to make a fist. A normal wrist will be kept in a neutral position due to the synkinetic contraction of both the wrist extensors and flexors. In radial nerve palsy, the "wrist drop" worsens when making a fist. This is due to the wrist and flexors being left unopposed as the synkinetic contraction of the wrist extensors is lost. On the contrary, synkinetic contraction in the case of a central wrist drop is preserved despite the weakened wrist extensors, resulting in a slight elevation of the fist at the wrist.[4]

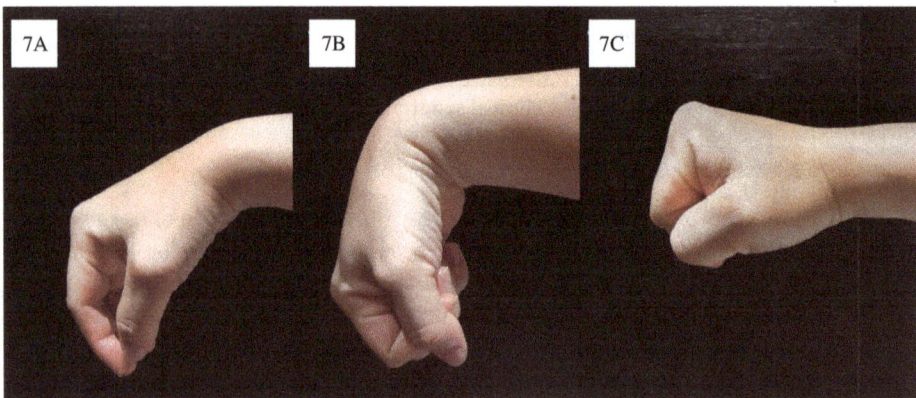

Figure 17.7.   When "wrist drop" (7A) occurs due to a peripheral cause such as radial nerve palsy, the "wrist drop" worsens when the patient attempts to make a fist (7B). A central "wrist drop" due to cerebral lesions (e.g., ischemic strokes — "cortical hand"), however, displays improvement of the "wrist drop" when attempting the same manoeuvre (7C).

Quick Reference	
Spinal roots	C5-T1
Motor function	The radial nerve innervates the extensors and flexors of the elbow as well as the extensors of the wrist, fingers, and thumb.
Sensory function	The radial nerve provides sensory innervation over the posterior and lower lateral aspects of the arm, the posterior forearm, and the dorsolateral aspect of the hand.

References

1. Abrams RA, Ziets RJ, Lieber RL, Botte MJ. (1997) Anatomy of the radial nerve motor branches in the forearm. *J Hand Surg Am* **22**(2): 232–237.
2. Chee YC, Ong BH. (2018) Finger drop sign — Characteristic pattern of distal weakness in Guillain-Barré Syndrome: A case report and review of the literature. *SAGE Open Med Case Rep* **6**: 2050313X18773649.
3. Ansari FH, Huergens AL. (2020) *Saturday Night Palsy*. StatPearls Publishing, Treasure Island.
4. Brigo F, Ragnedda G, Canu P, Nardone R. (2018) Synkinetic wrist in distinguishing cortical hand from radial nerve palsy. *Pract Neurol* **18**(6): 520–521.

18

Approach to a Patient with Parkinsonism

A. Introduction

The features of parkinsonism may be elicited through clinical history and neurologic examination. Although Parkinson's disease (PD) is the commonest cause, the list of differential diagnoses remains lengthy, such as other neurodegenerative disorders (e.g., the "Parkinson-plus syndrome" group of disorders), structural brain lesions (e.g., cerebrovascular disease, post-traumatic brain injury, etc.), and secondary causes (e.g., neuroleptic medications). It is thus crucial to have a systematic approach to a patient with parkinsonism.

B. 3-Step Approach

The approach may be broadly divided into 3 steps, similar to those described in the United Kingdom Parkinson's Disease Society Brain Bank (UKPDSBB) diagnostic criteria for Parkinson's disease.

Steps	Description	Comments
Step 1	Clinical features of parkinsonism	This initial step is to assess for the clinical features of parkinsonism. Bradykinesia and one or more of the following: • Muscular rigidity • 4-6Hz rest tremors • Postural instability not caused by primary visual, cerebellar, vestibular, or proprioceptive dysfunction **Bradykinesia** is the essential prerequisite for the diagnosis of parkinsonism. It is typically described as a progressive decline in speed and amplitude of quick and repetitive movements and may be demonstrated by asking the patient to rapidly and widely unclench and clench the hands or to tap the thumb and index fingers (Figure 18.2).

(Continued)

(Continued)

Steps	Description	Comments
		Muscular rigidity is a type of hypertonia that is characteristically independent of the velocity of the stretching force, a vital quality which can help to differentiate true rigidity from spasticity. Patients with parkinsonism may display rigidity over the appendicular and/or axial regions. Rigidity may be accentuated by voluntary movement of other body regions (Froment's manoeuvre) and may display a cog-wheel quality ("**cog-wheel rigidity**") when concomitant resting tremors are present.
		Asymmetrical **rest tremors** are classically described in PD and observed as involuntary rhythmic (4–6 Hz) oscillatory movements of varying amplitudes affecting a relaxed limb. These tremors attenuate with active movement, but can reappear with the arms outstretched after a delay of a few seconds (**re-emergent tremors**).[1] **The pill-rolling tremor** is perhaps the best known variant (thumb-flexion tremor whilst in contact with the other fingers, as though trying to roll a pill), although other variants have been described, such as flexion-extension of the fingers, tremors of the lower limbs, and those of the jaw.[1]
		Postural instability may be present due to the loss of postural reflexes. The "pull test" may be performed to demonstrate postural instability. After explaining the test to the patient, exert a pulling force on the patient's shoulders whilst standing behind him or her, allowing the patient to step back to regain balance. Patients with postural instability will likely fall without evident postural responses.
Step 2	"Red flags"	This step aims to look for clinical features that are unusual for PD, but are strongly suggestive of atypical causes of parkinsonism. The list of said features is lengthy and multifarious, but can be better remembered when grouped into the following categories: A. Neurodegenerative disorders B. Structural brain lesions C. Metabolic/endocrinologic disorders D. Drug-induced causes
		A. Neurodegenerative disorders: many diseases fall into this group, but this chapter will focus on diseases that are more pertinent to a non-neurologist. Rarer disorders such as spinocerebellar ataxias (SCAs) and dentate-rubro-pallido-luysian atrophy (DRPLA) will not be discussed here.

(Continued)

Steps	Description	Comments	

		Diseases	"Red Flags"[1,2]
		Corticobasal degeneration syndrome (CBS)[3]	Myoclonus Dystonia Alien hand Cortical sensory disturbances Motor apraxia
		Progressive supranuclear palsy (PSP)	Rapid progression Supranuclear gaze palsy Apathy, disinhibition Motor impulsivity Early falls Axial > appendicular rigidity Axial dystonia Motor apraxia
		Multiple system atrophy (MSA) • Parkinsonism (MSA-p) • Cerebellar (MSA-c)	Rapid progression Cerebellar signs Early severe autonomic dysfunction Dysphonia Orofacial, cervical, or axial dystonia Pyramidal involvement Nocturnal inspiratory stridor
		Dementia with Lewy bodies (DLB)[4]	Early/profound levodopa intolerance Early/profound cognitive dysfunction Visual hallucinations

B. Structural brain lesions

Diseases	"Red Flags"[2]
Cerebrovascular disease	History of repeated strokes Stepwise progression of parkinsonism
Post-traumatic, post-encephalitic, post-anoxic	History of repeated head trauma (dementia pugilistica) History of encephalitis History of prior hypoxic/anoxic brain injury
Toxic exposure	History of exposure to 1-methyl-4-phenyl-1,2,3,6-tetrahydropyridine (MPTP), cyanide, carbon monoxide, mercury, methanol, and manganese.
Intracranial tumours	Presence of cerebral tumours on brain imaging studies

(Continued)

(Continued)

Steps	Description	Comments
		C. Metabolic/endocrinologic disorders: common disorders include hypothyroidism and hypoparathyroidism, while rarer disorders include Wilson's disease, Huntington's disease, and Gaucher's diseases, to name a few. Focusing on the more frequent causes, it is important to ask for accompanying symptoms of **hypothyroidism** (i.e., cold intolerance, weight gain, loss of appetite, etc.) and **hypoparathyroidism** (i.e., paraesthesia of the peripheries, facial twitching, muscle cramps, etc.).[2]
		D. Drug-induced: medications can cause parkinsonism by antagonising the dopaminergic pathways of the central nervous system. Notorious groups of medications include:

Drug Class	Medications
Antipsychotics	Typical antipsychotics such as **haloperidol and chlorpromazine** harbour significant potential to cause drug-induced parkinsonism. The risk of extrapyramidal side effects is thought to be lower for atypical antipsychotics.
Anti-emetics	Metoclopromide
Calcium channel blockers	Flunarizine Cinnarizine Verapamil
Antiepileptic medications	Valproic acid
Others	Lithium

Steps	Description	Comments
Step 3	Features supportive of PD	The following features are supportive of PD, of which three or more are required to make a definite diagnosis of PD based on the UKPDSBB criteria:

Clinical symptoms, signs, and features	• Unilateral onset • Persistent asymmetry, affecting the side of onset more severely • Rest tremors present • Progressive disorder • Clinical course of 10 years or more
Levodopa-associated features	• Excellent response (70–100%) to levodopa • Levodopa response for 5 years or more • Severe levodopa-induced chorea

C. Parkinson's Disease

PD is one of the commonest neurodegenerative disorders, second only to Alzheimer's disease. A type of α-synucleinopathy, it is characterised by the typical features of parkinsonism due to dopaminergic denervation of the *substantia nigra pas compacta*. Intraneuronal Lewy bodies are typical pathologic findings. Although the cause of PD remains unknown, age remains a significant risk factor for sporadic PD, and the disease's prevalence is expected to increase in Singapore as the population continues to age. Motor features of PD are well-known to most, but non-motor features are increasingly recognised, each fully capable of significantly impairing the patient's quality of life. The clinical severity is described using the modified Hoehn and Yahr scale.[5]

Motor Features	Non-motor Features
Bradykinesia Muscular rigidity Rest tremors, 4–6 Hz Postural instability	**Neuropsychiatric features:** • Cognitive impairment • Anxiety • Depression • Psychosis (illusions, hallucinations, delusions) **Autonomic dysfunction** **Disorders of sleep:** • Insomnia • REM behaviour disorder • Excessive daytime sleepiness • Restless leg syndrome • Periodic leg movement **Sensory dysfunction** • Hyposmia • Paraesthesia • Decreased visual motion perception, visual contrast, color discrimination **Pain and fatigue**
Additional Comments	
The gait in PD is distinctive and readily recognisable. Early abnormalities include **slowing of speed**, **stooped posture**, and asymmetrically **decreased arm swing**. As the disease progresses, the length of stride and the step height become increasingly smaller, and **hesitation**, **festination** and **freezing** (inability to start walking, or sudden failure to continue forward whilst walking) can develop. A common mistake amongst medical students is the use of the term "festination" to describe freezing episodes, when it actually describes the increasingly rapid and small steps when the patient walks. Notably, the **gait remains narrow** even in advanced stages of PD. A patient with parkinsonism who walks with a broad-based gait should lead one to consider the atypical causes.[2]	

(Continued)

(Continued)

Modified Hoehn and Yahr (HY) Scale[5]
1.0: Unilateral involvement only
1.5: Unilateral and axial involvement
2.0: Bilateral involvement without impairment of balance
2.5: Mild bilateral disease with recovery on pull test
3.0: Mild to moderate bilateral disease; some postural instability but physically independent
4.0: Severe disability but still able to walk or stand unassisted
5.0: Wheelchair bound or bedridden unless aided
A simpler way to remember the modified HY scale is to note the following clinical "checkpoints":
• **A score of 2** is given when there are parkinsonian features **bilaterally**.
• **A score of 3** is given when **postural instability** is present.
• **A score of 5** is given when **mobility aids** are required.

The diagnosis of PD is largely based on the patient's clinical history and findings. Blood tests are rarely done beyond a serum thyroid panel. Depending on the likelihood, additional tests such as serum caeruloplasmin and 24H urinary copper levels may be appropriate when Wilson's disease is suspected. Genetic tests may be useful when heredodegenerative disorders are suspected. Although infrequent, hereditary forms of PD (i.e., autosomal-dominant PD, autosomal-recessive PD) should be suspected in young patients (<40 years old) with a family history of PD, for which genetic tests will be appropriate. Brain-imaging studies are seldom required unless features of atypical parkinsonism are present.

Being a chronic progressive disorder with significant potential for disability, a multidisciplinary approach is vital. **Levodopa-based medications** are the mainstay in managing the motor symptoms, although **dopamine agonists** (ergot and non-ergot derivatives), selective monoamine oxidase B inhibitors (**MAO-B-I**), catechol-O-methyltransferase inhibitors (**COMTI**), **anticholinergics**, and **amantandine** are regularly used, each with their own unique risk-benefit profile. Finally, **deep brain stimulation** is an effective but invasive procedure to control motor symptoms, especially in patients with advanced PD.[1]

D. Atypical Parkinsonism

Distinguishing PD from other causes of parkinsonism is quintessential component when assessing a parkinsonian patient. The need to identify the "Parkinson-plus syndromes" (PPS) is relevant for the following reasons:

The Need to Know	Clinical Implications	Treatment Implications	Prognostic Implications

The patient should know about his or her diagnosis.	Different causes of PPS have unique clinical complications:
	• MSA
	  o Dysautonomia
	  o Stridor
	• PSP
	  o Supranuclear gaze palsies
	  o Motor recklessness
	• DLB
	  o Visual hallucinations
		PD medications are generally less effective in patients with PPS.	Disease progression of PPS is generally faster than that of PD.

In this chapter, we will selectively discuss **CBS**, **PSP**, **MSA** and **DLB** in greater detail. Typical features of Magnetic Resonance Imaging (MRI) scans are shown in Figure 18.1.

	CBS[3]	PSP[7,8]
Pathogenesis	Tauopathy	Tauopathy
Age of onset (y)	60s	60s
Pattern of signs	Asymmetrical	Symmetrical
Atypical features	**Motor features:** • Akinetic-rigid syndrome • Dystonia • Focal or segmental myoclonus **Cortical sensorimotor features:** • Limb apraxia • Alien limb phenomenon • Orobuccal apraxia • Cortical sensory loss **Cognitive features:** • Dysphasia (usually non-fluent) • Frontal executive dysfunction • Visuospatial deficits	**Ocular motor dysfunction** • Supranuclear gaze palsy: vertical saccades are affected first* **Postural instability:** • Repeated falls early (within 3 years) of the disease **Akinesia:** • Early progressive gait freezing (within 3 years) • Predominantly axial akinetic-rigid parkinsonism **Cognitive dysfunction:** • Non-fluent or agrammatic variant of primary progressive aphasia • Progressive apraxia of speech • Frontal cognitive-behavioral abnormality

(Continued)

(Continued)

	CBS[3]	PSP[7,8]

		Others:
		• Dystonia
		  ○ Orofacial
		  ○ Axial
		  ○ Cervical (retrocollis)
		• Procerus sign
		
		Falling early is a prominent feature in patients with PSP. This is likely due to a combination of factors:
		• Early freezing and prominent postural instability
		• Axial rigidity, axio-cervical dystonia
		• Supranuclear gaze palsy
		• Motor recklessness

Response to dopaminergic medications	Generally poor response	Generally poor response
Progression and prognosis	Insidious onset Average survival at 7 years[3]	Rapid progression
Imaging features	Typical MRI findings include:[6] • Asymmetric **cortical atrophy**, especially over the superior parietal lobule, peri-Rolandic gyri, superior frontal gyri • Bilateral basal ganglia atrophy • Atrophy of corpus callosum	Reflecting **atrophy of the midbrain** (amongst other regions), the typical features on the MRI include the "**hummingbird**" and "**morning glory**" signs.

*While there is no dispute that the impairment of vertical saccades in PSP is both early and profound, whether up or downgaze (or both) is affected more severely remains controversial. A large retrospective study of PSP patients found no significant differences in limitations of saccadic speed and range in both up and downgaze, running contrary to older reports which emphasised predominant downgaze palsy in PSP patients.[7,8] The authors opined that the presence of biomechanical changes in the orbital fascia limiting upgaze in otherwise healthy elderly patients (Blickerschwernis) complicates the clinical assessment of gaze in PSP patients, driving the belief that downgaze is more severely affected.[7]

	MSA (MSA-p and MSA-c)	DLB
Pathogenesis	α-synucleinopathy	α-synucleinopathy
Age of onset (y)	55–60	>50
Pattern of signs	Symmetrical	Symmetrical

(*Continued*)

	MSA (MSA-p and MSA-c)	DLB
Atypical features	**Autonomic dysfunction:** • Orthostatic hypotension • Urinary incontinence • Erectile dysfunction (ED) (prominent early feature in males) **Parkinsonism** **Cerebellar dysfunction** **Corticospinal tract dysfunction** **Other features:** • Orofacial dystonia • Cervical dystonia (antecollis) • Axial dystonia (camptocormia, Pisa syndrome) • Vocal cord paralysis, causing high-pitched inspiratory stridor • REM sleep behavioral disorder (RBD) • Sleep apnea syndrome	**Early, profound and progressive cognitive decline**, plus the following features: • Fluctuating cognition with variations in attention and alertness • Well-formed and detailed visual hallucinations • Parkinsonism • RBD • Severe neuroleptic sensitivity
Response to dopaminergic treatment	One third show partial but unsustained response[2]	Early and profound intolerance
Progression and prognosis	Rapid progression	The average survival is about 8 years after diagnosis[4]
Imaging features (Figure 18.1)	MRI: the **"hot cross bun"** sign is associated with MSA-c, while the **putaminal rim sign** is associated with MSA-p.	MRI: Generalised cerebral atrophy, especially of the frontal and parietotemporal lobes, with focal atrophy of the midbrain and hypothalamus.

E. Examination of a Patient with Parkinsonism — the "Parkinsonian Dance"

This segment aims to augment candidates' examination techniques for the undergraduate and postgraduate medical examinations, with appreciation of the time limitations artificially imposed onto them. The candidates will likely be asked to examine the upper limbs of a patient with parkinsonism. Thus, we will concentrate on the additional steps needed when examining a patient with parkinsonism, on top of those already encompassed in the routine neurologic assessment of the upper limbs. The format described below are by no means doctrinal and may be modified to suit your practice. Because most undergraduate examinations evaluate their

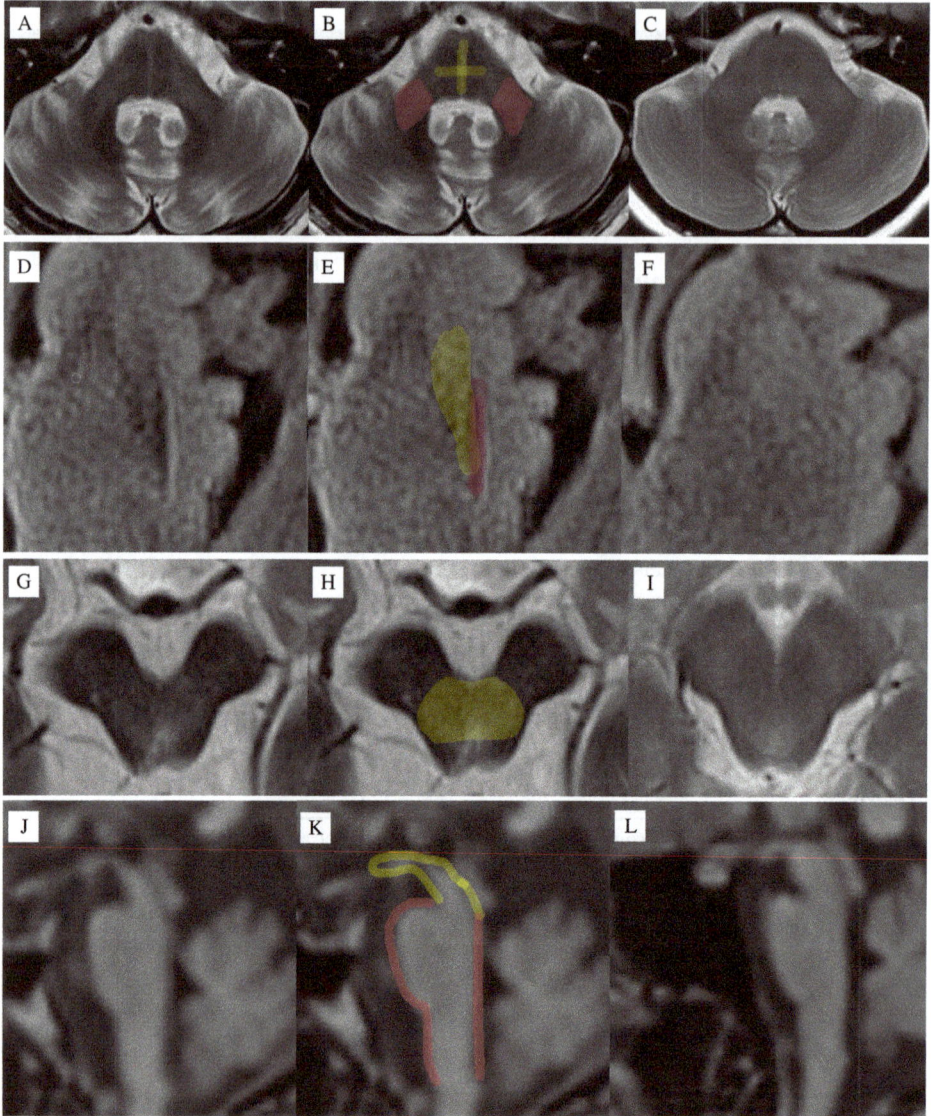

Figure 18.1.   MRI brain images of patients with MSA-c (A–C), MSA-p (D–F), and PSP (G–L). A: Axial T2-weighted (T2-W) sequences of the pons, showing the cruciform pontine T2-hyperintense abnormality (also known as the "hot cross bun" sign). B: The "hot cross bun" is coloured yellow, while the accompanying symmetric T2-W signal abnormalities seen in bilateral middle cerebellar peduncles are coloured red. C: A normal pons is shown here for comparison. D: Axial T2-W sequences (1.5T MRI) of the left lentiform nucleus, showing a linear region of T2 hyperintense abnormality over the lateral aspect of the left putamen (putaminal rim sign). E: The putaminal rim sign is coloured red, while the additional findings of a relatively hypointense putamen compared to the globus pallidus is coloured yellow. F: A normal left lentiform nucleus is shown here for comparison. The putamen is normally more hyperintense than the globus pallidus on T2-W sequences. G: Axial T2-W sequences of the midbrain showing significant midbrain atrophy, with loss of the lateral convexity of the tegmentum, giving it an appearance of a morning glory (PSP's "morning glory" sign). H: The atrophic midbrain is coloured yellow. I: A normal midbrain is shown here for comparison. J: Sagittal T2-W sequences of the brainstem showing significant midbrain atrophy, with flattening and thinning of the midbrain, giving it an appearance similar to the hummingbird's long beak and small head (PSP's "hummingbird" sign). K: The atrophied midbrain (head of the hummingbird) and the beak are coloured yellow, while the normal pons (belly of the bird) is coloured red. L: A normal midbrain is shown here for comparison.

students against a checklist, the student may therefore be required to sequentially complete the routine examination steps when examining the upper limbs, before proceeding to the targeted components pertinent to the assessment of patients with parkinsonism.

	Steps	What to Look Out for?	Comments

ROUTINE	Inspection	• Hypomimia, with decreased eye blink
		• Hypophonia
		• Sitting or standing posture
		  o Stooped posture
		  o Antecollis/retrollis
		  o Camptocormia, "Pisa" sign
		• Rest tremors
		• Spontaneous eye movement
		• Functional aids
		  o Mobility aids
		  o Nasogastric tube
		  o Indwelling catheter, etc.
			Diminished eye-blink may provide the first clue. A PD patient's blink rate is at 4–12 blinks/min, far lower than normal (>24 blinks/min).[9]
			
			Rest tremors are better observed with the patient distracted but fully relaxed.

	Tone	• Appendicular rigidity, with or without cog-wheel quality	Distraction (Froment's manoeuvre) may be helpful in eliciting subtle rigidity.
	Deep tendon reflexes, power, and sensation to pinprick are usually preserved and normal in PD.		The presence of brisk reflexes and a pyramidal pattern of weakness suggest another diagnosis other than PD, or that a concomitant upper motor neuron pathology is present.

	Cerebellar	• Cerebellar dysfunction
		  o Dysmetria
		  o Dysdiadochokinesia
			The presence of bilateral cerebellar deficits is atypical for PD, and may suggest a diagnosis of MSA-c.

ADDITIONAL	Rapidly alternating movements (Figure 18.2)	• Bradykinesia o Progressive decline in speed and amplitude of quick and repetitive movements	Bradykinesia is an essential component in the 3-step approach and should thus be properly demonstrated (Figure 18.2).
	Ocular movement (Figure 18.3)	• Impairment of voluntary saccades • Doll's manoeuvre, when appropriate	This step aims to demonstrate the ocular features of PSP. If ocular movements are limited, **Doll's manoeuvre must be performed**. Due to the supranuclear pathology in PSP, ocular movements are relatively preserved during Doll's manoeuvre.

(Continued)

(Continued)

Steps	What to Look Out for?	Comments
Motor apraxia (Figure 18.4)	• Pantomime of meaningful gestures • Pantomime of tool use	This step aims to demonstrate the various motor apraxias, which when present are suggestive of PPS (PSP and CBS). This may be demonstrated by having the patient perform gestures with their hands or mimic the hand actions required when manipulating tools (Figure 18.3).
Gait	• Posture • Width of the gait • Step height and stride length • Hesitation, festination, freezing	A PD patient typically adopts a stooped posture with asymmetrically diminished arm swing. His gait is narrow and shuffling.
Requests	N/A	At the end of your examination, request for the following: 1. Vital parameters 2. Postural blood pressure measurements 3. Medication chart

Additional Comments

Dressing apraxia tests the integrity of tactile and visuospatial coordination, rather than the inability to use tools. The culprit lesion usually lies in the right parietal lobe. I have observed medical trainees test for dressing apraxia by having the patient undo and redo the first button on his or her shirt. This is erroneous, and the proper assessment involves more complex processes, such as having the patient wear a shirt with the sleeves deliberately turned inside out.[10]

A positive glabellar tap (Myerson's sign) is observed when the patient cannot resist blinking when tapped repeatedly on the glabella. Although seen in early PD, this sign is poorly specific for the disease, and may be seen in other dementia syndromes. As such, it has limited utility when assessing a patient with parkinsonism.[11]

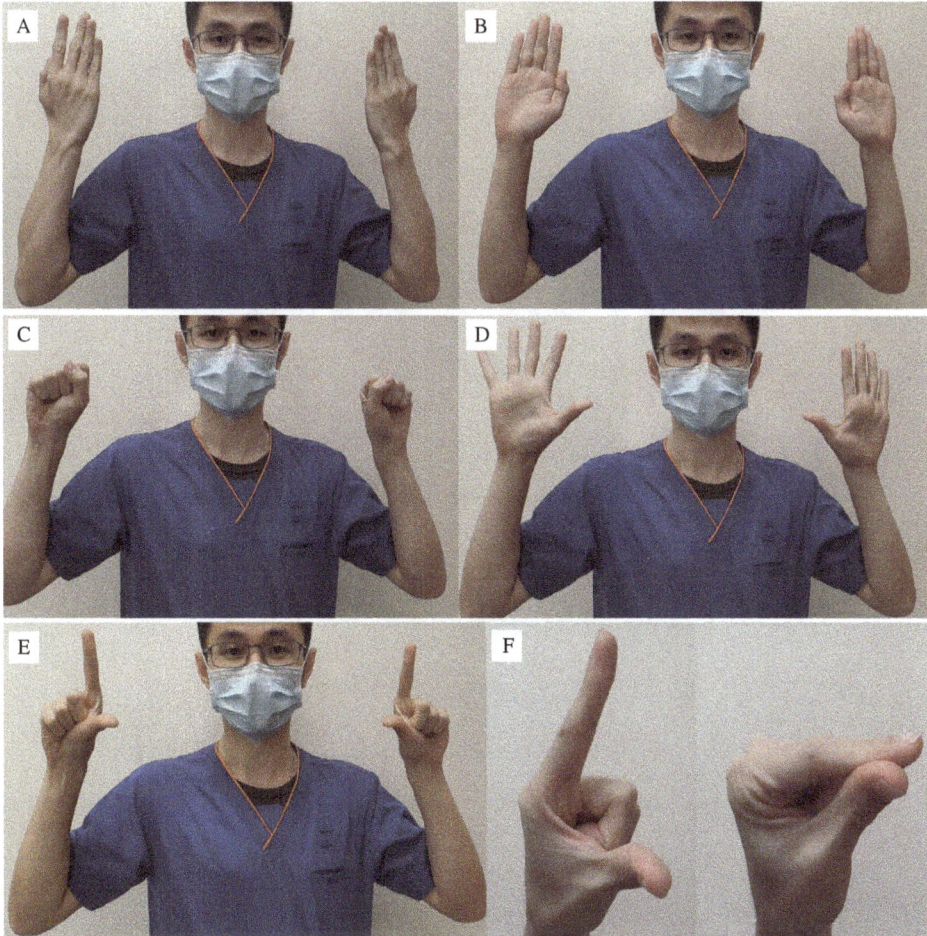

Figure 18.2. Bradykinesia may be demonstrated through rapidly alternating movements. A–B: twisting of the hands; C–D: rapid opening and closing of the fists; E–F: finger tapping or pinching. Observe for progressive decline of the speed and amplitude, which may be asymmetrical in patients with PD.

Tips for Examination Candidates

The first clue that your patient at the examination station has parkinsonism usually lies in the case vignette — "This patient has frequent falls. Examine his upper limbs." Why are you asked to examine the upper limbs when the intuitive thing to do is to examine the lower limbs? In such scenarios, observe for features of hypomimia hypophonia and bradykinesia during your initial interaction with the patient.

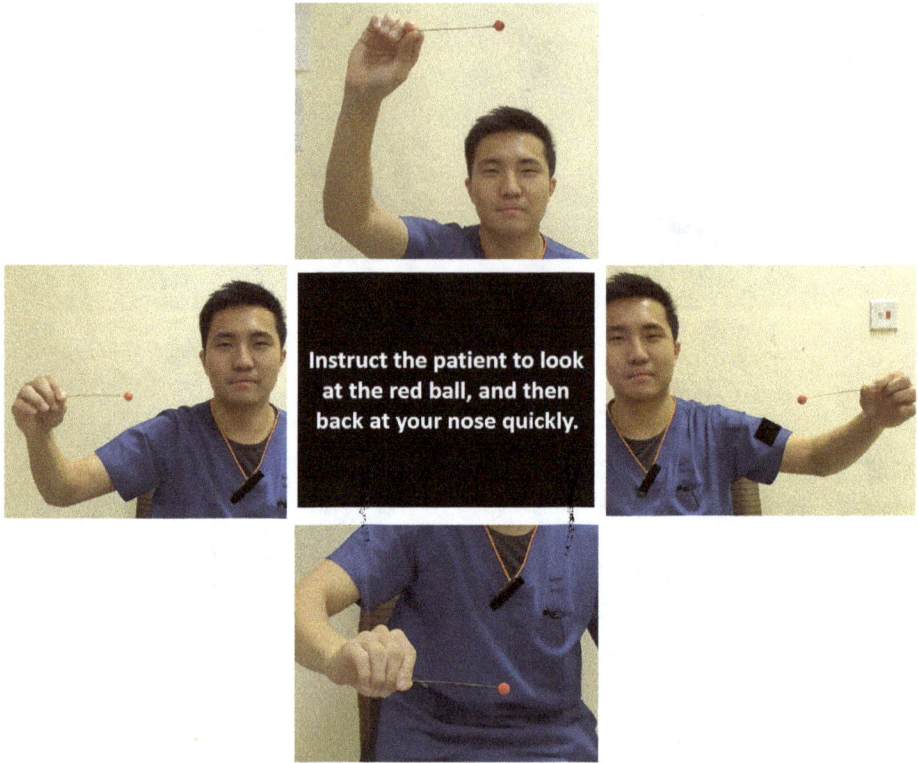

Figure 18.3.   Testing of saccades. Begin by having the patient fixate on your nose. Next, instruct the patient to quickly shift his or her gaze to the object of interest (a red hat pin is shown here), and then back to your nose. Repeat these steps along the vertical and horizontal axes.

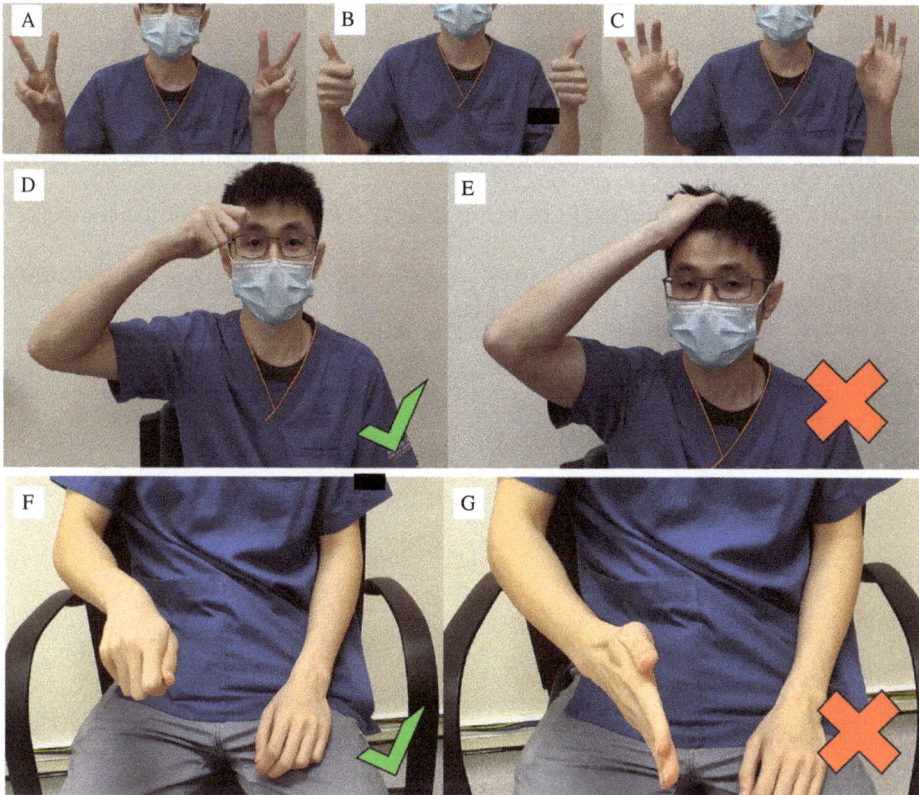

Figure 18.4. Assessment of limb apraxia using pantomime. A–C: Gestural pantomime may be tested using meaningful gestures such as the "victory" sign (A), the "thumbs up" (B), and the "okay" sign (C). D–G: Limb apraxia can also be tested through the demonstration of tool use (transitive pantomime), such as to comb one's hair with an imaginary comb (D) or to cut a cake with an imaginary knife (F). Patients with ideomotor apraxia may demonstrate "body-part-as-object" error (E and G).[12]

References

1. Massano J, Bhatia KP. (2012) Clinical approach to Parkinson's disease: features, diagnosis, and principles of management. *Cold Spring Harb Perspect Med* **2**(6): a008870.

2. Aerts MB, Esselink RA, Post B, van de Warrenburg BP, Bloem BR. (2012) Improving the diagnostic accuracy in parkinsonism: a three-pronged approach. *Pract Neurol* **12**(2): 77–87.

3. NINDS Corticobasal Degeneration Information Page. *National Institute of Neurological Disorders and Stroke.* February 6, 2015; https://www.ninds.nih.gov/disorders/all-disorders/corticobasal-degeneration-information-page.

4. Dementia with Lewy bodies information page. *National Institute of Neurological Disorders and Stroke.* March 27, 2019; Dementia-Lewy-Bodies-information-page.

5. Goetz CG, Poewe W, Rascol O, Sampaio C, Stebbins GT, Counsell C, Giladi N, Holloway RG, Moore CG, Wenning GK, Yahr MD, Seidl L. (2004) Movement Disorder Society Task Force report on the Hoehn and Yahr staging scale: status and recommendations. *Mov Disord* **19**(9): 1020–1028.

6. Tokumaru AM, O'uchi T, Kuru Y, Maki T, Murayama S, Horichi Y. (1996) Corticobasal degeneration: MR with histopathologic comparison. *Am J Neuroradiol* **17**(10): 1849–1852.

7. Chen AL, Riley DE, King SA, Joshi AC, Serra A, Liao K, Cohen ML, Otero-Millan J, Martinez-Conde S, Strupp M, Leigh RJ. (2010) The disturbance of gaze in progressive supranuclear palsy: implications for pathogenesis. *Front Neurol* **1**: 147.

8. Williams DR, Lees AJ, Wherrett JR, Steele JC. (2008) J. Clifford Richardson and 50 years of progressive supranuclear palsy. *Neurology* **70**(7): 566–573.

9. Karson CN, Burns RS, LeWitt PA, Foster NL, Newman RP. (1984) Blink rates and disorders of movement. *Neurology* **34**(5): 677–678.

10. Fitzgerald LK, McKelvey JR, Szeligo F. (2002) Mechanisms of dressing apraxia: a case study. *NNBN* **15**(2): 148–155.

11. Shah RC. (2010) Glabellar reflex. In: Kompoliti K, Metman LV (eds), *Encyclopedia of Movement Disorders*, pp. 549–550.

12. Goodglass H, Kaplan E. (1963) Disturbance of gesture and pantomime in aphasia. *Brain* **86**: 703–720.

19

Approach to the Patterns
of Weakness

A. Introduction

The patterns of weakness are important to recognise. Coupled with the character of weakness, i.e., upper (UMN) or lower motor neuron (LMN), the pattern of motor deficits can provide vital clinical clues. As this book aims to augment the neurologic foundations of non-neurologists, the esoteric and rarely encountered conditions will not be discussed in detail.

B. The Patterns of Weakness

This segment discusses the "geographical" patterns of weakness. Because of the significant neurolocalising implications behind each pattern, the terminologies should be carefully and eruditely used. There are four basic descriptors of weakness, depending on the extent of involvement — monoparesis, hemiparesis, tetraparesis and paraparesis (Figure 19.1). While not able to describe all the known patterns of weakness, they nevertheless provide a basic framework when presenting your clinical findings to a listener, and can help guide your neurolocalisation processes.

Monoparesis — Weakness of a limb

Hemiparesis — Weakness of one half of the body

Tetraparesis — Weakness of all four limbs

Paraparesis — Weakness of both legs

UMN weakness — **Proximal > distal**

LMN weakness — **Distal > proximal**

Mixed — **Proximal = distal**

UMN: upper motor neuron
LMN: lower motor neuron

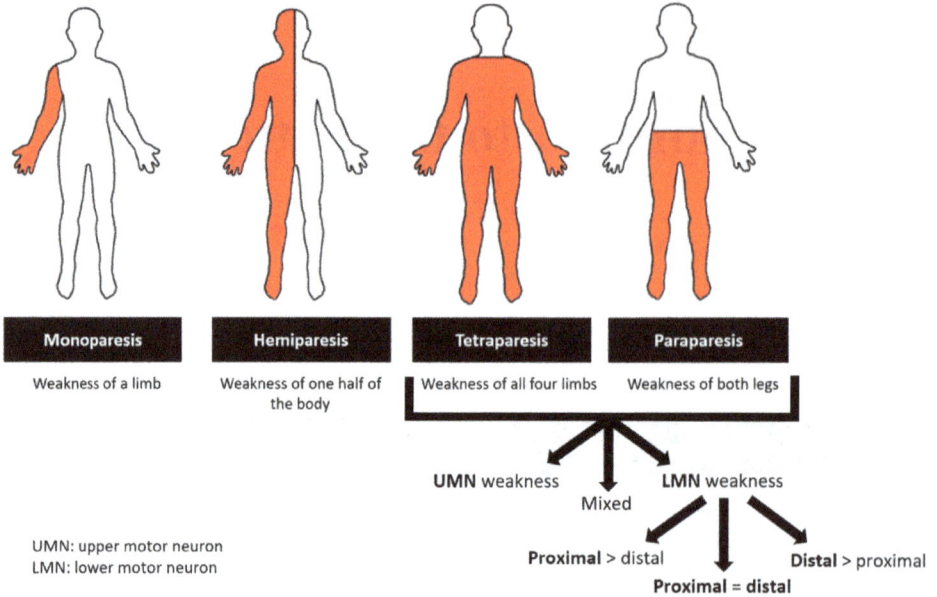

Figure 19.1.   Four main patterns of weakness — monoparesis, hemiparesis, tetraparesis and paraparesis. Within tetraparesis and paraparesis, the character of weakness (UMN vs. LMN) and its predilection for proximal or distal musculature have significant neurolocalising value.

Pattern of Weakness	Description and Localisation
 Monoparesis	**Monoparesis** describes weakness affecting **only one limb**. Common causes of focal weakness include: 1. Radiculopathies 2. Plexopathies 3. Neuropathies (single nerve or multiple nerves of the same limb) Roots ⎯ Plexus ⎯ Nerve Roots ⎯ Nerve Roots ⎯ Nerve However, generalised but asymmetric disease processes can also cause "monoparesis", especially during the early phases of the disease. Amyotrophic lateral sclerosis (ALS), for example, can present with monoparesis early in the disease, despite being a motor neuron disorder.[1,2] Of course, there are other diseases of the anterior horn cell that specifically cause monoparesis (e.g., Hirayama disease). Due to their rarity, they will not be discussed in this book.

(*Continued*)

Pattern of Weakness	Description and Localisation
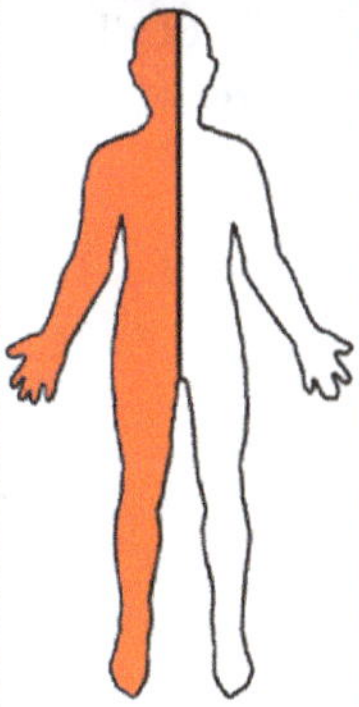 **Hemiparesis**	**Hemiparesis** describes weakness affecting **one half of the body**, and usually reflects an underlying UMN disease process. As such, the neurolocalisation of a hemiparetic patient is relatively simple, as the lesion likely lies within the following regions: 1. Contralateral cerebrum 2. Contralateral brainstem 3. Ipsilateral hemicord The UMN pattern of weakness, also known as the "pyramidal pattern", describes the relatively stronger flexors of the upper limbs and the extensors of the lower limbs when examined against their antagonistic muscles. Its presence indicates disease along the first-order neurons of the corticospinal tracts. 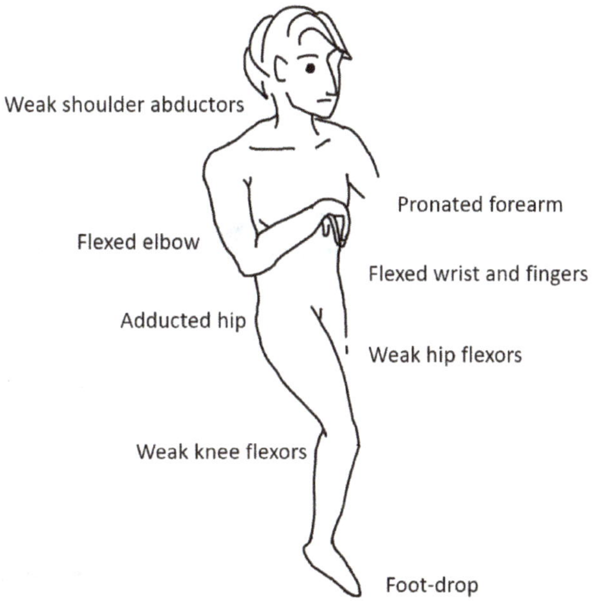 Figure 19.2. Posturing in a patient with right hemiparesis from a stroke. Common examples include hemiparesis from infarctions of the contralateral lentiform nucleus or the contralateral hemipons. Hemiparesis due to disease of the ipsilateral hemicord (e.g., Brown-Sequard syndrome) is comparatively rarer.

(*Continued*)

(Continued)

Pattern of Weakness	Description and Localisation
 Tetraparesis	**Tetraparesis**, also known as **quadriparesis**, describes weakness **of all four limbs** and may be further described based on the **character**, **symmetry** and predilection for **proximal** or **distal** musculature. Tetraparesis, when present, is usually suggestive of a diffuse disease process (e.g., muscular dystrophies, myasthenia gravis, etc.), although focal processes such as cervical myelopathies can also result in tetraparesis as well.

Tetraparesis	Examples

UMN	• **Cervical myelopathies:** likely to have co-existing sensory deficits.
	 ○ **Extramedullary**
	 ○ **Intramedullary**, inclusive of:
	  ▪ **Nutritional deficiencies** (subacute combined degeneration of the spinal cord)
	  ▪ **Demyelination of the central nervous system** (multiple sclerosis)
	  ▪ **Infections** (HSV, VZV, syphilis)
	  ▪ **Hereditary myelopathies** (hereditary spastic paraplegia, spinocerebellar ataxias)
	• **Primary lateral sclerosis:** without sensory deficits

Mixed	A mixed pattern likely implies concomitant UMN and LMN disease processes, e.g.: • Myeloradiculopathies • Syringomyelia • Amyotrophic lateral sclerosis

(Continued)

Pattern of Weakness	Description and Localisation	
	Tetraparesis	**Examples**
	LMN	Diseases causing LMN patterns of tetraparesis usually reside within one of the following four "levels", each with their own predilection for either proximal or distal musculature:

Pattern	Location of the Disease Process
Proximal > distal	Muscle Neuromuscular junction (NMJ)
Distal > proximal	Nerve Anterior horn cell (AHC)

Paraparesis describes weakness of both lower limbs. Certain generalised disease processes can cause paraparesis rather than diffuse weakness, especially during the early stages. Acute inflammatory demyelinating polyradiculoneuropathy (AIDP), for example, predominantly affects the lower limbs in the early stages of the disease, before progressing to the upper limbs as the disease progresses (ascending weakness).

Paraparesis

Tetraparesis	Examples

UMN	• Thoracic myelopathies
	  o Intramedullary diseases
	  o Extramedullary diseases
	• Parasagittal lesions

Mixed	There are many diseases that can result in mixed UMN and LMN features in a paraparetic patient. Patients with these conditions may display the odd combination of extensor plantar responses and absent ankle reflexes, and they may be remembered by a local mnemonic "**M**y **F**riend **C**an **S**ing **D**irty **T**rendy **S**ongs":[3] • Multiple sclerosis • Friedreich ataxia • Conus medullaris syndrome • Syringomyelia • Diabetes mellitus • Tabes dorsalis • Subacute combined degeneration of the spinal cord

(Continued)

Pattern of Weakness	Description and Localisation	
	Tetraparesis	**Examples**
	LMN	Diseases causing LMN patterns of paraparesis usually reside within one of the following four "levels", each with their own predilection for either proximal or distal musculature:

Pattern	Localisation
Proximal > distal	Muscle NMJ
Distal > proximal	Nerve AHC

C. Flaccid Weakness of Both Lower Limbs During an Examination: Localisation Principles

Patients with flaccid paraparesis are commonly encountered in clinical practice. However, the underlying causes are aplenty, varying from muscular disorders, to diseases of the anterior horn cell. Thankfully, there are a couple of ways to create order amidst a sea of chaos. Herein, we describe a method for use during the professional examinations when facing a patient with flaccid weakness of both legs:

- Step 1: Is there a "**sensory level**" pattern of sensory loss?
- Step 2: If there is no "sensory level" pattern of sensory loss, is the weakness predominantly **proximal** or **distal**?

In patients with bilateral flaccid weakness without a "sensory level" pattern of sensory deficits to pinprick, the lesion lies within one of these four structures, listed in order of their proximity to the spinal cord — AHC, neuron, NMJ, and muscle. Interestingly, diseases affecting the more "proximal" structures (AHC and neurons) tend to cause distal weakness, while those affecting the "distal structures" (NMJ and muscles) tend to cause proximal weakness. I will list a few examples:

Site of Disease Process		Weakness	Example(s) of Diseases/Diagnoses
Proximal	AHC	**Distal**	Motor neuron disease (e.g., ALS)
	Motor neuron		Multifocal motor neuropathy
Distal	NMJ	**Proximal**	Myasthenia gravis Lambert-Eaton myasthenic syndrome
	Muscle		(Most) inflammatory myopathies Corticosteroid-induced myopathy (Most) muscular dystrophies

Flaccid Weakness of the Lower Limbs

Without "sensory level" pattern of sensory loss

With "sensory level" pattern of sensory loss

Proximal Weakness (Usually)

Distal Weakness (Usually)

Muscle | Neuromuscular Junction (NMJ) | Peripheral Nerve (PN) | Anterior Horn Cell (AHC)

A few exceptions:

Muscle	NMJ	PN	AHC
Predominantly distal weakness: • Myotonic dystrophy • Distal myopathies • Inclusion body myositis (distal upper limb weakness)	N/A	Different patterns of weakness may be observed in different variants of AIDP and CIDP.	Predominantly proximal weakness: • Kennedy's disease • Spinal muscular atrophy

Additional helpful defining features:

Features	Muscle	NMJ	PN	AHC
Prominent wasting	Yes	No	Yes	Yes
Sensory deficits	No	No	Variable	No
Reflexes	Normal	Normal	Reduced	Variable, dependent on the variant of disease
Fasciculations	No	No	Variable	Yes

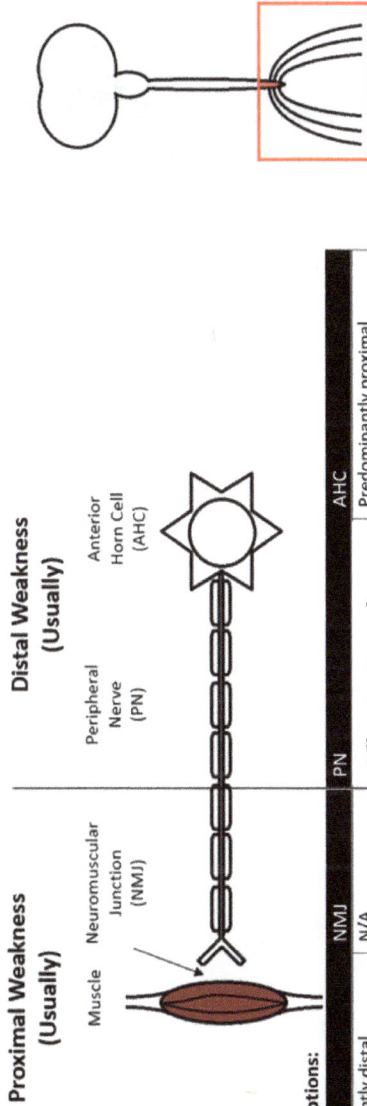

• **Conus medullaris** (mixed upper and motor neurone pattern)
• **Cauda equina**

Figure 19.3. Approach to bilateral flaccid weakness.

Co-existing clinical signs of wasting, sensory deficits, and fasciculations can be helpful in distinguishing the diseases from each other and should be taken into account (Figure 19.3). I should clarify that the method described above is meant to aid your approach to bilateral flaccid weakness, and its application should not be stubbornly doctrinal. There are multiple exceptions to the above-mentioned pattern, and their individual specificities are important to recognise (Figure 19.3).

References

1. Ferguson TA, Elman LB. (2007) Clinical presentation and diagnosis of amyotrophic lateral sclerosis. *NeuroRehabilitation* **22**(6): 409–416.
2. Hulisz D. (2018) Amyotrophic lateral sclerosis: disease state overview. *Am J Manag Care* **24**(15 Suppl): S320–S326.
3. Tey HL, Lim ECH, Lim JWK. (2009) *The Black Book of Clinical Examination*, McGraw-Hill, Singapore.

20

Approach to Unilateral Foot Drop

A. Introduction

In this chapter, we discuss the approach to patients with unilateral weakness of ankle dorsiflexion but without hemiparesis. Thankfully, unilateral foot drop is particularly acquiescent to the anatomical approach. We will begin by acquainting ourselves with the essential neuroanatomy of the lower limb.

B. Neuroanatomy

The innervation of the lower limbs spans extensively from the lumbosacral nerve roots to the distal branches of the tibial and peroneal nerves, traversing through the lumbosacral trunk and the sciatic nerve. The "wiring" is relatively easier to remember, and a degree of familiarity is helpful when assessing a patient with unilateral foot drop.

Anatomical Structures	Description
Sacral plexus	The **sacral plexus** is formed by the sacral roots **S1, S2, S3** and **S4**, with contributions from **L4** and **L5** roots via the lumbosacral trunk. It passes through the greater sciatic foramen, giving off branches to supply the **pelvic and gluteal muscles,** and to the skin over the inferomedial parts of the buttocks (**perforating cutaneous nerve**) and the posterior aspects of the thigh and upper calf (**posterior cutaneous nerve of the thigh**). It then "continues" as its largest branch — the **sciatic nerve** (Figures 20.1 and 20.2).

(Continued)

(Continued)

Anatomical Structures	Description
	Important nerves in the region of the sacral plexus include:

Nerves	Function and Significance
Superior gluteal nerve	The superior gluteal nerve innervates three muscles: • **Gluteus minimus** muscle • **Gluteus medius** muscle • **Tensor fascia latae** muscle These muscles **abduct** the hip. Additionally, the **gluteus medius** and **gluteus minimus** muscles **internally rotate** the hip when the hip is flexed. Hip abduction and internal rotation are predominantly served by the **L5 myotomes**.
Inferior gluteal nerve	The inferior gluteal nerve innervates the **gluteus maximus** muscle, which is the main **extensor** of the hip. Hip extension is predominantly served by the **L5, S1 myotomes**.
Posterior cutaneous nerve of the thigh	This nerve provides sensory innervation over the **posterior aspect of the thigh and upper calf**. Sensory deficits over this area in the presence of ipsilateral foot drop may help localise the pathology at the sacral plexus, with the differential diagnosis of S2 radiculopathy.
Sciatic nerve	The sciatic nerve is the largest branch of the sacral plexus and is often described as being "continuous" with the plexus. The sciatic nerve is discussed in detail below.

Anatomical Structures	Description
Sciatic nerve	The sciatic nerve is the largest branch of the sacral plexus and is often described as being "continuous" with the plexus. Functionally, it consists of **two separate divisions**: • Common peroneal division • Tibial division The sciatic nerve at the thigh provides motor innervation to the **hamstring** muscles and is thus important for knee flexion: • Medially, the **semimembranosus** and **semitendinosus** muscles • Laterally, the **biceps femoris** muscles (short and long heads) Because the origins of the hamstring muscles (except the short head of the biceps femoris) attach across the hip at the ischial tuberosity (the origin), they also assist in **extension of the hips**. At the **apex of the popliteal fossa**, the sciatic nerve formally divides into the **common peroneal** and **tibial** nerves.

(*Continued*)

Anatomical Structures	Description
Tibial nerve	The tibial nerve provides motor innervation to the **plantar flexors, ankle invertors** and **toe flexors**: • **Plantar flexors:** predominantly S1 myotome[1] o Gastrocnemius muscle o Soleus muscle • **Ankle invertors:** predominantly L4 and L5 myotomes o Predominantly the **tibialis posterior** muscle • **Toe flexors** Through its branches at the foot (the **medial and lateral plantar nerves**), the tibial nerve also provides sensory innervation to the soles.
Common peroneal nerve	The common peroneal nerve divides from the sciatic nerve at the apex of the popliteal fossa and descends along the medial border of the biceps femoris muscle, giving off the **lateral sural cutaneous nerve** before leaving the popliteal fossa by winding around the **fibular neck**. Here, it divides into the **deep** and **superficial peroneal nerves**. The lateral sural cutaneous nerve supplies the lateral surfaces of the knee and upper calf (Figure 20.3).
Superficial peroneal nerve	A branch of the common peroneal nerve, it primarily provides: • **Sensory innervation** over the (Figure 20.3): o Lateral aspect of the lower calf o Dorsum of the foot (except the first web space) • Motor innervation to the **ankle evertors**, (S1 myotome)[1] o Peroneus longus muscle o Peroneus brevis muscle
Deep peroneal nerve	A branch of the common peroneal nerve, it primarily provides: • **Motor innervation** to: o The ankle dorsiflexors/extensors (L4 and L5 myotomes)[1-4] ▪ Tibialis anterior muscle (primary) ▪ Extensor hallucis longus muscle (contributory) ▪ Extensor digitorum longus muscle (contributory) ▪ Pronator tertius muscle (contributory) o Toe extensors ▪ Extensor hallucis longus (L5 myotome)[1,2] and brevis muscles ▪ Extensor digitorum longus and brevis muscles • **Sensory innervation** to the first webspace over the dorsum of the foot (Figure 20.3).

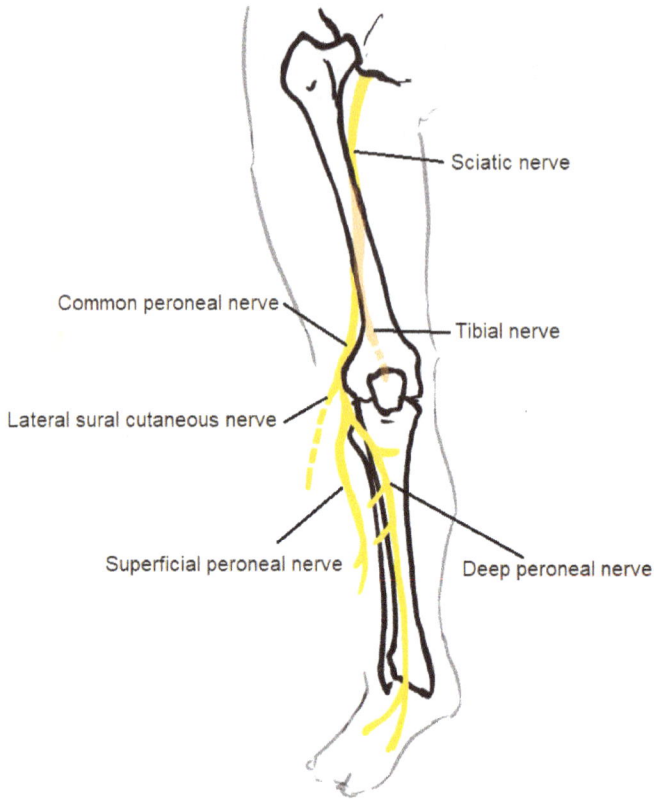

Figure 20.1. The major nerves of the lower limbs.

C. Clinical Assessment and Neurologic Examination

Whichever the cause, foot drop is the clinical manifestation of a weakened tibialis anterior muscle (Figure 20.4). "All foot drops lead to the tibialis anterior". As we recall, the tibialis anterior is innervated by the deep peroneal nerve, followed by a branch of the common peroneal nerve, the sciatic nerve, and so on, up till to the lumbar roots (L4, L5). A search for accompanying sensorimotor deficits provides valuable clues in localising the level where the culprit resides. We must not forget the possibility of an insult at the motor cortex causing a "cortical foot drop". Also, we should remain mindful of causes of bilateral foot drop, which may falsely appear to be unilateral in the early stages of the disease due to marked asymmetry. Amyotrophic lateral sclerosis is one good example.

The clinical approaches to unilateral foot drop are varied in complexity and applicability, with most methods designed to quickly discern whether the pathology lies within or without the peroneal nerve. I find the **"milestone"** and **"matrix table" methods** easier to learn and apply. I should highlight that **"simple foot drop"** and **"complex foot drop"** are not universally accepted terminologies, and, as such, should not be used.

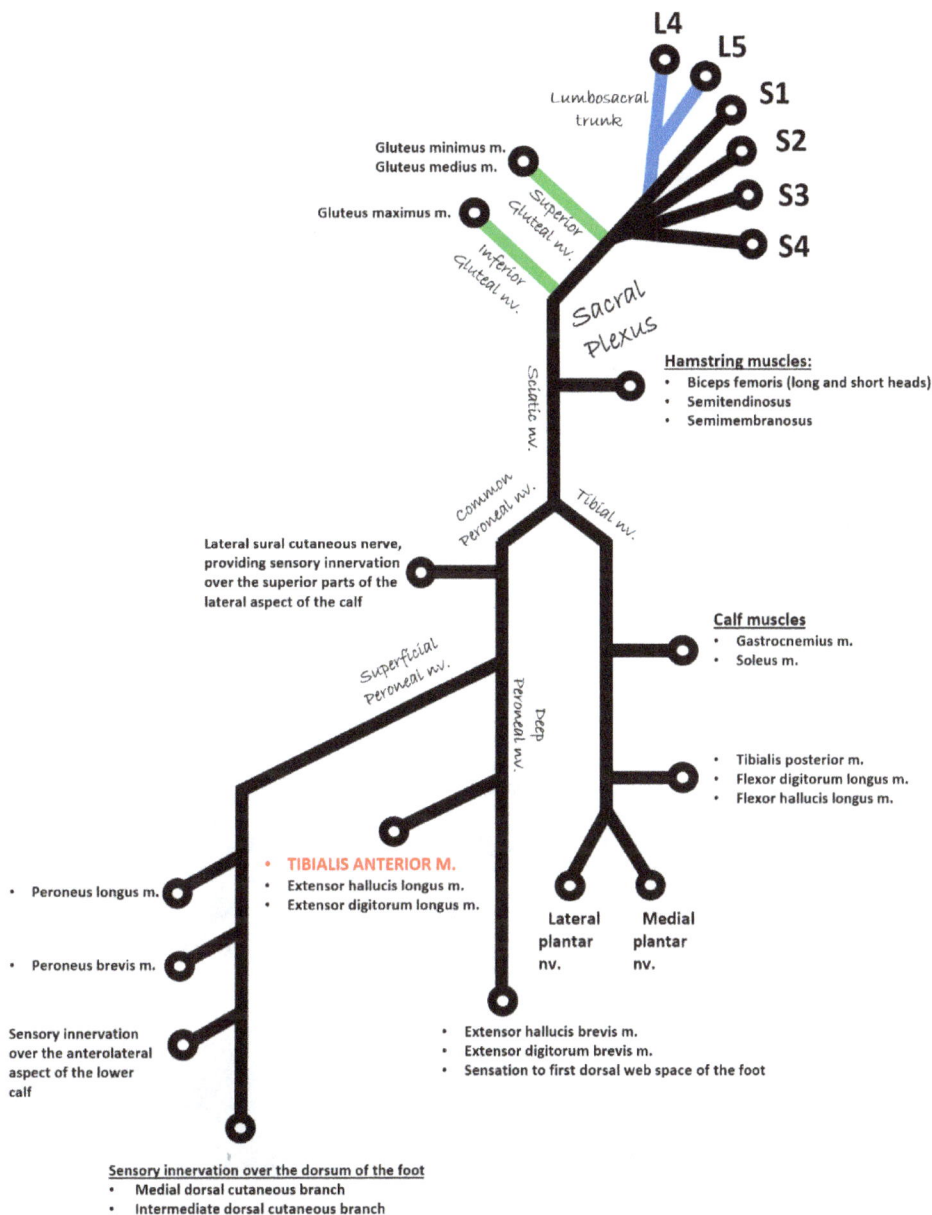

Figure 20.2. Schematic drawing of the major nerves, their branches and corresponding muscles to which they innervate. This drawing mimics a circuit board, simplifying the nervous structures of the lower limbs. The tibialis anterior muscle is bolded and coloured in red.

The **"milestone" method** utilises a series of vital checkpoints to localise the lesion as you examine the patient. These "milestones" are vital motor examination steps, such that weakness elicited during these "milestones" have immense localising value when evaluating a patient with unilateral foot drop. The order of these milestones may be modified to suit your **preferred sequence of motor examination**.

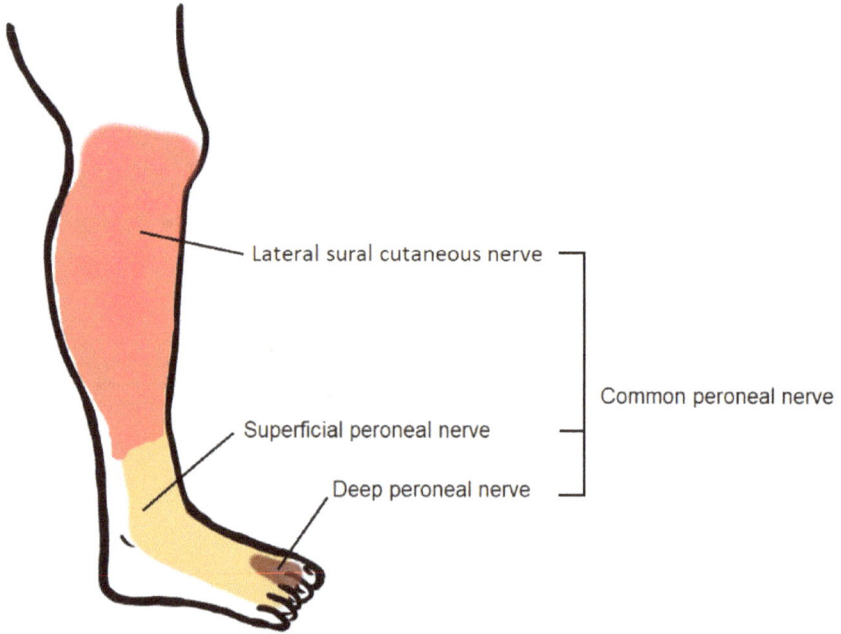

Figure 20.3.　Sensory territories of the lateral sural cutaneous, superficial peroneal and deep peroneal nerves.

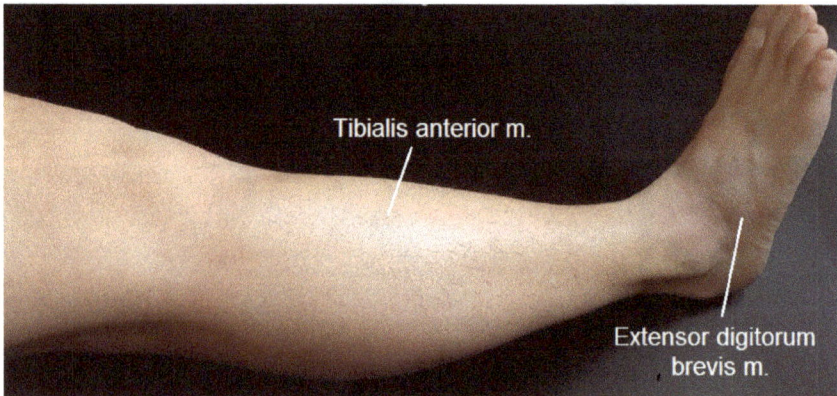

Figure 20.4.　The tibialis anterior and extensor digitorum brevis muscles are shown here. Both muscles are supplied by the deep peroneal neve.

(Continued)

Milestones	Implications When Weak	Details
Hip extension	Weakness of **gluteus maximus** muscle	The gluteus maximus muscle is innervated by the **inferior gluteal nerve** and is served by the L5, S1 and S2 myotomes. Weakness suggests a localisation beyond the peroneal nerve and may reside within the following: a. Sacral plexus b. Sciatic nerve c. Sacral roots (radiculopathy), which may co-exist with L4 and L5 radiculopathy due to degenerative spinal diseases A sacral plexus localisation should be considered strongly if the hip abductors are weak as well. Hip abductors (gluteus medius and minimus muscles) are supplied by the superior gluteal nerve, a branch of the sacral plexus.
Hip abduction and internal rotation	Weakness of **gluteus medius** and **minimus** muscles	These muscles are innervated by the **superior gluteal nerve**, and are served by the L5 myotome. Weakness of these muscles suggests that the lesion lies beyond the peroneal nerve, and may reside within the following: a. Sacral plexus b. L4, L5 lumbar roots (radiculopathy)
Knee flexion	Weakness of **hamstrings**: • Biceps femoris • Semitendinosus • Semimembranosus	These muscles are innervated by the **sciatic nerve**. Weakness of knee flexion suggests a localisation beyond the peroneal nerve, and may reside along the sciatic nerve.
Ankle plantar flexion and/or inversion	Weakness of **gastrocnemius, soleus** and **tibialis posterior** muscles	These muscles are innervated by the **tibial nerve**, and are served by the L4, L5 (inversion) and S1 (plantarflexion) myotomes.[1] In the presence of unilateral foot drop, co-existing plantar flexion weakness localises the lesion at the sciatic nerve, and weakness of knee flexion is likely to be present as well. Simultaneous lesions along the common peroneal and tibial nerves are a plausible, though less likely, differential diagnosis.

Milestones	Implications When Weak	Details
Ankle eversion	Weakness of **peroneus longus** and **brevis** muscles	These muscles are supplied by the **superficial peroneal nerve**, a branch of the common peroneal nerve. As such, weakness of eversion on top of ankle dorsiflexion weakness implies a lesion at or proximal to the common peroneal nerve. It is noteworthy that the tibialis anterior muscle (innervated by the deep peroneal nerve) inverts the ankle too. However, significant ankle inversion weakness is only observed when there is involvement of the tibial nerve.

Applying this to a hypothetical case of a patient with a left foot drop, we observe these findings in the following sequence of examination steps:

Examination Steps	Findings	Details
Hip flexion	Normal	N/A
Hip extension	Normal	The gluteus maximus muscle is uninvolved. Localisation at the sacral plexus is less likely.
Hip abduction or internal rotation	Normal	The gluteus medius and miminus muscles are uninvolved. Localisation at the sacral plexus or L5 nerve root is less likely.
Knee extension	Normal	N/A
Knee flexion	Normal	The hamstring muscles are mainly supplied by the sciatic nerve, and in this case are spared. Localisation along the sciatic nerve is less likely.
Ankle dorsiflexion	**Weak**	Weakness of ankle dorsiflexion at this point, may be the result of neuropathy of the common or deep peroneal nerves. Proceed to the next step.
Ankle eversion	**Weak**	Weakness of the peroneus longus and brevis muscles implies the involvement of the superficial peroneal nerve, a branch of the common peroneal nerve. As such, the localisation of the lesion is likely to be along the common peroneal nerve.
Ankle plantar flexion	Normal	The tibial nerve is uninvolved.
In Summary		
The lesion likely lies along the left common peroneal nerve. Sensory testing of the calf and foot can further assist in supporting your diagnosis.		

The **matrix table method** may be more useful in routine practice, as there will be ample opportunity to consolidate and interpret the signs without the time limitations of professional examinations. The common localisations are listed together with the expected clinical deficits

Table 20.1. Matrix table for the approach to unilateral foot drop.

	Hip		Knee	Ankle				Hallux	Sensory Deficits
	Extension	Abduction and Internal Rotation	Flexion	Dorsiflexion	Eversion	Plantar Flexion	Inversion	Dorsiflexion	
DPN				Weak				Weak	1st dorsal web space
CPN				Weak	Weak			Weak	Lateral aspect of the calf and the dorsum of the foot
Sciatic nerve	Weak*		Weak	Weak	Weak	Weak	Weak	Weak	Sensory territories of the common peroneal and tibial nerves
Sacral plexus	Weak*	Weak	Weak	Weak	Weak	Weak	Weak	Weak	Variable
L4 and L5 roots	May be weak**	Weak		Weak		Weak	Weak	Weak	L4/L5 dermatome
Cortical foot drop				Weak	Weak	Weak	Weak	Weak	Variable

Abbreviations: DPN: deep peroneal nerve; CPN: common peroneal nerve.

*: The hamstrings (except for the short head of biceps femoris) assist in hip extension, in tandem with the gluteus maximus muscle. The gluteus maximus is supplied by the inferior gluteal nerve, which branches directly from the sacral plexus. As such, the weakness of hip extension in sacral plexopathy is likely to be more profound than in sciatic neuropathy due to the additional involvement of the gluteus maximus, on top of the weak hamstrings.

**: The gluteus maximus is served by the L5, S1 and S2 myotomes. As such, disease of the L5 root may mildly affect hip extension.

appropriate for that localisation. Table 20.1 is an example of a matrix table. Feel free to modify the columns and rows if it helps optimise your learning.

Both methods have been found useful by undergraduate and postgraduate trainees. Identify the one that you find easiest to remember, and practice often!

D. L4 or L5 Radiculopathy (or Both?)

Various myotomes have been described to serve the tibialis anterior muscle. Proponents of the L4 myotome have gone further to describe how the relative weakness of ankle dorsiflexion (L4, deep peroneal nerve) compared to hallux extension (L5, deep peroneal nerve) can clinically discern lumbar radiculopathy from that of a deep peroneal neuropathy: in deep peroneal neuropathy, both ankle dorsiflexion and hallux extension are equally weak, while hallux extension is relatively weaker than ankle dorsiflexion in patients with L5 radiculopathy.[2–4,6] This, however, remains a controversial topic, and I would advise candidates to consider a localisation of L4-5 radiculopathy rather than L4 or L5 radiculopathy in isolation.

E. High Steppage Gait vs. Circumduction (Spastic) Gait

The patient's gait may yield useful clues in differentiating between upper and lower motor neuron pathologies. Patients with foot drop due to hemiparesis from a stroke, for example, will **circumduct** on the symptomatic side (Figure 20.5). This is due to the **spasticity, pyramidal pattern** of weakness (weakness of hip and knee flexors lead to greater difficulty in clearing the foot off the

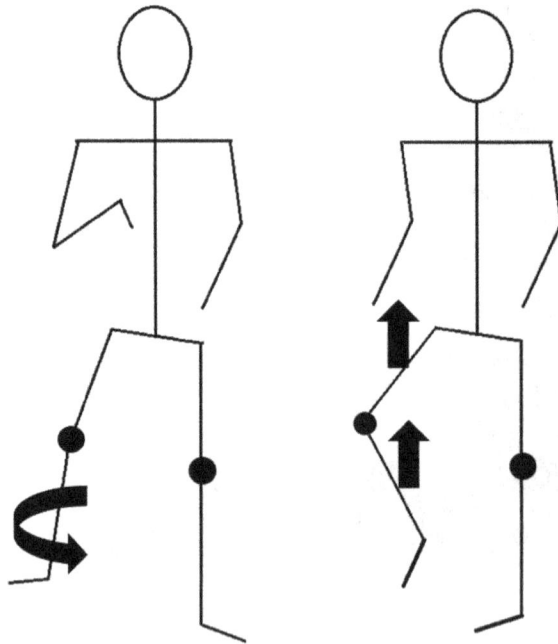

Figure 20.5.   Circumduction gait (left) and high-steppage gait (right).

ground), and presence of **Strümpell's tibialis phenomenon**.[5] Strümpell's phenomenon describes the dorsiflexion and inversion of the ankle when a patient with upper motor neuron deficits flexes the knee. The resultant ankle inversion renders it harder for the patient to clear his or her foot off the ground, causing the patient to adopt a circumduction gait to overcome these difficulties.

In comparison, patients with unilateral foot drop due to lower motor neuron pathologies will adopt a high steppage gait, as flexing the hip helps to elevate the symptomatic foot off the ground (Figure 20.5).

Tips for Examination Candidates
The purpose of bringing a patient with unilateral foot drop to the examination hall is to test your ability to: a. localise the level of the lesion, b. discuss the possible aetiologies resulting in the deficits, and c. discuss the diagnostic work up as guided by the list of possible aetiologies. I have had the privilege of examining a patient with unilateral food drop during my MRCP PACES examination. The localisation process was uneventful, as the patient clearly displayed features consistent with palsy of his left common peroneal nerve: • weakness of ankle dorsiflexion and eversion, • weakness of hallux extension and extension of the other toes, and • sensory deficits over the lateral aspect of the calf and the dorsal surface of the foot.

References

1. Magee DJ. (2009) *Orthopaedic Physical Assessment*, 4th ed. Elsevier, St. Louis.
2. Bryce T. (2009) *Spinal Cord Injury*. Demos Medical Publishing, New York.
3. Thage O. (1965) The myotomes L2–S2 in man. *Acta Neurol Scand* **41**(S13): 241–244.
4. Kawano O, Shiba K, Ueta T, Shirasawa K, Ohta H, Mori E, Rikimaru S, Kaji K, Akune H, Mihara T, Matsukura Y, Yoshikane K. (1996) Study of lower extremity myotomes by compound muscle action potential. *Orthop Traumatol* **45**(4): 1255–1258.
5. Engmann B, Wagner A, Steinberg H. (2012) Adolf von Strümpell: a key yet neglected protagonist of neurology. *J Neurol* **259**(10): 2211–2220.
6. Yue Q, Hale T, Knecht A, Laidacker J. (2017) Intraoperative loss of tibialis anterior transcranial electrical motor evoked potentials predicted postoperative footdrop. *World Neurosurg* **97**: 755.e1–755.e3.

21

Approach to Headaches

A. Introduction

Headache is a common symptomatic complaint, both in primary and specialist care. In Singapore, the lifetime prevalence of headaches is at 82.7%, with significant detrimental impact on health and well-being.[1,2] The underlying causes span a wide spectrum, ranging from the benign to the sinister. The role of the physician during the initial encounter is to identify the red flag signs and symptoms in the given clinical history and physical examination findings, and subject the patient to appropriate investigative evaluations as required.

The evaluation of an adult with headache involves a **3-step process**:

- Step 1: Is this a primary headache disorder?
- Step 2: Are there red flag symptoms or signs?
- Step 3: Are there any features in the patient's clinical background which may suggest a worrisome cause of the headaches?

B. Step 1: Primary Headache Disorder?

Primary headache disorders are common causes of chronic headaches, and are categorised based on their clinical phenotype as determined by the character, site, frequency and severity of the headaches and accompanying signs and symptoms. Within this group are the better-known headache disorders such as migraine headache, tension-type headache (TTH) and trigeminal autonomic cephalalgias (TACs). A good degree of familiarity with these common conditions is vital, and the International Classification of Headache Disorders (3rd edition), otherwise known as ICHD-3, is a useful reference (Tables 21.1 and 21.2)[2].

Table 21.1. The ICHD-3 classification of primary headache disorders.[3]

1. Migraine
2. Tension type headache (TTH)
3. Trigeminal autonomic cephalalgias (TACs)
a. Cluster headaches
b. Paroxysmal hemicranias
c. SUNCT/SUNA*
4. Other primary headache disorders:
a. Primary cough headache
b. Primary exercise headache
c. Primary headache associated with sexual activity
d. Primary thunderclap headache
e. Cold-stimulus headache
f. External-pressure headache
g. Primary stabbing headache
h. Nummular headache
i. Hypnic headache
j. New daily persistent headache

SUNCT: short-lasting unilateral neuralgiform headache with conjunctival injection; SUNA: short-lasting unilateral neuralgiform headache with autonomic features.

Table 21.2   Selected primary headache disorders and their ICHD-3 diagnostic criteria.[3]

	Migraine Without Aura	Tension-type Headache	Cluster Headache
A	≥5 attacks, fulfilling criteria B-D	Episodic: ≥10 episodes, occurring on less than 1 day/month on average Chronic: ≥15 days/month for more than 3 months on average	≥5 attacks, fulfilling criteria B-D
B	Headaches lasting 4–72 hours	Headaches lasting 30 minutes to 7 days	Severe or very severe unilateral orbital, supraorbital and/or temporal pain lasting 15 minutes to 3 hours (when untreated)

C	≥2 of the following:
	a. Unilateral location
	b. Pulsatile
	c. Moderate to severe intensity
	d. Aggravated by or causes avoidance of routine physical activities
		≥2 of the following:
		a. Bilateral location
		b. Pressing or tightening quality (non-pulsatile)
		c. Mild to moderate intensity
		d. Not aggravated by routine physical activities
			Either or both of the following:
			a. ≥1 of the following, ipsilateral to the headache:
			  i. Conjunctival injection and/or lacrimation
			  ii. Eyelid oedema
			  iii. Miosis and/or ptosis
			  iv. Nasal congestion and/or rhinorrhoea
			  v. Forehead and facial perspiration
			b. Sense of restlessness or agitation

D	≥1 of the following during headaches: a. Nausea and/or vomiting b. Photophobia and phonophobia	Both of the following: a. No nausea or vomiting b. No more than one of photo-phobia or phonophobia	Occurs with a frequency of between once every other day and 8 attacks per day
E	Not attributable to another disorder	Not attributable to another disorder	Not better accounted for by another ICHD-3 diagnosis

I was taught a simpler way to remember the diagnostic criteria for migraine without aura — the 5/4/3/2/1 rule:

- 5 or more attacks
- Lasting 4 hours to 3 days
- 2 or more of unilaterality, pulsatile character, moderate to severe intensity and aggravation by routine physical activities
- 1 or more of nausea or photophobia and phonophobia

I found this easy to remember and apply, so this may also be beneficial for your revision.

C. Step 2: The Sinister "Red Flags"

A large part of the assessment involves looking out for "red flag" symptoms. These symptoms, when present, often imply a deeper, more sinister cause of headaches, for which urgent investigations and treatment may be required. As these "red flag" symptoms are diverse and varied, it may be difficult to recall most of them. Thankfully, there are mnemonics out there to assist you, and the SNOOP4 mnemonic is a good example (Table 21.3).[1]

	Clinical Symptoms or Features	Significance
S	**S**ystemic symptoms (fever, chills, anorexia, loss of weight etc.)	Inflammation (infective and non-infective) Malignancies
N	Focal **n**eurologic deficits	Focal structural abnormality of the brain due to ischemia, haemorrhage, tumours, or infection (encephalitis or cerebral abscesses)
O	**O**lder age (>50 years old)	Giant cell arteritis (temporal arteritis), tumours of the brain, glaucoma
O	**O**nset that is sudden (thunderclap)	Intracranial bleeds, pituitary apoplexy, cerebral vasoconstriction syndromes
P	**P**apilloedema	Raised ICP
P	**P**ositional variation	Raised ICP or intracranial hypotension
P	**P**recipitated or exacerbated by exertion or Valsalva manoeuvres	Raised ICP
P	**P**rogressive or associated with significant change in **p**attern and character	Secondary causes of headache

Abbreviations: ICP, intracranial pressure

In essence, these mnemonics (and by extrapolation, the "red flag" features) aim to represent the following aetiologic groups of sinister conditions that can cause secondary headaches — the sinister 6 "I"s:

(*Continued*)

Groups	Conditions	Clinical Symptoms and Features
Intracranial bleed	• SAH • SDH • EDH • Parenchymal haemorrhage	Patients with SAH may complain of headaches of **"thunderclap"** nature. A history of preceding **head trauma,** or concurrent use of **anticoagulants** or **antiplatelet** therapy should prompt the consideration of intracranial bleeds in a patient with headaches.
Inflammation (infective)	• Meningitis • Encephalitis • Cerebral abscess	These conditions are commonly associated with **constitutional symptoms** such as fever, chills and loss of appetite. Features of **meningeal irritation** (neck stiffness and photophobia) may be present in meningitis, while **clouding of sensorium and focal neurologic deficits** may be present in patients with encephalitis or cerebral abscesses.
Inflammation (non-infective)	• Vasculitis (e.g., giant cell arteritis) • Systemic connective tissue diseases	These conditions are commonly associated with **constitutional symptoms** such as fever, loss of weight and loss of appetite. Dependent on the underlying disease, **photosensitivity, rash, ulcerations or joint inflammation** may be present. **Giant cell arteritis (temporal arteritis)** is of especial concern in older patients, and accompanying features of **jaw claudication** on mastication, and symptoms of **polymyalgia rheumatica** may be present.
Infarctions	• Ischemic strokes • Cerebral venous thrombosis (+/− venous infarctions) • Pituitary apoplexy Headaches in ischemic strokes may appear in close temporal relation to the stroke, and may persist for months after the stroke.[4,5]	The symptoms in patients with cerebral venous thrombosis may vary, depending on the presence of complications such as venous infarctions, haemorrhage and cerebral oedema. Presence of risk factors such as a history of **venous thromboembolic disease, autoimmune diseases** (e.g., antiphospholipid syndrome), consumption of **oral contraceptive pills,** or ongoing **hormone replacement therapy** may be present. Patients with pituitary apoplexy can present with severe **"thunderclap"** headaches, and may have a history of pituitary adenoma.

(Continued)

Groups	Conditions	Clinical Symptoms and Features
Infiltrative disease	This category includes both **primary brain tumours**, and **secondary metastasis** to the brain and surrounding structures.	The symptoms experienced by patients with tumorous brain lesions depend greatly on the site, size and complications. A large lesion, or one complicated by significant oedema, may result in **raised ICP**. Symptoms of raised ICP include **morning headaches** and **nausea, exacerbated by recumbency** and **Valsalva manoeuvres**. Lesions within the brain and/or brainstem may cause **focal neurologic deficits.** Additionally, concomitant **constitutional symptoms** due to active malignancies may be present.
Injury	• Soft tissue injury to head and neck • Injury to the vessels (cervical artery dissection)	Dissection of the cervical artery is of particular concern, especially when **stroke-like deficits** are present. A preceding history of **neck manipulations or injuries** may be supportive.

Abbreviations: SAH, subarachnoid haemorrhage; SDH, subdural haemorrhage; EDH, extradural haemorrhage; CNS, central nervous system.

D. Step 3: Patient's Clinical Background

While we often base our clinical judgement on the patient's symptoms and signs, information on the patient's background and medical history have significant influence on the subsequent diagnostic and management processes. For example, a history of metastatic breast carcinoma in a patient with headaches may prompt you to send the patient for a contrasted Magnetic Resonance Imaging (MRI) scan of the brain to exclude intracranial metastasis. This quintessential step forces us to appreciate the patient in entirety, so that we may refine our diagnostic and management decisions.

E. Thunderclap Headache

"Thunderclap headache" is a descriptive term for a **severe** headache of **instantaneous** onset, peaking in intensity within a minute.[6-8] Thunderclap headaches may occur spontaneously, on exertion (sports or sexual activity), with stress, or when performing the Valsalva manoeuvre. The presence of the "thunderclap" nature warrants urgent evaluation of sinister secondary causes, especially subarachnoid haemorrhage.[6-8] Other worrisome diagnoses include cervical artery dissections, pituitary apoplexy and reversible cerebral vasoconstriction syndrome (RCVS).

F. Medication Overuse Headache

Medication overuse headache (MOH) is a secondary headache disorder caused by excessive and chronic use of acute analgesics. Symptoms are chronic, frequent, and potentially disabling. It is more common in middle-aged people, with a 3:1 female to male ratio.[9] MOH should be suspected in patients with chronic headaches that are difficult to treat, especially when the characteristics of the prevailing headache differ from those at its initial stage. Once MOH is suspected, a referral to a neurologist may be warranted to better manage the patient's headache symptoms.

Based on the ICHD-3 clinical diagnostic criteria, MOH may be diagnosed if the following are present:[3]

A. **Headache** present on ≥15 days/month in a patient with a pre-existing headache disorder
B. **Regular overuse** of one or more drugs that can be taken for acute or symptomatic treatment of headache for >3 months*
C. Not better accounted for by another ICHD-3 diagnosis

*The threshold defining overuse varies between the class of medications:
- Usage of **simple analgesics** such as non-steroidal anti-inflammatory drugs on ≥**15 days/month**
- Usage of **combination analgesics, triptans, ergotamines or opioids** on ≥**10 days/month**

G. Conclusion

The 3-step approach is simple to remember and apply when evaluating patients with headaches. Only after going through **all three steps** can you make learned and appropriate diagnostic and management decisions. A degree of familiarity with the common primary headache syndromes remains important, as patients with migraines and tension-type headaches are frequently encountered in our routine practice. The ICHD-3 is a good online reference, boasting an expansive list of clinical criteria for the many headache syndromes.

Tips for Examination Candidates

The ability to safely and proficiently assess patients with headaches is quintessential to all physicians. As such, professional examinations often include patients with headaches. The examiners aim to test the candidate's ability to:
- Recognise the primary headache syndromes
- Elicit "red flag" symptoms and signs
- Subsequently make decisions with regards to:
  - Referring the patient to a neurologist
  - Referring the patient to the emergency department for urgent evaluation
  - Diagnostic tests and scans

A common recurring scenario in MRCP is that of a patient with recurring thunderclap headaches. Further questioning will reveal a family history of kidney disease, and that a close relative died from a brain haemorrhage. The candidate is then expected to consider the diagnosis of subarachnoid haemorrhage in a patient with possible polycystic kidney disease, and to have the patient undergo urgent imaging studies such as a brain computed tomography (CT) scan.

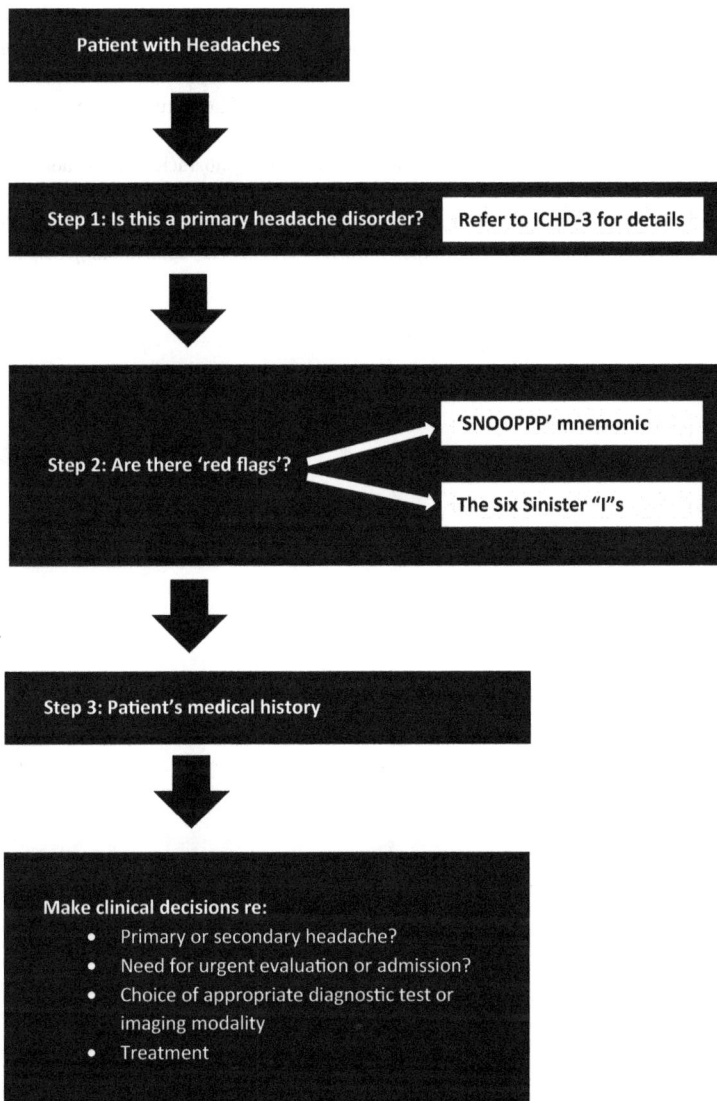

Patient with Headaches

Step 1: Is this a primary headache disorder? | **Refer to ICHD-3 for details**

Step 2: Are there 'red flags'?

'SNOOPPP' mnemonic

The Six Sinister "I"s

Step 3: Patient's medical history

Make clinical decisions re:
- Primary or secondary headache?
- Need for urgent evaluation or admission?
- Choice of appropriate diagnostic test or imaging modality
- Treatment

References

1. Lee VME, Ang LL, Soon DTL, Ong JJY, Loh VWK. (2018) The adult patient with headache. *Singapore Med J* **59**(8): 399–406.

2. Ho KH, Ong BK. (2003) A community-based study of headache diagnosis and prevalence in Singapore. *Cephalalgia* **23**(1): 6–13.

3. The international Classification of Headache Disorders, 3rd Edition (2019). Retrieved from http://ichd-3.org.

4. Paciaroni M, Parnetti L, Sarchielli P, Gallai V. (2001) Headache associated with acute ischemic stroke. *J Headache Pain* **2**(1): 25–29.

5.   Lai J, Harrison RA, Plecash A, Field TS. (2018) A narrative review of persistent post-stroke headache — a new entry in the International Classification of Headache Disorders, 3rd edition. *Headache* **58**(9): 1442–1453.

6.   Day JW, Raskin NH. (1986) Thunderclap headache: symptom of unruptured cerebral aneurysm. *Lancet* **2**: 1247–1248.

7.   Al-Shahi R, White PM, Davenport RJ, Lindsay KW. (2006) Subarachnoid haemorrhage. *BMJ* **333**: 235–240.

8.   Schwedt TJ, Matharu MS, Dodick DW. (2006) Thunderclap headache. *Lancet Neurol* **5**(7): 621–631.

9.   Kristoffersen ES, Lundquist C. (2014) Medication-overuse headache: epidemiology, diagnosis and treatment. *Ther Adv Drug Saf* **5**(2): 87–99.

22

Approach to a Patient with Vertigo

A. Introduction

Acute giddiness is a common symptomatic complaint, but many face difficulty when assessing a patient with acute vertigo. Misdiagnoses are not uncommon, with up to half of the initial diagnoses being "completely changed" upon subsequent neurological reviews.[1] With three simple steps, we hope to provide some structure to your diagnostic processes when evaluating a patient with acute vertigo. These were taught to me by my seniors and peers, which I find easy to remember and apply.

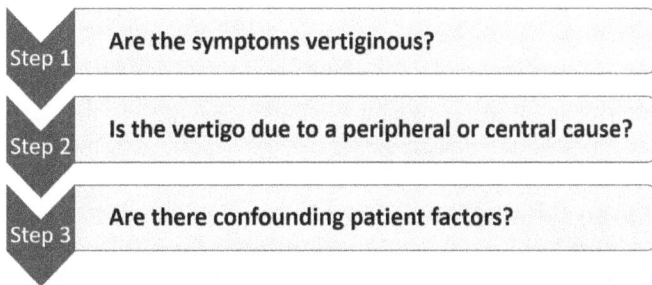

Step 1 | Are the symptoms vertiginous?

Step 2 | Is the vertigo due to a peripheral or central cause?

Step 3 | Are there confounding patient factors?

B. Step 1. Are the Symptoms Vertiginous?

Vertigo is defined as an illusion of motion. Although classically described as "spinning", the sense of motion may be linear, with the patient experiencing more of a "tilt" or "slant". When assessing a patient with giddiness, it is necessary for us to determine what the patient meant when he or she "feels giddy", as most patients are unfamiliar with the terminologies that accurately describe their symptoms, and may describe the symptoms of light-headedness, disequilibrium, head-heaviness, and even headaches as "giddiness". This is made worse by the inappropriately-restrictive description of vertigo used by some, limiting it to the presence of "spinning" motions.

The following recommendations can help in your clinical interview of a patient with vertigo:

1. **Ask open-ended questions:**
   - "What do you mean by giddiness?"
   - "Are you able to describe your symptoms in your own words?"
   - "Does it feel similar to those times when you're on a boat (or something equivalent)?"

2. **Explore beyond that of a "spinning" sensation** and ask for other non-rotational sensations (e.g., swaying, tilting) as these may also be experienced by patients with vertigo.

C. Step 2. Is the Vertigo Due to a Peripheral or Central Cause?

The aetiologies of vertigo may be grouped into central and peripheral causes.

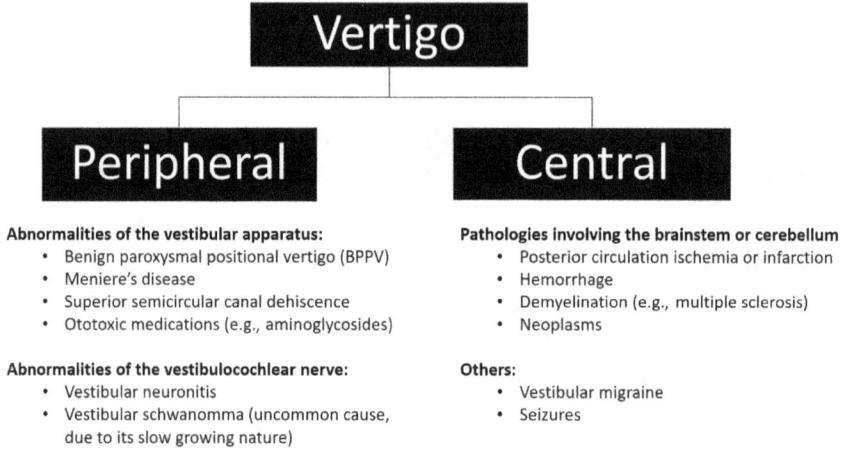

Vertigo

Peripheral

Abnormalities of the vestibular apparatus:
- Benign paroxysmal positional vertigo (BPPV)
- Meniere's disease
- Superior semicircular canal dehiscence
- Ototoxic medications (e.g., aminoglycosides)

Abnormalities of the vestibulocochlear nerve:
- Vestibular neuronitis
- Vestibular schwanomma (uncommon cause, due to its slow growing nature)

Central

Pathologies involving the brainstem or cerebellum
- Posterior circulation ischemia or infarction
- Hemorrhage
- Demyelination (e.g., multiple sclerosis)
- Neoplasms

Others:
- Vestibular migraine
- Seizures

Benign paroxysmal positional vertigo (BPPV) is by far the most common cause of peripheral vertigo.[2] The characteristic paroxysms of vertigo triggered by positional changes of the head make it relatively easy to diagnose, especially when aided by provocative tests. BPPV, vestibular neuronitis, and Meniere's disease are discussed in detail below.

Vestibular neuronitis is of particular concern, as it can be difficult to distinguish from central causes of vertigo such as posterior circulation ischemia or infarctions, especially when the latter occur without other neurologic deficits. 10% of patients with cerebellar infarcts, especially when only the medial branch of the posterior inferior cerebellar artery is involved, can have vertigo alone without additional deficits.[3]

The **HiNTs (head impulse, nystagmus, and test of skew) examination** is a useful screening tool for distinguishing vestibular neuronitis from a central cause of vertigo. Notably, the **test should only be used in persistently symptomatic patients**, and should not be performed in patients with BPPV.

The HiNTs test has three components:

Test	Description	Interpretation
Head impulse test (HIT)	• Ensure that there are no contraindications (e.g., neck trauma, arterial dissection etc.). • Ask the patient to relax his or her neck. • Have the patient fixate his or her gaze on your nose. • Gently but briskly rotate the patient's head to the side (Figure 22.1).	The head impulse test examines the integrity of the **vestibulo-ocular reflex**, and is positive if a significant lag that is followed by corrective saccades is observed. This reflects a defective vestibular apparatus or nerve on the side where the head was turned to.

(Continued)

Test	Description	Interpretation
Nystagmus	• Observe if nystagmus is present in primary gaze and in lateral gaze. • If nystagmus is present, note the direction of the fast phase. • Observe for changes in direction and intensity of the fast phase as the patient changes his direction of gaze.	A horizontal unidirectional nystagmus that obeys **Alexander's law** is likely to be of peripheral origin. A **multidirectional nystagmus** (fast phase changes with the direction of gaze), or one that is purely vertical or torsional, is likely to be due to central pathologies.
Test of skew	• Have the patient fixate his gaze on your nose. • Cover one eye first. • Uncover the first eye and cover the other eye. • Observe the now-uncovered eye for vertical and/or diagonal movement. • Repeat the manoeuver on the now-covered eye (Figure 22.2).	The presence of **vertical and/or diagonal corrective movements** of the uncovered eye implies the presence of vertical ocular mis-alignment, and is indicative of a central cause of vertigo.

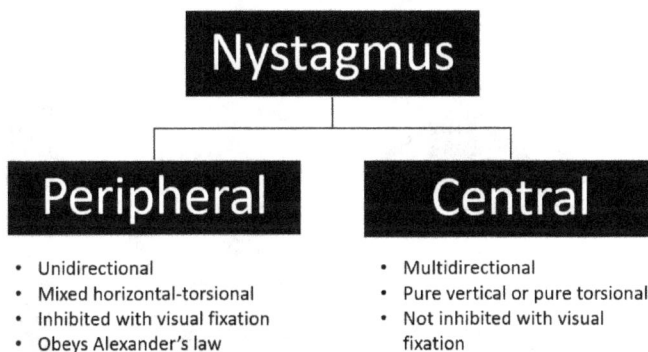

Nystagmus

Peripheral

- Unidirectional
- Mixed horizontal-torsional
- Inhibited with visual fixation
- Obeys Alexander's law

Central

- Multidirectional
- Pure vertical or pure torsional
- Not inhibited with visual fixation

When **all three components are entirely consistent with a peripheral cause** of vertigo (i.e., positive head impulse test, horizontal unidirectional nystagmus and absent skew deviation), the test enjoys high sensitivity and specificity of 100% and 96% respectively for a peripheral aetiology, although not without certain caveats.[4] Otherwise, brain imaging in the form of a magnetic resonance imaging (MRI) scan will likely be warranted.

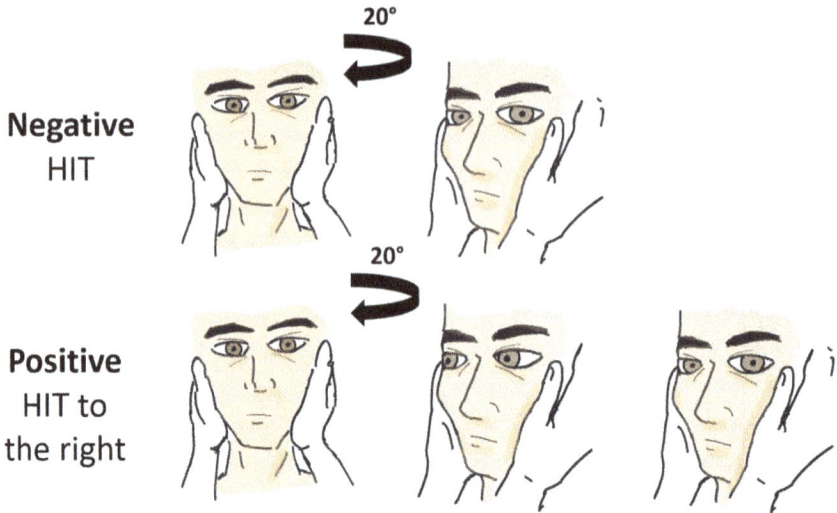

Figure 22.1. Head impulse test, with demonstrations of a negative (top panel) and a positive (bottom panel) test. Positive HIT to the right lateralises the pathology to the right.

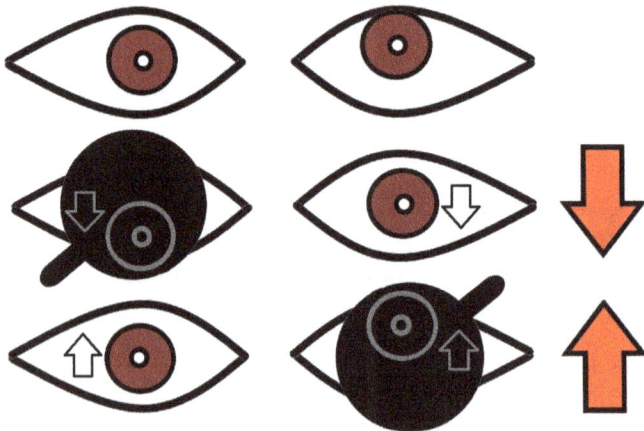

Figure 22.2. Demonstrating vertical misalignment using the alternating cover test on a patient with a hypertropic left eye due to skew deviation.

D. Step 3: Are there Confounding Patient Factors?

Is the patient known to have cardiovascular risk factors such hypertension, hyperlipidaemia, diabetes mellitus or chronic smoking? Does he or she have a history of previous strokes? These factors are significant, as they increase the patient's inherent risk of cerebrovascular accidents, thus inclining the physician to search and evaluate for a central cause of the patient's vertigo.

E. BPPV, Vestibular Neuronitis, and Meniere's Disease

Peripheral Causes	Details
BPPV	BPPV, as the name suggests, describes the recurrent paroxysms of vertigo, induced by changes in head position, lasting less than a minute (usually seconds). Although benign in its clinical course, patients may describe the attacks of vertigo as severe, uncomfortable and disabling.[5] Classical triggers include turning in bed, bending over and straightening up and looking up.[6] Significant relief is often achieved when the patients remain still and immobile.
	BPPV is thought to be the result of displaced otoliths or calcium debris within the semicircular canal, with the posterior canal being most commonly affected (80–90%).[7] The diagnosis is further supported by provocative manoeuvres (e.g., Dix-Hallpike test, Semont's manoeuvre, etc.). Treatment with therapeutic manoeuvres (e.g., Epley and BBQ manoeuvre) can help to relocate these otoliths and provide relief.
	The **Dix-Hallpike Manoeuvre (DHP)** is commonly used to induce the symptoms and signs of BPPV and is regarded as an important diagnostic test. However, the DHP is not 100% sensitive, as the symptoms and signs may not be elicited during asymptomatic periods (Figure 22.3).[8]
	In patients with posterior canal BPPV, the nystagmus induced by DHP displays the following characteristics: 1. **Latency:** The latency period refers to the time between the lowering of the patient's head and the advent of vertigo and nystagmus, usually lasting between 5 to 20 seconds.[9] 2. **Duration:** The nystagmus and vertigo typically increases and declines in intensity within a period of 60 seconds. 3. **Character of nystagmus:** The nystagmus is typically described as mixed torsional-vertical, increasing and then decreasing in intensity over time (crescendo-decrescendo nystagmus). 4. **Fatigability:** Severity and intensity of nystagmus typically reduces with repeated performance of the manoeuvre.
Vestibular Neuronitis	Vestibular neuronitis is thought to be an inflammatory disorder affecting the vestibular portion of the vestibulocochlear nerve, causing acute vertigo, nausea and vomiting without accompanying cochlear deficits (deafness and tinnitus). The vertigo is often severe in the early stage, subsequently subsiding over a period of days or weeks. Reflecting an underlying inflammatory process, the symptoms and signs are often persistent. Preceding or concurrent infectious illness is present in 43–46% of patients.[10] Unsteadiness is a common complaint, and patients often fall to the side of the lesion.[10]

(Continued)

Peripheral Causes	Details
	Vestibular neuronitis gives rise to nystagmus with the following characteristics: 1. Spontaneous 2. Jerky: slow phase towards the side of the lesion 3. Unidirectional 4. Horizontal or horizontal-torsional 5. Suppressed with visual fixation 6. Alexander's law: nystagmus increases in intensity when the patient gazes towards the direction of the fast phase Although vestibular neuronitis is a self-limiting disease that may be treatable with symptomatic medications and steroids, the sinister differential diagnosis of a posterior circulation stroke poses a significant diagnostic challenge. The HiNTs examination is an especially helpful bedside screening tool for distinguishing a peripheral cause of vertigo (e.g., vestibular neuronitis) from a central cause (i.e., a posterior circulation stroke) and is explained in detail above.
Meniere's disease	Meniere's disease (idiopathic endolymphatic hydrops) is a disease of the inner ear. Multiple aetiologies have been theorised, with the common end-result of endolymphatic sac distension, increase in pressure and rupture of the inner membrane, with resultant decreased vertigo and hearing loss. The disease typically affects patients in their 20s to 50s, and is characterised by the following triad: • Recurrent rotatory vertigo • Fluctuating sensorineural hearing loss • Tinnitus Ear fullness is a common complaint, and the chronic deterioration of inner ear function will ultimately result in progressive sensorineural hearing loss, affecting the lower frequencies early.

Tips for Examination Candidates

A patient with acute vestibular syndrome can appear in clinical OSCES and in PACES Station 5. You will likely be tested on your ability to:
• Clinically assess a patient with vertigo
• Decide if the vertigo is of a central or peripheral cause
• Perform the HiNTs test
• Offer reasonable management:
  ○ Does the patient require admission?
  ○ Is brain MRI required?
 	
The 3-step approach is something I learned from an esteemed senior of mine during my training days. It provides a structured approach to a person with acute vestibular syndrome, and is easy to remember and apply.

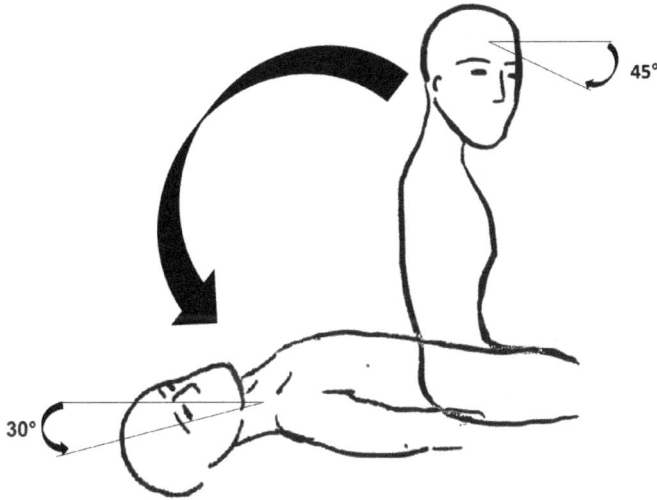

Figure 22.3.   Before performing the Dix-Hallpike manoeuvre, you should warn the patient that vertigo may be triggered. Begin with the patient sitting upright and turn the patient's head 45° yaw to the side of interest. With the patient's eyes kept open, quickly lie the patient supine while allowing the neck to hyperextend slightly at 30° pitch by hanging off the edge of the couch or bed, and observe for nystagmus. Because of the characteristic latency of the nystagmus in BPPV, do observe the patient's eyes for at least 20 seconds.

References

1. Seemungal BM, Bronstein AM. (2008) A practical approach to acute vertigo. *Pract Neurol.* **8**(4): 211–221. doi:10.1136/jnnp.2008.154799.

2. Jahn K, Lopez C, Zwergal A, *et al.* (2019) Vestibular Rehabilitation Research Group in the European DIZZYNET. Vestibular rehabilitation therapy in Europe: Chances and challenges. *J Neurol* **266**(Suppl 1):9–10.

3. Nelson JA, Viirree E. (2009) The Clinical differentiation of cerebellar infarction from common vertigo syndromes. *West J Emerg Med* **10**(4): 273–277.

4. Kattah JC, Talkad AV, Wang DZ, Hsieh H, Newman-Toker DE. (2009) HINTS to diagnose stroke in the acute vestibular syndrome: Three-step bedside oculomotor examination more sensitive than early MRI diffusion-weighted imaging. *Stroke* **40**(11): 3504–3510.

5. Epley JM. (1993) Benign Paroxysmal Positional Vertigo (Canalithiasis). Diagnosis and non-surgical management. In: Arenberg IK, editor. Dizziness and balance disorders. Amsterdam: Kugler Publishers; pp. 545–549.

6. Fife TD, Iverson DJ, Lempert T, Furman JM, Baloh RW, Tusa RJ, *et al.* (2008) Practice parameter: Therapies for benign paroxysmal positional vertigo (an evidence-based review): Report of the Quality Standards Subcommittee of the American Academy of Neurology. *Neurology* **70**: 2067–2074.

7. Korres S, Balatsouras DG, Kaberos A, Economou C, Kandiloros D, Ferekidis E. (2002) Occurrence of semicircular canal involvement in benign paroxysmal positional vertigo. *Otol Neurotol* **23**: 926–932.

8. Beynon GJ. (1997) A review of management of benign paroxysmal positional vertigo by exercise therapy and by repositioning maneuvers. *Br J Audiol* **31**: 11–26.

9. Bhattacharyya N, Baugh RF, Orvidas L, Barrs D, Bronston LJ, Cass S, Chalian AA, Desmond AL, Earll JM, Fife TD, Fuller DC, Judge JO, Mann NR, Rosenfeld RM, Schuring LT, Steiner RW, Whitney SL,

Haidari J. (2008) American Academy of Otolaryngology-Head and Neck Surgery Foundation. Clinical practice guideline: benign paroxysmal positional vertigo. *Otolaryngol Head Neck Surg* **139**(5 Suppl 4): S47–S81. doi:10.1016/j.otohns.2008.08.022. PMID: 18973840.

10. Cooper CW. (1993) Vestibular neuronitis: a review of a common cause of vertigo in general practice. *Br J Gen Pract* **43**(369): 164–167.

23

Pictorial Maps of the Brainstem

A. Introduction

The brainstem anatomy can be daunting to many trainees. A somewhat cylindrical 3D structure, packed tightly with important traversing tracts and structures, its actual anatomical layout is confusing to most. To make matters worse, the projection of the brainstem in most anatomy textbooks differ greatly from those encountered in brain scans, discombobulating even the most enthusiastic of students. As such, we have included a series of hand-drawn images of selected levels, which we think will be useful to help you remember the anatomy of the brainstem.

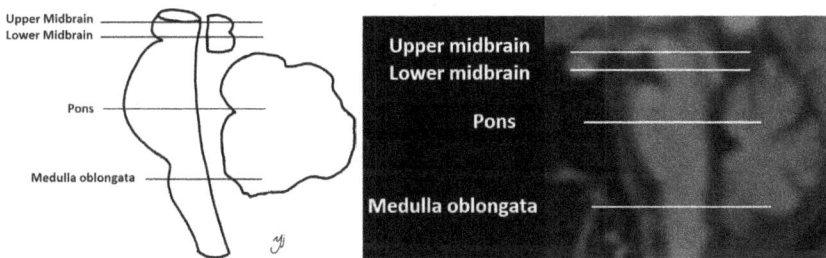

Figure 23.1. A schematic drawing of the brainstem and cerebellum with its corresponding sagittal Magnetic Resonance Imaging (MRI) projection, showing the levels that we have selected for inclusion in this chapter.

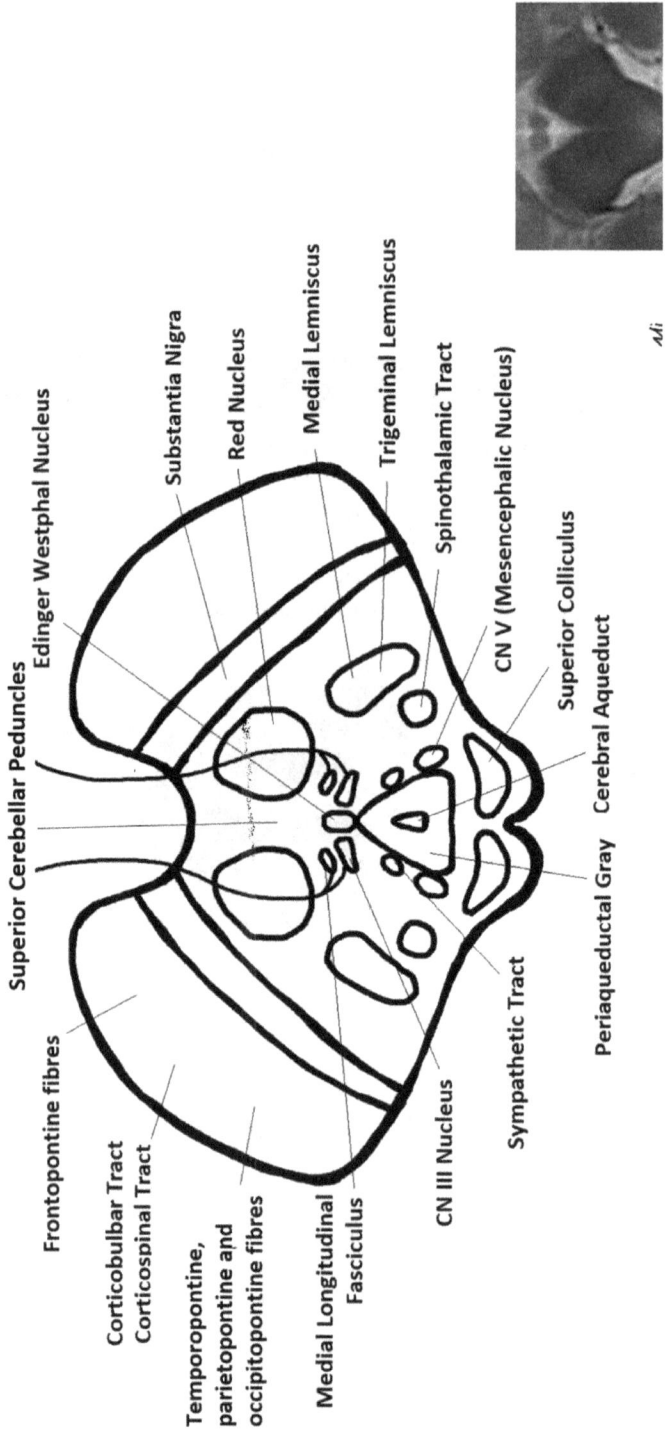

Figure 23.2.   A schematic drawing of the superior midbrain at the level of the superior colliculus. A corresponding axial MRI image is included for comparison.

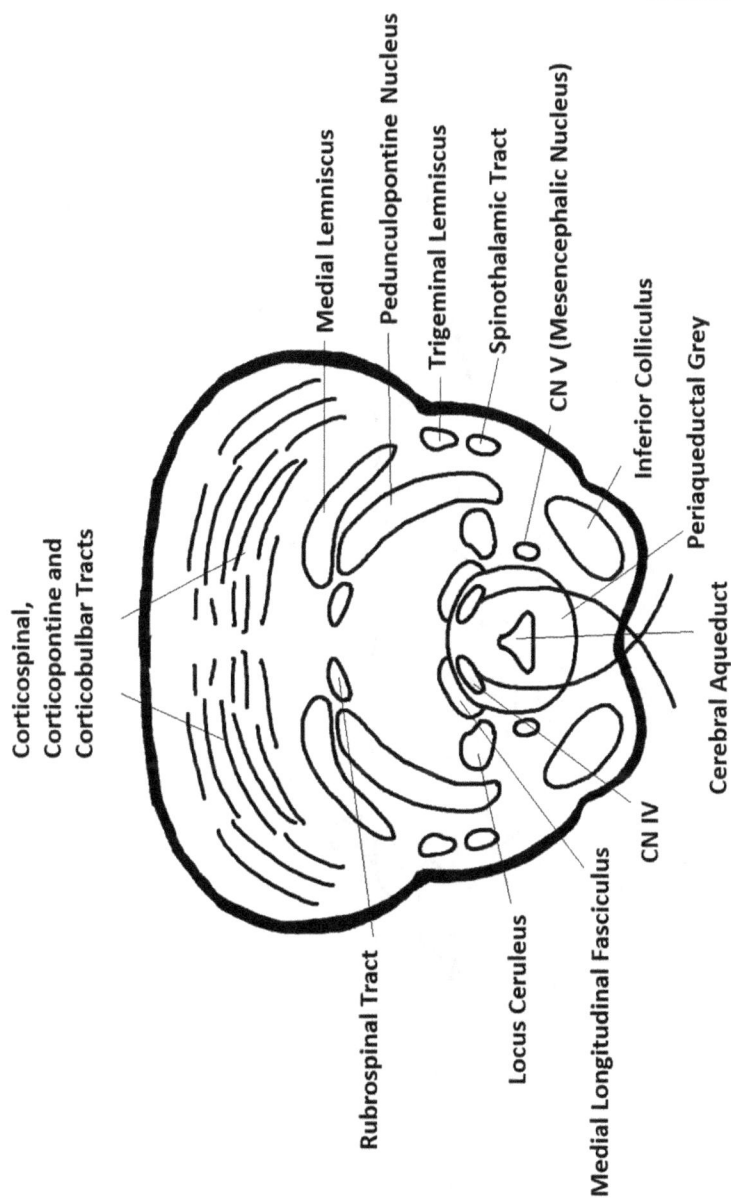

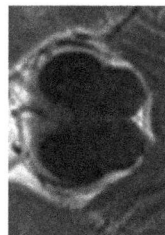

Figure 23.3.   A schematic drawing of the inferior midbrain at the level of the inferior colliculus. A corresponding axial MRI image is included for comparison.

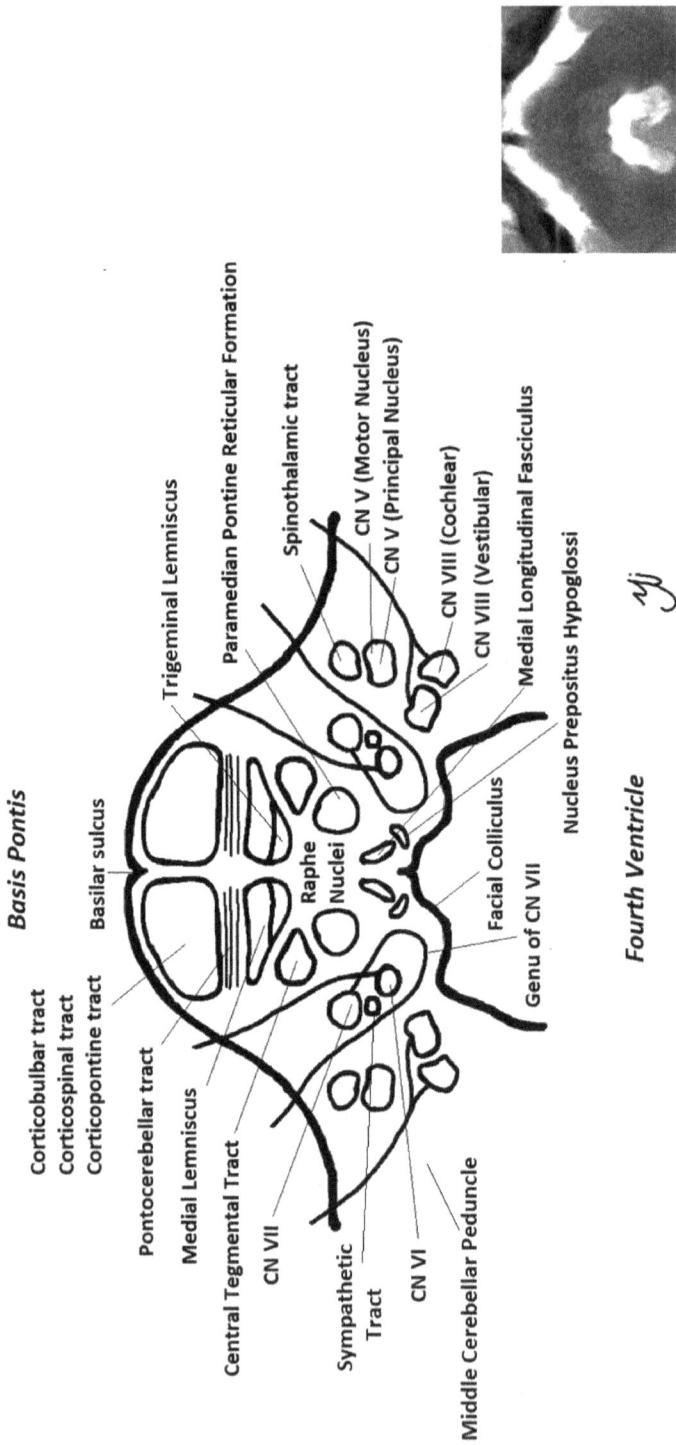

Figure 23.4.   A schematic drawing of the pons. A corresponding axial MRI image is included for comparison.

Basis Pontis

Corticobulbar tract
Corticospinal tract
Corticopontine tract

Basilar sulcus

Pontocerebellar tract

Medial Lemniscus

Central Tegmental Tract

CN VII

Sympathetic Tract

CN VI

Middle Cerebellar Peduncle

Trigeminal Lemniscus

Paramedian Pontine Reticular Formation

Spinothalamic tract

CN V (Motor Nucleus)

CN V (Principal Nucleus)

CN VIII (Cochlear)

CN VIII (Vestibular)

Medial Longitudinal Fasciculus

Nucleus Prepositus Hypoglossi

Facial Colliculus

Genu of CN VII

Raphe Nuclei

Fourth Ventricle

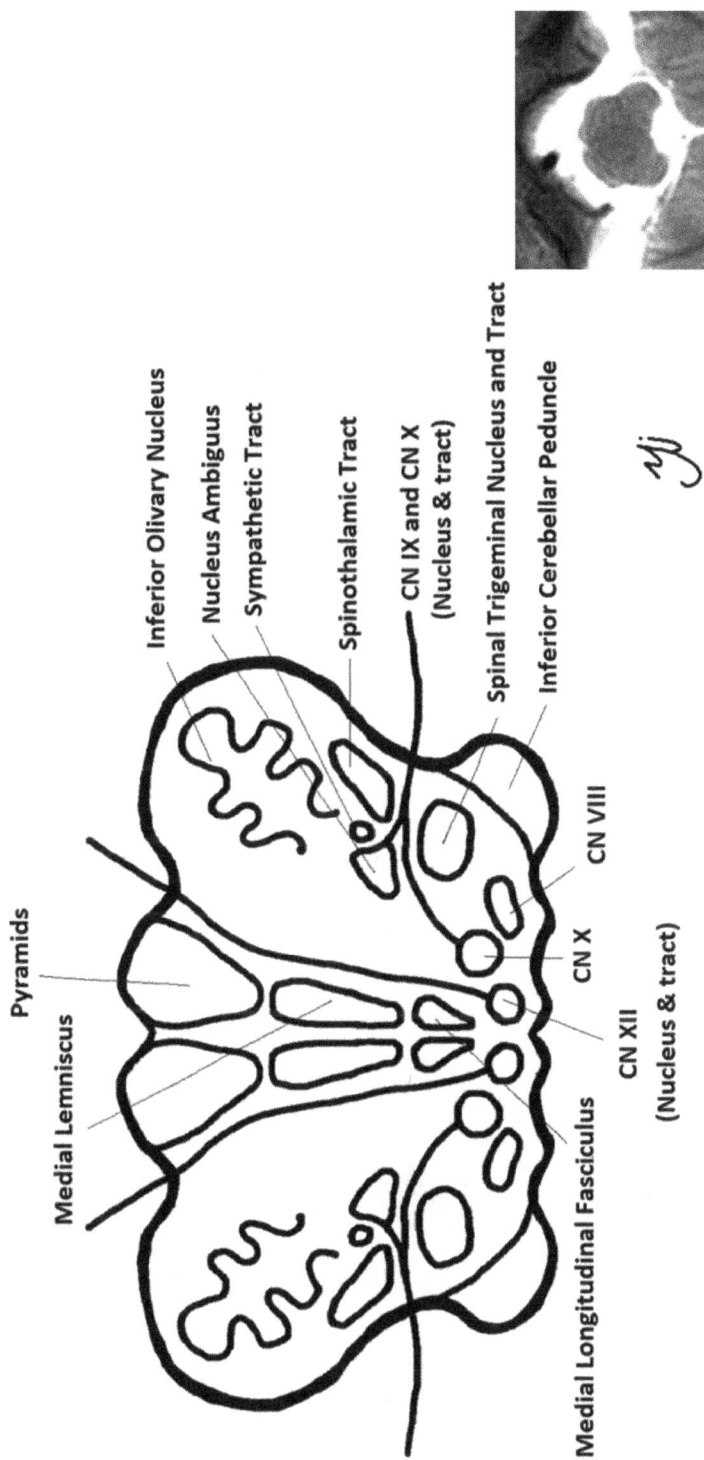

Figure 23.5. Schematic drawing of the medulla oblongata. A corresponding axial MRI image is included for comparison.

Index

www.ingramcontent.com/pod-product-compliance
Lightning Source LLC
Chambersburg PA
CBHW081056220326

41598CB00038B/7122